Science-based Rehabilitation

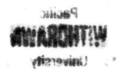

For Butterworth-Heinemann:

Senior Commissioning Editor: Heidi Harrison
Associate Editor: Robert Edwards
Project Manager: Anne Dickie
Design Direction: George Ajayi

Science–based Rehabilitation

Theories into Practice

Edited by

Kathryn Refshauge PhD (UNSW) MBiomedE (UNSW) GradDipManipTher DipPhty

Louise Ada PhD MA GradDipPhty

Elizabeth Ellis PhD MHL GradDipPhty

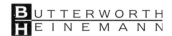
BUTTERWORTH HEINEMANN

EDINBURGH   LONDON   NEW   YORK   OXFORD   PHILADELPHIA   ST LOUIS   SYDNEY   TORONTO   2005

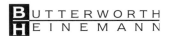

An imprint of Elsevier Limited

First published 2005

ISBN 0 7506 5564 X

British Library Cataloguing in Publication Data
A catalogue record for this book is available from the British Library

Library of Congress Cataloging in Publication Data
A catalog record for this book is available from the Library of Congress

Notice
Medical knowledge is constantly changing. Standard safety precautions must be followed, but as new research and clinical experience broaden our knowledge, changes in treatment and drug therapy may become necessary or appropriate. Readers are advised to check the most current product information provided by the manufacturer of each drug to be administered to verify the recommended dose, the method and duration of administration, and contraindications. It is the responsibility of the practitioner, relying on experience and knowledge of the patient, to determine dosages and the best treatment for each individual patient. Neither the Publisher nor the author assumes any liability for any injury and/or damage to persons or property arising from this publication.

Neither the publishers nor the author will be liable for any loss or damage of any nature occasioned to or suffered by any person acting or refraining from acting as a result of reliance on the material contained in this publication.

The Publisher

 your source for books, journals and multimedia in the health sciences

www.elsevierhealth.com

Printed in China

The publisher's policy is to use **paper manufactured from sustainable forests**

Contents

Preface

In the last 30 years, the physiotherapy profession has faced significant challenges, resulting in unprecedented changes in our professional role. In particular, these years encompass the period when physiotherapists developed independent reasoning and professional practice. For the first time in Australia and around the world, physiotherapists were developing career paths in scholarship and learning as well as in the clinic. Entry programmes were increasingly located in universities, and therefore academic pathways became possible, leading to the proliferation of higher degrees and research within the profession. This period was particularly significant for us as we were students in the mid-1970s and began our academic careers in the early 1980s.

The move from hospital-based to university-based education resulted in the physiotherapy profession changing from an art to a science. There was strong recognition of the importance of deriving clinical implications from the literature, particularly the related sciences, and of conducting research on human function. More recently there has been a rapid development of interventions based on a wider and sounder theoretical basis, the development of reliable measurement tools and the vigorous testing of outcomes.

Professors Janet Carr and Roberta Shepherd have been at the forefront of many of these changes over the last two to three decades. This drive for change is particularly evident in their scholarly work and academic leadership. A marker of the early stage of their influence was the publication in the early 1980s of one of their first internationally available textbooks, *A Motor Relearning Programme for Stroke*. This textbook was extensively referenced to support their arguments, particularly unusual at that time and which, in fact, still contrast with some textbooks published today.

This book has been designed to provide a lasting tribute to the enormous contribution of Professors Carr and Shepherd to clinical practice through their academic work and professional leadership. They also stimulated passionate debate and the development of ideas within the broad physiotherapy community, and between physiotherapy and other professions. They conducted their own research and scholarly work, while encouraging and mentoring young researchers and clinicians. We particularly wanted to honour their contribution to our profession, because Janet and Roberta provided a very important influence for each of us in our formative academic years, and have remained our great friends.

The book is also a collection of works about various aspects of rehabilitation by invited contributors. The authors were included because they are colleagues of Professors Carr and Shepherd, have contributed significantly to their field and share a passion for scholarship. They are colleagues from within the physiotherapy profession, some of whom have been mentored by Professors Carr and Shepherd over the years as fellow academics or research students, and others of whom have been collaborators. In addition, the authors share a vision of translating theory into practice.

The book captures the evolution of knowledge in the area of rehabilitation from an international perspective. It is a collection of work that provides some insight into the physiotherapy profession today. The various contributions follow an unintended but logical progression, from assessment, through the nature and contribution of impairments, to disability and finally handicap. *Science-based Rehabilitation: Theories into Practice* not only draws on related sciences but also reflects the research outcomes of physiotherapists. It is a clear illustration of where we are now and where we have come from.

Kathryn Refshauge
Louise Ada
Elizabeth Ellis
March 2004

Contributors

Louise Ada PhD MA BSc GradDipPhty
*School of Physiotherapy, University of Sydney,
NSW, Australia*

Julie Bernhardt PhD BSc
*National Stroke Research Institute, Heidelberg
West, Victoria, Australia*

Suzann K. Campbell PT PhD FAPTA
*Professor and Head, Department of Physical
Therapy, University of Illinois at Chicago,
Chicago, Illinois, USA*

Colleen Canning BPhty MA PhD
*School of Physiotherapy, University of Sydney,
NSW, Australia*

Janet Carr EdD FACP
*Associate Professor, School of Physiotherapy,
University of Sydney, NSW, Australia*

Glen M. Davis BPE(Hons) MA PhD
*Associate Professor, Rehabilitation Research
Centre, University of Sydney, NSW, Australia*

Karen Dodd PhD
*School of Physiotherapy, La Trobe University,
Bundoora, Victoria, Australia*

Elizabeth Ellis PhD MSc MHL BSc GradDipPhty
*School of Physiotherapy, University of Sydney,
NSW, Australia*

Robert Herbert BAppSc MAppSc PhD
*School of Physiotherapy, University of Sydney,
NSW, Australia*

Keith Hill BAppSc(Physio) Grad Dip Physio PhD
*National Ageing Research Institute, Parkville,
Victoria, Australia*

Frances Huxham Dip Physio Grad Dip (Health Research
Methods)
*School of Physiotherapy, La Trobe University,
Bundoora, Victoria, Australia*

Victoria Jayalath BA(Hons)
*School of Physiotherapy, La Trobe University,
Bundoora, Victoria, Australia*

Sharon L. Kilbreath BSc(PT) MClSc(PT) PhD
*School of Physiotherapy, University of Sydney,
NSW, Australia*

Francine Malouin PhD
*Professor, Department of Rehabilitation, Faculty
of Medicine, Laval University, Ste Foy, Quebec,
Canada*

Meg Morris BAppSc Grad Dip(Gerontol) MAppSc PhD
MAPA
*Professor, School of Physiotherapy, La Trobe
University, Bundoora, Victoria, Australia*

Di J. Newham PhD MCSP
*Professor of Physiotherapy and Director of the
Centre for Applied Biomedical Research, GKT
School of Biomedical Science, Kings College,
London, UK*

Jennifer Oates BAppSc (Sp Path) MAppSc PhD
*School of Human Communication Sciences, La
Trobe University, Bundoora, Victoria, Australia*

Sandra J. Olney PhD MEd P&OT BSc
*Professor, School of Rehabilitation Therapy,
Queens University, Kingston, Ontario, Canada*

Kathy Refshauge PhD MBiomedE GradDipManipTher
DipPhty
*Professor, School of Physiotherapy, University of
Sydney, NSW, Australia*

Carol L. Richards PhD DU pht
*Professor, Department of Rehabilitation, Faculty
of Medicine, Laval University, Ste Foy, Quebec,
Canada*

Roberta Shepherd EdD FACP
*Professor, School of Physiotherapy, University of
Sydney, NSW, Australia*

Chapter 1

Bridging the gap between theory and practice

Roberta Shepherd and Janet Carr

Understanding the history of physiotherapy practice enables us to reflect on the concept of change and development in clinical practice and to feel more comfortable about the notion that clinical practice quite naturally responds and adapts as new scientific knowledge emerges. The history of neurological physiotherapy exemplifies the process of change. Practitioners early in the 20th century used forms of corrective exercise and muscle re-education, the latter involving exercises directed at individual muscles, with consideration of the roles of other muscles that act as synergists. The knowledge that clinicians applied in their practice reflected an early focus on structural anatomy and the principles of exercise. Many of the patients were individuals with muscle weakness and paralysis from poliomyelitis.

In the 1950s, a major conceptual shift in neurological physiotherapy was evident as the neurophysiological, or 'facilitation', approaches were developed. The focus changed from the muscle to non-muscular elements. Methods were directed primarily at the nervous system, with movement facilitated by stimulation of the nervous system. Major developments were those of the Bobaths (Bobath 1965, 1970), called Bobath therapy or neurodevelopmental therapy (NDT), and of Kabat (1961) and Knott and Voss (1968), whose methods of facilitation were referred to as 'proprioceptive neuromuscular facilitation' (PNF). Other therapists also developed their ideas for therapy around this time, including Rood (1956), Ayres (1977) and Brunnstrom (1970).

These approaches to therapy are often referred to as eponymous because they were named after their originators. Methods were based largely on interpretations of the neurophysiological literature of the time. By and large, most of these methods fitted within the scientific understanding of the first half of the 20th century, with its experimental paradigms in neurophysiology of stimulus–response mechanisms, much of it based on animal models. Many of the therapeutic methods developed focused on facilitating movement by stimulating sensory receptors, specifically muscle and joint proprioceptors and tactile receptors.

These therapy approaches, particularly of Bobath and PNF, dominated the second half of the 20th century, and are still currently in use in many countries. However, during this time there were newer developments as physiotherapists and others who had access to the scientific literature sought ways of transferring new scientific findings to clinical practice. These developments utilized experimental work that focused, for example, on how humans acquire skill in movement or motor learning (Carr and Shepherd 1980, 1987, 2000), on muscle biology and muscle adaptability (Gossman et al 1982, Rose and Rothstein 1982) and on psychology (Anderson and Lough 1986). These developments reflected to a large extent the increasing opportunity for physiotherapists to enrol in postgraduate courses, developing research skills and engaging in intensive study of specific fields. Not surprisingly, they saw the clinical implications.

The clinical thinking underlying these new developments reflected a change from approaches to therapy that were developed inductively, that is, clinical findings of interest leading to a search for a theoretical explanation (Gordon 2000). Early attempts at developing therapy methods to improve functional movement were largely inductive, and this was partly due to the lack of a scientific body of knowledge on human movement from which clinical implications could be derived. Over the last few decades, however, technological developments together with changes in the conceptualizing of how the human nervous system might function to produce skilled movement are producing an increasing volume of movement-related research that has obvious relevance to clinical practice. Experimental paradigms have shifted from a reductionist approach, in which the focus was on, for example, stretch reflex mechanisms using animal models, to an exploration of mechanisms of movement control in humans from the perspectives of performance as well as of physiological mechanisms. Technological developments in motion analysis and electromyography (EMG) enabled biomechanical studies of balance and of actions such as walking, standing up and reaching to pick up an object. Recently, new brain imaging methods are enabling an examination of organizational changes occurring within the brain itself.

The increase in clinically relevant research findings related to movement made possible the development of movement rehabilitation by a deductive process, clinical implications being derived from a theoretical science base. As an example, for the action of sit-to-stand (Carr et al 2002, Shepherd and Koh 1996), there is now a rational biomechanical base that enables the development of standardized guidelines for training this action (Carr and Shepherd 1998, 2003).

Increasing scientific knowledge about motor control processes and motor performance, the effects of lesions and recovery processes enables us to question the assumptions underlying both clinical theorizing and current practice (Gordon 2000). Scrutiny of theoretical assumptions can enable us to move on from old methods of practice to methods more congruent with contemporary scientific understanding. Furthermore, clinical research is enabling us to test the efficacy of interventions.

The process of change can be difficult for the practitioner, and there is a temptation to combine newer methods with those already in use. In the history of scientific endeavour there have always been attempts to integrate new methods with old at times of major change (Abernethy and Sparrow 1992). In some fields this mixing is called hybridization. The move towards hybridization can be compelling and, as Abernethy and Sparrow (1992) point out, 'the case for reconciliation of competing paradigms is superficially attractive'. Hybridization or eclecticism can also seem attractive to a physiotherapist clinician. There can be a reluctance to let go of familiar therapeutic methods and move on.

However, competing paradigms have philosophical and conceptual differences (Abernethy and Sparrow 1992) because they are based on different views of, for example, how the system is organized or the nature of impairments after a lesion. Hybridization can become a problem when new methods are added into a therapy approach that is based on contradictory theoretical assumptions, particularly if there is lack of evidential support.

The need for practice to move on by responding to new knowledge is well illustrated by examining research over the last few years that is changing the way in which we view impairments following a lesion of the upper motor neuron system. A re-evaluation of the relative contributions of muscle weakness, of adaptive changes in muscle such as increased stiffness and of spasticity is requiring significant changes in clinical practice. The view that spasticity is the major impairment underlying movement dysfunction led to the development of methods based on the premise that spasticity had to be decreased or inhibited in order to facilitate more normal movement (Bobath 1965, 1990). This view has been very influential over the past few decades. Muscle weakness was not a primary focus in physiotherapy because spasticity was considered the cause of weakness and disability. Congruent with this view, therapists avoided exercise that required effort (as in strength training) because this effort was assumed to increase spasticity.

Of major significance to the planning of interventions, therefore, are contemporary research findings that support the view that the major impairments interfering with functional performance after lesions of the motor system (upper motor neuron lesions) are paralysis and weakness (absent or reduced muscle force generation) and loss of dexterity (disordered motor control) (Landau 1980). In addition, soft-tissue adaptations occurring in response both to muscle weakness and to post-lesion inactivity and disuse impact negatively on the potential for regaining function. These adaptations include increased muscle stiffness (defined as a mechanical response to load on a non-contracting muscle and decreased soft-tissue length) and structural and functional reorganization of muscle and connective tissue (Sinkjaer and Magnussen 1994).

The significance of spasticity (defined as velocity-dependent stretch reflex hyperactivity – Lance 1980) for the regaining of motor function remains equivocal. There is little to support the view that reflex hyperactivity is a significant contributor to movement dysfunction. Some reports indicate stretch reflex hyperactivity can develop some time after the lesion, suggesting that it may be an adaptive response to non-functional, contracted, stiff muscles (Gracies et al 1997). In clinical practice, increased resistance to passive movement is typically referred to as spasticity, although mechanical and functional changes to muscle are likely to be major contributors. Clinical tests, such as the Ashworth Scale, that are commonly used in clinical research are not able to distinguish the relative contributions of increased stiffness of muscles and reflex hyperactivity.

Our own collaborative theoretical and investigative work has developed over the years, being broadly based on research related to human movement, and updated as new developments emerge in science and as evidence of the effects of intervention slowly began filtering into the literature from clinical studies. Principal research areas driving our work include motor control mechanisms, muscle biology, biomechanics, skill acquisition and exercise science (Carr and Shepherd 1987, 1998, 2000, 2003). A point of interest is that the focus is strongly on the importation of theories and data from fields other than physiotherapy, illustrating the nature of physiotherapy as an applied clinical science.

Attempts to illustrate how to bridge the gap between scientific research in other fields and clinical practice have led to the formulation and testing of hypotheses related to clinical practice.

Systematic collection of objective data in clinical practice is critical not only as an important step in establishing best practice but also in making changes to practice as more effective methods of training are developed and tested.

As a result of both the theoretical and the clinical evidence, intervention is increasingly focusing on task-oriented exercise and motor training, together with strength and fitness training, as a means of improving the patient's capacity to learn motor skills and optimize functional motor performance. An increasing number of studies have shown positive effects in individuals with brain lesions of task-oriented training and strength training on muscle strength and functional performance (e.g. Brown and Kautz 1998, Butefisch et al 1995, Dean et al 2000, Dean and Shepherd 1997; Sharp and Brouwer 1997, Teixeira-Salmela et al 1999, 2001, Visintin et al 1998). Strength training does not appear to result in increases in resistance to passive movement (hypertonus) or reflex hyperactivity (spasticity). Training that is sufficiently intensive can also produce a cardiovascular training effect (Macko et al 1997). Methods of stimulating activation in poorly innervated muscles are also being developed and include electromyography (EMG)-triggered electrical stimulation and computer-aided training.

Important insights into mechanisms mediating motor recovery after injury to the sensorimotor cortex are now beginning to emerge. Neurophysiological and neuroanatomical studies in animals and neuroimaging and other non-invasive mapping studies in humans are providing substantial evidence that the adult cerebral cortex is capable of significant functional reorganization (e.g. Barbro 2000, Nudo et al 2001). These studies have demonstrated plasticity in functional topography and anatomy of intact cortical tissue adjacent to the injury and of more remote cortical areas. Of critical importance for rehabilitation is that experience, learning and active use of the affected limbs appear to modulate the adaptive reorganization that inevitably occurs after cortical injury. It seems likely from current research that, for rehabilitation to be effective in optimizing neural reorganization and functional recovery, increased emphasis needs to be placed on motor learning using intensive and repetitive task-oriented exercise and training (e.g. Liepert et al 2001, Nelles et al 2001, Nudo and Friel 1999).

As physiotherapists, we are becoming increasingly aware of patients as active participants in intervention rather than as passive recipients of therapy. This is due partly to our increasing knowledge of how people learn and relearn motor skills. The idea that motor learning research can provide a rich source of scientific information to guide clinical practice has been available to the profession for several decades. Our own textbooks have discussed motor learning research and its obvious relevance to physiotherapy. In 1980 we suggested that training methods shown to be associated with improvement in motor skills in able-bodied populations are also likely to be effective in a person with disability who must regain skill in everyday actions and learn new skills such as wheelchair locomotion.

Performance of an action that is effective in consistently achieving a specific goal with some economy of effort is said to be skilled. We assume that the acquisition or learning of skill, involving practice and exercise, is a manifestation of internal processes making up what is called motor learning. Motor learning itself cannot be directly observed. It is a set of complex internal processes that can only be inferred from a relatively consistent improvement in performance of an action, that is, a relatively stable change in motor behaviour as a result of practice of that action (Magill 2001, Schmidt 1988). It can only be inferred from the behaviour we observe when we measure certain characteristics of motor performance over a period of time (see Magill 2001). To know whether or not performance has improved, the therapist has, therefore, to measure the person's performance at the start of training, at various stages throughout rehabilitation and periodically after discharge home.

For several decades, scientists have investigated the process of acquiring skill, typically with young healthy adults as they learn a novel task or train to improve a specific skill, and increasingly with people with motor disability. Gentile (2000) describes the stages of learning as first getting the idea of the movement, then developing the ability to adapt the movement pattern to environmental demands. In the initial stages the person learns to pay attention to the critical features of the action/task and is actively engaged in practice. Considering the patient as a learner involves setting up conditions under which skill learning can take place.

Awareness of the characteristics of each stage of learning enables the therapist to provide appropriate practice conditions to optimize performance (Carr and Shepherd 2003). In clinical practice, the learner's focus of attention shifts as muscle strength, motor control and skill increase. In walking, for example, it may shift from the feet to the surrounding environment; star billing for sit-to-stand may change from initial foot placement and increasing the speed of forward rotation of the upper body to the need to steady a glass of water while standing up.

As part of the training process, the therapist may direct the patient's focus of attention away from an internal body-oriented focus (the feet, upper body movement) to an external focus that is directly related to the goal (avoiding obstacles on the floor). Some recent findings with healthy subjects have shown what a difference it can make to performance and skill development if the learner directs attention toward the effect of the movement (an external focus) instead of to the movement itself (an internal focus) (Wulf et al 1998).

Skilled performance is characterized by the ability to perform complex movements, with the flexibility to vary movement to meet ongoing environmental demands with economy of effort. This applies as much to everyday actions such as walking and standing up from a seat, as it does to recreational, sporting or work-related actions. Skill is task-specific. Although such actions as level walking and stair walking may share similar biomechanical characteristics, the demands placed on the individual by each action are different. The individual learns to reshape and adapt the basic movement pattern according to different contexts; crossing the street at pedestrian lights may require an increase in walking speed, negotiating obstacles in the house requires other changes in the walking pattern.

Improvement in a particular action therefore requires practice of that action; that is, the learner has to practise in order for performance to become effective in achieving the specific goal. For some individuals, speeding up the action and improving power generation may be major performance goals. However, for those whose muscle strength and motor control are below a certain threshold, such practice may not be possible. Exercises to increase strength and control may be necessary, together with practice of the action under modified conditions, for example, standing up from a higher seat, which requires less muscle force generation. Many repetitions of an action are required to increase strength and for the patient to develop an optimal way of performing the action (Bernstein in Latash and Latash 1994). Traditional physiotherapy has neglected the repetitive element of skill acquisition that probably forms an essential prerequisite in motor rehabilitation (Butefisch et al 1995).

In training functional tasks, the therapist sets the goals in consultation with the individual and based on evaluation of the patient's capabilities. As 'coach', the therapist may point out how a movement is organized based on knowledge of crucial biomechanical characteristics; provide verbal instructions, feedback or demonstration; direct the person's visual attention; or highlight regulatory cues in the environment (e.g. height of an obstacle). However, it is the patient who must learn to organize movement that matches the environment in order to achieve these goals.

Goal-setting involves organizing the environment to be functionally relevant; that is, by providing meaningful objects of different sizes, weight, graspability, which allow for different tasks to be trained. Goals are concrete rather than abstract, for example: 'Reach out and take the glass from the table' rather than 'Raise your arm'; 'Reach sideways to pick up the glass from the floor' rather than 'Shift your weight over to the left'. Recent research has illustrated well the different outcomes when individuals after stroke work with concrete goals linked to real objects rather than with more abstract goals (van Vliet et al 1995, Wu et al 2000). Wu and colleagues examined a task in which participants used one hand to scoop coins from a table into the other hand. Able-bodied persons and persons with stroke took part, sometimes with coins, sometimes mimicking the movement without coins. Both groups of participants demonstrated faster movements, with smoother and straighter reaches, all characteristics of well-learned coordinated movement, when they scooped the coins compared with when they mimicked the action.

If brain reorganization and functional recovery from brain lesions is dependent on use and activity, then the environment in which rehabilitation is carried out is likely to play an important role in patient outcomes. The rehabilitation environment is made up of: the physical or built environment (the physical setting); the methods used to deliver rehabilitation (type of intervention, intensity, dosage); and the staff (their knowledge, skill, attitudes and their ability to teach).

Evidence from animal experiments suggests that the nature of the environment, its physical structure together with the opportunities it offers for social interaction and physical activity, can influence outcome after a lesion. In animal research, the aspects of the enriched environment that appear to be critical as enhancers of behaviour are social stimulation, interaction with objects that enable physical activity (Bennett 1976) and an increased level of arousal (Walsh and Cummins 1975).

Observational studies of rehabilitation settings provide some insights into how patients spend their days. The results suggest that the rehabilitation environment may not be sufficiently geared to facilitating physical and mental activity or social interaction, and that it may not function as a learning environment (Ada et al 1999). Other studies suggest that a large percentage of the patient's day is spent in passive pursuits rather than in physical activity.

The issue of how much time is spent in physical activity, including practice of motor tasks, and how this time is organized, is therefore a critical one for rehabilitation.

Focusing on task-oriented training has required some changes in physiotherapy practice, not only in methods used but also in delivery. Physiotherapists are exploring different ways to organize the delivery of physiotherapy to enable the patient to be an active learner; for example, examining the effects of a more interactive relationship between patient and therapist, of small group training sessions during circuit training, of sessions where patients work in partnership with each other (McNevin et al 2000). Technological innovations are aiding the development of computer-aided training methods that foster independent practice.

However, what the patient is actually doing in physiotherapy must itself be effective if increasing the amount of time spent practising is to improve outcome. Important evidence is emerging that cortical reshaping depends on the nature and intensity of practice, rather than simply on its presence (Small and Solodkin 1998). Furthermore, what the patient does outside time allotted for supervised training is also likely to impact significantly on progress. For example, self-propulsion in a one-arm-driven wheelchair using non-paretic limbs is at odds with goals to increase strength and control of paretic limbs (Esmonde et al 1997). If the patient spends more time in this activity than in exercising the impaired limbs, it is not hard to guess the probable outcome.

An aspect of therapy for neural lesions that has received little attention until recently is the intensity of exercise and the extent of cardiovascular stress induced during physical activity. The detrimental effect of low exercise capacity and muscle endurance on functional mobility and resistance to fatigue can be compounded by the high metabolic demand of adaptive movements. Stroke patients are often unable to maintain comfortably their most efficient walking speed, indicating that the high energy cost of walking and poor endurance further compromise functional performance (Olney et al 1986, Wade and Hewer 1987).

There are several reports of improved aerobic capacity in chronic stroke with appropriate training such as bicycle ergometry (Potempa et al 1995), with graded treadmill walking (Macko et al 1997) and with a combination of aerobic and strengthening exercises (Teixeira-Salmela et al 1999). As might be expected, the effects are exercise-specific. Generalization occurs, however, in the improvements noted in general health and well-being. Teixeira-Salmela and colleagues (1999) assessed participants' general level of physical activity on the Human Activity Profile, a survey of 94 activities that are rated according to their required metabolic equivalents. The results indicated that participants were able to perform more household chores and recreational activities after strength and aerobic training.

It is interesting to consider that despite the common risk factors and pathophysiology of stroke and cardiac disease, physical rehabilitation for these conditions varies considerably. It is well documented that stroke patients have low physical endurance when discharged from rehabilitation. Deconditioning has been shown to occur within the first six weeks after stroke in a study that measured exercise capacity in the early post-stroke period. Patients performed incremental maximal effort tests on a semirecumbent cycle ergometer (Kelly et al 2003). This deconditioning may be a consequence of the relatively static nature of typical rehabilitation programmes and indicates that intensity of training needs to be addressed specifically and early after an acute brain lesion.

Recently MacKay-Lyons and Makrides (2002) investigated the aerobic component of physiotherapy and occupational therapy for stroke patients by monitoring heart rate (using heart-rate monitors) and therapeutic activities biweekly over a 14-week period without influencing the content. The major finding was that the therapy sessions involved low-intensity exercise and activity that did not provide adequate metabolic stress to induce a training effect. Although one might expect progressively higher exercise intensities over time as functional status improves, any increase in mean heart rate (HR_{mean}) and peak heart rate (HR_{peak}) did not reach statistical significance.

It should be noted that the benefits of task-oriented skill training and strength training are also being reported in studies of children with cerebral palsy (Blundell et al 2003, Damiano et al 1995). Although the primary deficit is injury to the brain, adaptive changes in the musculoskeletal and cardiorespiratory systems also impose severe limitations on the gaining of functional motor performance (Booth et al 2001, Rimmer and Damiano 2001). Many of these changes are preventable or reversible (Damiano 2003).

CONCLUDING COMMENTS

The regaining of skill in critical tasks requires specific training, with intensive practice of actions in the appropriate contexts. In addition, the individual must be fit enough to perform the tasks of daily life, including taking part in social and recreational activities. Participation in regular exercise and training appears to have significant effects on reducing disability and improving quality of life. Post-discharge services for individuals with chronic disability, however, are poor or non-existent, and there are reports of high levels of patient dissatisfaction (Tyson and Turner 2000) and loss of rehabilitation gains (Paolucci et al 2001). The provision of facilities such as strength and fitness centres directed at all age groups and degrees of disability requires collaboration between public health and community services. Physiotherapists can play a significant role in this collaborative process.

Entry-level physiotherapy curricula have also to respond to evidence of the importance of exercise and training for individuals with chronic disability, with the inclusion as core knowledge of subjects such as biomechanics, exercise science and motor learning. The skills required for training individuals with disability, including how to adapt training and exercise to the patient's level of performance, should also form a significant part of the education of physiotherapy students as well as of skill upgrading in continuing professional education.

References

Abernethy B, Sparrow W A 1992 The rise and fall of dominant paradigms in motor behaviour research. In: Summers J J (ed) Approaches to the study of motor control and learning. Elsevier Science, North Holland, pp 3–45.

Ada L, Mackey F, Heard R et al 1999 Stroke rehabilitation: does the therapy area provide a physical challenge? Australian Journal of Physiotherapy 45:33–38.

Anderson M, Lough S 1986 A psychological framework for neurorehabilitation. Physiotherapy Practice 2:74–82.

Ayres A J 1977 Sensory integration and learning disorders. Western Psychological Services, Los Angeles.

Barbro J (2000) Brain plasticity and stroke rehabilitation: The Willis lecture. Stroke 31:223–230.

Bennett E L 1976 Cerebral effects of differential experience and training. In: Rosenzweig MR, Bennett EL (eds) Neural mechanisms of learning and memory. MIT Press, Cambridge, MA, pp 279–287.

Blundell S W, Shepherd R B, Dean C M et al 2003 Functional strength training in cerebral palsy: a pilot study of a group circuit training class for children aged 4–8 years. Clinical Rehabilitation 17:48–57.

Bobath B 1965 Abnormal reflex activity caused by brain lesions. Heinemann, Oxford.

Bobath B 1970 Adult hemiplegia: evaluation and treatment. Butterworth-Heinemann, Oxford.

Bobath B 1990 Adult hemiplegia: evaluation and treatment, 3rd edn. Butterworth-Heinemann, Oxford.

Booth C M, Cortina-Borja M J, Theologis T N 2001 Collagen accumulation in muscles of children with cerebral palsy and correlation with severity of spasticity. Developmental Medicine and Child Neurology 43:314–320.

Brown D A, Kautz S A 1998 Increased workload enhances force output during pedalling exercise in persons with poststroke hemiplegia. Stroke 29:598–606.

Brunnstrom S 1970 Movement therapy in hemiplegia: a neurophysiological approach. Harper and Row, New York.

Butefisch C, Hummelsheim H, Mauritz K-H 1995 Repetitive training of isolated movements improves the outcome of motor rehabilitation of the centrally paretic hand. Journal of Neurological Science 130:59–68.

Carr J H, Shepherd R B 1980 Physiotherapy in disorders of the brain. Butterworth-Heinemann, Oxford, pp 71–93.

Carr J H, Shepherd R B 1987 A motor relearning programme for stroke, 2nd edn. Butterworth-Heinemann, Oxford.

Carr J H, Shepherd R B 1998 Neurological rehabilitation optimizing motor performance. Butterworth-Heinemann, Oxford.

Carr J H, Shepherd R B 2000 A motor learning model for rehabilitation. In: Carr J H, Shepherd R B (eds) Movement science foundations for physical therapy in rehabilitation, 2nd edn. Aspen Publishers, Rockville, MD, pp 33–110.

Carr J H, Shepherd R B 2003 Stroke rehabilitation: guidelines for exercise and training. Butterworth-Heinemann, Oxford.

Carr J H, Ow J E G, Shepherd R B 2002 Some biomechanical characteristics of standing up at three different speeds: implications for functional training. Physiotherapy Theory and Practice 18:47–53.

Damiano D I 2003 Strength, endurance, and fitness in cerebral palsy. Developmental Medicine and Child Neurology 45 Suppl 94:8–10.

Damiano D I, Vaughan C L, Abel M F 1995 Muscle response to heavy resistance exercise in children with spastic cerebral palsy. Developmental Medicine and Child Neurology 37:731–739.

Dean C M, Shepherd R B 1997 Task-related training improves performance of seated reaching tasks after stroke: a randomized controlled trial. Stroke 28:722–728.

Dean C M, Richards C L, Malouin F 2000 Task-related training improves performance of locomotor tasks in chronic stroke. A randomized controlled pilot study. Archives of Physical Medicine and Rehabilitation 81:409–417.

Esmonde T, McGinley J, Goldie P et al 1997 Stroke rehabilitation: patient activity during non-therapy time. Australian Journal of Physiotherapy 43:43–51.

Gentile A M 2000 Skill acquisition: action, movement, and neuromotor processes. In: Carr J H, Shepherd R B (eds) Movement science foundations for physical therapy in rehabilitation, 2nd edn. Aspen Publishers, Rockville, MD, pp 111–187.

Gordon J 2000 Assumptions underlying physical therapy interventions: theoretical and historical perspectives. In: Carr J H, Shepherd R B (eds) Movement science foundations for physical therapy in rehabilitation, 2nd edn. Aspen Publishers, Rockville, MD, pp 1–31.

Gossman M R, Sahrmann S A, Rose S J 1982 Review of length-associated changes in muscle. Physical Therapy 62:1799–1808.

Gracies J-M, Wilson L, Gandevia S C et al 1997 Stretched position of spastic muscles aggravates their co-contraction in hemiplegic patients. Annals of Neurology 42:438–439.

Kabat H 1961 Proprioceptive facilitation in therapeutic exercise. In: Licht S (ed) Therapeutic exercise. E. Licht, New Haven.

Kelly J, Kilbreath S L, Davis G M et al 2003 Cardiorespiratory fitness and walking ability in acute stroke patients. Archives of Physical Medicine and Rehabilitation 84:1780–1785.

Knott M, Voss D E 1968 Proprioceptive neuromuscular facilitation, 2nd edn. Harper and Row, New York.

Lance J M (1980) Symposium synopsis. In: Feldman R G, Young R R, Koella W P (eds) Spasticity: disorder of motor control. Year Book Medical, Chicago, pp 485–494.

Landau W M 1980 Spasticity: What is it? What is it not? In: Feldman R G, Young R R, Koella W P (eds) Spasticity: disorder of motor control. Year Book Medical, Chicago, pp 17–24.

Latash L P, Latash M L 1994 A new book by NA Bernstein: 'On Dexterity and its Development'. Journal of Motor Behavior 26:56–62.

Liepert J, Uhde I, Graf S et al 2001 Motor cortex plasticity during forced-use therapy in stroke patients: a preliminary study. Journal of Neurology 248:315–321.

MacKay-Lyons M J, Makrides L 2002 Cardiovascular stress during a contemporary stroke rehabilitation program: is the intensity adequate to induce a training effect? Archives of Physical Medicine and Rehabilitation 83:1378–1383.

Macko R F, De Souza C A, Tretter L D et al 1997 Treadmill aerobic exercise training reduces the energy and cardiovascular demands of hemiparetic gait in chronic stroke patients. Stroke 28:326–330.

McNevin N H, Wulf G, Carlson C 2000 Effects of attentional focus, self-control, and dyad training on motor learning: implications for physical therapy. Physical Therapy 80:373–385.

Magill R A 2001 Motor learning concepts and applications, 6th edn. McGraw-Hill, New York.

Nelles G, Jentzen W, Jueptner M et al 2001 Arm training induced brain plasticity in stroke studied with serial positron emission tomography. NeuroImage 13:1146–1154.

Nudo R J, Friel K M 1999 Cortical plasticity after stroke: implications for rehabilitation. Revista Neurologia 9:713–717.

Nudo R J, Plautz E J, Frost S B 2001 Role of adaptive plasticity in recovery of function after damage to motor cortex. Muscle Nerve 8:1000–1019.

Olney S J, Monga T N, Costigan P A 1986 Mechanical energy of walking of stroke patients. Archives of Physical Medicine and Rehabilitation 67:92–98.

Paolucci S, Grasso M G, Antonucci G et al 2001 Mobility status after inpatient stroke rehabilitation: 1 year follow-up and prognosis factors. Archives of Physical Medicine and Rehabilitation 82:2–8.

Potempa K, Lopez M, Braun L T et al 1995 Physiological outcomes of aerobic exercise training in hemiparetic stroke patients. Stroke 26:101–105.

Rimmer J H, Damiano D L 2001 Maintaining or improving fitness in children with disabilities. In: Carr J, Shepherd R (eds) Topics in Pediatrics. American Physical Therapy Association, Alexandria, pp 1–16.

Rood M S 1956 Neurophysiological mechanisms utilised in the treatment of neuromuscular dysfunction. American Journal of Occupational Therapy 10:220–225.

Rose S J, Rothstein J M (1982) Muscle mutability Part 1. General concepts and adaptations to altered patterns of use. Physical Therapy 62:1773–1785.

Schmidt R A 1988 Motor and action perspectives on motor behavior. In: Meijer O G, Roth K (eds) Complex motor behavior: the motor-action controversy. Elsevier, Amsterdam, pp 3–44.

Sharp S A, Brouwer B J (1997) Isokinetic strength training of the hemiparetic knee: effects on function and spasticity. Archives of Physical Medicine and Rehabilitation 78:1231–1236.

Shepherd R B, Koh H P (1996) Some biomechanical consequences of varying foot placement in sit-to-stand in young women. Scandinavian Journal of Rehabilitation Medicine 28:79–88.

Sinkjaer T, Magnussen I 1994 Passive, intrinsic and reflex-mediated stiffness in the ankle extensors of hemiparetic patients. Brain 117:355–363.

Small S L, Solodkin A 1998 The neurobiology of stroke rehabilitation. Neuroscientist 4:426–434.

Teixeira-Salmela L F, Olney S J, Nadeau S et al 1999 Muscle strengthening and physical conditioning to reduce impairment and disability in chronic stroke survivors. Archives of Physical Medicine and Rehabilitation 80:1211–1218.

Teixeira-Salmela L F, Nadeau S, McBride I et al 2001 Effects of muscle strengthening and physical

conditioning training on temporal, kinematic and kinetic variables during gait in chronic stroke survivors. Journal of Rehabilitation Medicine 33:53–60.

Tyson S, Turner G (2000) Discharge and follow-up for people with stroke: what happens and why. Clinical Rehabilitation 14:381–392.

Visintin M, Barbeau H, Korner-Bitensky N et al 1998 A new approach to retrain gait in stroke patients through body weight support and treadmill stimulation. Stroke 29:1122–1128.

van Vliet P, Kerwin D G, Sheridan M et al 1995 The influence of goals on the kinematics of reaching following stroke. Neurology Report 19:11–16.

Wade D T, Hewer R L (1987) Functional abilities after stroke: measurement, natural history and prognosis. Journal of Neurology, Neurosurgery and Psychiatry 50:177–182.

Walsh R N, Cummins R A (1975) Mechanisms mediating the production of environmentallly induced brain changes. Psychology Bulletin 82:986–1000.

Wu C, Trombly C A, Lin K et al 2000 A kinematic study of contextual effects on reaching performance in persons with and without stroke: influences of object availability. Archives of Physical Medicine and Rehabilitation 81:95–101.

Wulf G, Hoß M, Prinz W 1998 Instruction for motor learning: differential effects of internal vs external focus of attention. Journal of Motor Behavior 30:169–179.

Chapter 2

We only treat what it occurs to us to assess: the importance of knowledge-based assessment

Julie Bernhardt and Keith Hill

PRINCIPLES OF ASSESSMENT

As Emily Keshner once said, 'We only treat what it occurs to us to assess' (Keshner 1991). That is why assessment is a vital part of rehabilitation. Assessment is used in this context to include selection of appropriate measurement instruments, the effective conduct of the assessment and correct interpretation of assessment outcomes. In this chapter, we explore how choice of assessment impacts on treatment. It is not our intention to provide a comprehensive review of measurement instruments used in rehabilitation. This information is already available from a range of sources (Cole et al 1994, Hill et al 2001, Wade 1992). Instead we wish to examine how research contributes to our understanding of what we should assess and how, in turn, this impacts on clinical practice.

Following a brief review of levels of assessment and measurement instruments, we provide two examples of how assessment can be shaped by knowledge derived from clinical research. In the first example, improving assessment of the upper limb after stroke is examined. This area has received very little attention to date. The focus of the second example is on balance dysfunction. In this example, we look at how choice of measurement instrument influences choice of training.

Effective assessment – the key to effective practice

The purpose of assessment is to help us determine the best intervention. Assessment differs from measurement in that it represents a process that includes both diagnosis and interpretation of what has been measured (Wade 1992). There are two main levels at which clinical assessment is conducted. At one level, assessment serves to establish the patient's functional status, that is, the extent to which the patient is able, with or without assistance, to perform aspects of everyday function. Functional assessment is conducted at selected time points throughout rehabilitation. It provides patients and therapists with information about recovery, and can be used to identify the effectiveness of rehabilitation programmes (Hamilton and Granger 1994, Vanclay 1991).

Assessment of functional abilities alone, however, is insufficient for the development of treatment plans (Atkinson 1992, Carr and Shepherd 1990a, Charlton 1992, Sawner and La Vigne 1992). The second level of assessment provides therapists with information about the impairments that contribute to the loss of ability to perform previously well-learned actions. This level of assessment focuses on the way in which movements are performed, noting how movement patterns differ from normal, and whether the critical features or essential movement components are present (Atkinson 1992, Carr and Shepherd 1990a, Higgins and Higgins 1995). Inferences about the underlying causes of impaired movements are then made, and treatments directed at restoring normal movement patterns are commenced (Figure 2.1). This form of assessment is also used to monitor response to interventions and redirect treatments until such time as the rehabilitation episode is complete. Information derived from assessment of both movement pattern and function contributes to the development of treatment strategies (Carr and Shepherd 1987, 1990b, Lynch and Grisogono 1991). A poor choice of assessment has the potential to undermine the effectiveness of our intervention. But how do we choose what to assess?

Figure 2.1   Clinical decision-making process outlining diagnosis, reassessment and management phases. (After Thomas 1989, with permission of Nelson Wadsworth.)

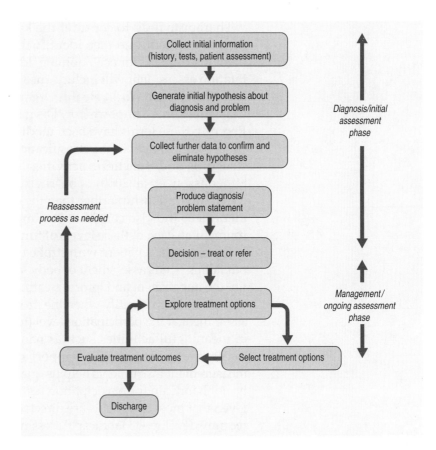

Deciding what to assess

In each clinical setting and for each patient population, choices about the most appropriate, useful and practical measurement instruments must be made. The general purpose of measurement is to detect differences, for example, whether patient performance is different from normal or has changed from one occasion to the next. There are some generic instruments that have utility across a range of clinical groups. These include:

- quality of life measures – e.g. the Assessment of Quality of Life, or AQoL (Hawthorne et al 1999);
- mobility measures – e.g. speed of walking (Friedman et al 1988) and Timed Up and Go (Podsiadlo and Richardson 1991);
- functional measures – e.g. the Functional Independence Measure (Granger et al 1993) and the Frenchay Index (Bond et al 1992).

Others are specific to a clinical group, for example the Unified Parkinson's Disease Rating Scale (UPDRS; Richards et al 1994) and the Extended Disability Status Scale for Patients with Multiple Sclerosis (Kurtzke 1983).

Therapists need to consider the key domains to be included in their assessment, and then identify the most appropriate measurement instruments for each domain. Ideally, a comprehensive rehabilitation assessment will include measurement across the key areas identified by the World Health Organization (WHO) International Classification of Impairment, Disability and Handicap (ICIDH). Recently, these terms have been modified to incorporate substantial conceptual changes in the classification of function, to include body structure and function, activities and participation (ICIDH2; Simeonsson et al 2000). The revised classification describes a dynamic relationship rather than the linear relationship previously identified, and also considers the important influence of the environment on each of these levels of function.

For example, a patient with stroke unable to reach forwards without falling needs assessment of body structure and function (to identify the impairment and inform treatment options), assessment at the activity level (to identify when the problem may affect function) and assessment at the participation level (to facilitate patient engagement in meaningful activities such as hanging out the washing, either through retraining or other support strategies). Most rehabilitation measurement instruments help us quantify impairment and disability, not handicap (or participation restriction). This is not surprising given that most treatments are directed at these levels. However, the recently developed Handicap Assessment and Resource Tool (HART; Vertesi et al 2000) could prove to be a useful addition that may help inform both our treatment decisions and discharge planning.

Over the past 20 years there have been an enormous number of measurement instruments developed for use in rehabilitation. Wherever possible, we should utilize existing instruments, rather than spending our energies developing new ones, or falling into the trap of modifying existing instruments without testing how changes have altered the measurement properties of the instrument. Most importantly, however, when choosing a measure we must be clear about what we hope to gain from measurement (detecting differences). Therapists need to be aware of the range of measurement instruments available, their reliability, validity, sensitivity and other measurement properties, as well as the time, training and equipment necessary for their use. Only then can informed decisions about the most appropriate measurement instrument for a specific need be made. Fortunately a number of books and manuals are available to help therapists make decisions about measurement (Cole et al 1994, Hill et al 2001).

Assessment options

Movement dysfunction is primarily assessed using observation (Carr et al 1987, Davies 1985, Patla and Clouse 1988). Observational assessment relies on accurate detection of movement kinematics such as the linear and angular displacements, velocities and accelerations of body segments. Observation is not only a convenient and cheap method, but may sometimes be the only way to gather clues about the nature of a movement problem (Herbert et al 1993). Therapists are trained to observe, and it is generally believed that training enables us accurately to infer the muscle activations and kinetics that underpin observable kinematics (Carr et al 1987, Herbert et al 1993, Malouin 1995, Perry 1992). At present, however, there is still much we do not know about the accuracy and limitations of observation.

We know more about the reliability and validity of measurement scales. Many, if not most, measurement scales used in rehabilitation are made up of ordered tasks or items with unequal intervals between them (Wade 1992). That is, they are ordinal in nature. The Motor Assessment Scale (Carr et al 1985) and the Functional Ambulation Categories (Holden et al 1986) provide just two examples of ordinal scales. Ordinal scales provide a useful framework for assessment of movement dysfunction on a wide range of tasks. When considering use of these scales it is sometimes helpful for therapists to understand not only the measurement properties of the scale, but also how and why the scale was developed in the first place. Understanding what drives instrument development helps us determine whether we share the same theoretical base for our practice and consequently whether the instrument will provide us with the information we require. It is also important to understand that there are limitations in how data from such instruments can be analysed and reported (Rothstein 1985).

Performance-based measurement that tests the capacity of patients to complete tasks in both closed and open environments (Gentile 1987) is also useful in rehabilitation. These measurement instruments provide information about how far a patient can go – e.g. Functional Reach (Duncan et al 1990), 6-minute walk test (Guyatt et al 1985) – or how fast they can move – e.g. 10-m walk (Dean et al 2001). Performance-based measurement provides continuous measurement (ratio, with true zero), allowing greater capacity for detecting differences between individual patients, or in the same patient over time when compared with ordinal measures for the same domain.

Finally, although we may encounter instruments such as electrogoniometers (Craik and Oatis 1985), load cells and force platforms (Condron and Hill 2002, Smith 1990) and perhaps electromyography (Craik and Oatis 1985) in the clinical setting, they are generally out of reach of the average therapist and largely restricted to the research environment.

In summary, good assessment is fundamental to the development of successful treatment programmes. Making the right choices about what and how to assess, including the selection of appropriate measurement instruments, can lead to the development of better treatment plans and improved evaluation of treatment outcomes.

ASSESSING THE HEMIPLEGIC UPPER LIMB

Earlier we said that simply measuring whether a patient can do a task generally provides insufficient information to guide hypothesis generation and the development of treatment plans. Therapists also need to assess the way in which movements are performed. This level of assessment is primarily conducted using observation. What is observed when we watch patients move is the kinematics of the movement, in other words, the focus of the observation is on how a performer's body segments are coordinated in space and time (Charlton 1994). That is to say, we look for movement cues that help generate hypotheses about the nature of dysfunction. These hypotheses must then be systematically tested.

One of the challenges of upper limb assessment is that the arm and hand are able to perform a vast array of complex activities. An important question is whether observation of upper limb movements can be conducted and recorded in a systematic or standardized fashion. Without this, observation will continue to be classed as 'subjective', the implication being that it is neither reliable nor accurate. There has been very little explicit discussion in physiotherapy literature about precisely what should be observed during movement performance (Herbert et al 1993). Carr and Shepherd (1990a) have developed a useful list of critical components of successful upper limb movements together with common adaptive behaviours after stroke. We also need to determine the critical cues or features of patients' movements that help us decide what to treat if a standardized process of observation is to be developed. The next step is to determine whether therapists are capable of making accurate visual judgements about these critical cues. Although this sounds simple, deciding what to observe is far from straightforward.

What characteristics of upper limb performance do therapists observe?

One method of gathering potentially important cues for upper limb assessment is to ask a group of therapists what cues they think they use when assessing movement. In 1994, experienced neurological therapists were surveyed in an effort to establish therapists' views about important visual cues for upper limb assessment (Bernhardt et al 1998a, 2003). The questionnaire asked therapists to think about watching a patient with stroke grasping and transporting an object from a table to place it on a shelf. They were then asked to list 10 visual cues they would use to make decisions about the quality of the movement or to decide whether performance had changed from one occasion to the next. In total, 584 cues were identified by the 67 therapists. Seventeen of these were classed as uninterpretable by two independent raters; the remaining 567 cues were coded. These were collapsed into 10 categories and the number of therapists with cues in each of the categories was determined (Table 2.1). The majority of therapists recorded at least one cue in the abnormal function, speed, effort, temporal control, spatial accuracy and smoothness categories. Over 98% of therapists recorded at least one cue in category 1. In this category, lack of essential components was noted at least once by 78.6% of therapists. Sixty-eight per cent of therapists had at least one cue pertaining to grasp/object manipulation, and 30.4% of therapists noted signs of compensation as a visual cue for movement dysfunction. It was clear, however, that therapists with a special interest in neurology had a range of opinions about important cues for assessment, with no common cue set in evidence.

In summary, general patterns in the cues proposed were found. For example, it was clear that cues related to abnormal muscle function, effort, speed, smoothness, timing and directness were most common, with over 50% of therapists noting at least one cue in each of these categories. This finding suggests that completing an upper limb task using essential components (normal function), without

Table 2.1   Coding categories, their cue characteristics and proportion of therapists using cue.

Coding category		Cue characteristics (subcategories)	Therapists using cue (%)
1	Muscle function	Impaired action; unable to do, or repeat the task Lack of essential movement components; shoulder, elbow, wrist, grasp, control of object Actions to compensate for impaired function	98.2
2	Effort	Evidence of effort: in active limb in other limb/trunk face	78.6
3	Speed	Time taken or pattern of speed	80.4
4	Smoothness	Jerkiness	55.4
5	Timing	Of joints (timing of, synchronicity of) Of movement phases	66.1
6	Directness	Path indirectness Overshooting/undershooting target	60.7
7	Posture	Head/trunk alignment Ability to balance, weight shift Symmetry	41.1
8	Different from normal	Contrasted with normal model Compared with non-hemiplegic side	12.5
9	Visual behaviour	Where vision is directed	8.9
10	Anticipatory	For example, sensory loss, cognitive status, painful shoulder	7.1

compensation, in a smooth, well-timed, accurate (direct) and well-paced manner and without undue effort are well-recognized characteristics of optimal upper limb performance. It follows that seeing slow, poorly timed, inaccurate or indirect, jerky and effortful movement when a patient attempts a task would furnish cues of suboptimal upper limb performance. These findings provide promising support for the use of observational assessment.

One problem that needs to be addressed, however, is whether the following characteristics differentiate suboptimal from optimal upper limb performance:

- lack of essential components;
- slowness;
- poor timing;
- indirectness;
- jerkiness;
- effort.

Looking at experimental studies of upper limb function for cues that discriminate performance by healthy subjects from those with neurological conditions may help to answer this question.

What characteristics differentiate suboptimal from optimal upper limb performance?

Studies of normal and abnormal performance were examined to answer two questions:

1. In what way do the upper limb movement characteristics of people with and without neurological impairment differ?
2. What changes in motor performance occur with recovery after stroke?

Research with healthy participants has focused mainly on the study of the reach-to-grasp movement. This task has provided a relatively simple model for the study of how movement is planned, produced and coordinated. We know that the reach-to-grasp movement in healthy participants is characterized by smooth, well-timed movements, with hand opening occurring soon after movement onset and maximum hand aperture closely linked to the size and properties of the object being picked up; see van Vliet and Turton (2001) for review. Relatively little is known about patients with stroke. In Table 2.2a movement characteristics (mostly derived from two-dimensional or three-dimensional motion analysis) that distinguish neurologically impaired performers from healthy subjects are summarized. From this we see that, compared with healthy individuals, patients with stroke exhibit movements that:

- are slower (reduced peak velocities, increased movement times);
- are more jerky;

Table 2.2a   Differences in kinematic characteristics of patients with stroke and control subjects performing upper limb tasks.

Reference	Subjects	Task	Characteristics of stroke compared with control
Single joint studies			
Jones et al 1989	8 stroke 36 control	Computer tracking tasks	Movement speed reduced in both hemiplegic (by 63%) and non-hemiplegic (by 19.5%) upper limbs Steadiness reduced in both hemiplegic and non-hemiplegic upper limbs
Lough 1987	4 stroke 1 control	Pointing task	Reduced speed Increased jerkiness (discontinuities) Without vision, performance deteriorated
Reaching			
Fisk and Goodale 1988	17 L hem stroke 11 R hem stroke 13 control	Reach to point at target illuminated on screen, fast and accurate	Reduced accuracy of reach Slower initiation of reach to target Reduced PV Increased MT
Levin 1996	10 stroke 6 control	Pointing arm movements to targets in horizontal plane, self-paced	Prolonged MT Reduced MA Marked deviations from straight path (up to 32 mm) Increased segmentation (jerkiness) Reduced coordination between shoulder and elbow
Karnath et al 1997	5 stroke + neglect 5 stroke 6 control	Pointing movements with and without vision	Increased variability of performance under no vision condition (neglect), 2 patients deviating from direct path by 20 cm
Chieffi et al 1993	1 stroke 6 control	Reach to grasp with visual distractors	Hand path longer in presence of distractor
Goodale et al 1990	9 R hem stroke 13 age-matched control	Reach to point at target illuminated on screen, fast and accurate	Marked early path deviations to right, particularly for contralateral targets
Cirstea and Levin 2000	9 stroke 9 control	Pointing to object in contralateral space, self-paced	Different pattern of reach, increased variability of performance Increased MT and reduced PV Less precise with greater segmentation (jerkiness) Disrupted inter-joint coordination Increased trunk involvement
Wu et al 2000	14 stroke 25 control	Reach to scoop real or imagined coins	Increased jerkiness Decreased MT and PV Longer hand path Using real objects improved reach in both groups

table continues

Table 2.2a   Continued

Reference	Subjects	Task	Characteristics of stroke compared with control
Transport			
Bernhardt (Study 3 in Boucher et al 1995); Bernhardt 1998, Bernhardt et al 1998b[*]	11 stroke 3 control	Raise object from table and transport to shelf	PV reduced by 41–74% Increased jerkiness: 3–10 times more jerks Less direct path of object to shelf
Scroggie 1998[*]	11 stroke 3 control	Raise object from table and transport to shelf	Longer MT More variability in timing of PV Increased jerkiness Trunk extension prior to lift in stroke patients, not in controls Poorer timing between trunk, shoulder and elbow
Reach and transport			
van Vliet et al 1995a	8 stroke 8 control	Reach to pick up, move or drink from cup	More variable timing of PV Increased MT (up to 5 times) and lower PV Less able to adapt to different task conditions Opening hand wider than necessary

L hem, left hemisphere; R hem, right hemisphere; MA, movement amplitude; MT, movement time; PV, peak velocity.
*Data from same subjects. Three-dimensional motion analysis of wrist (Bernhardt, 1998) and trunk, shoulder and elbow (Scroggie, 1998).

- exhibit less direct movement paths;
- are less well timed;
- are more likely to include trunk movement with the reach;
- are more likely to have wider hand aperture than required for object size.

The timing of peak velocity (PV), reflecting the point at which speed is greatest during the movement, and the overall movement pattern are similar to those of control subjects in most neurologically impaired performers and may reflect an invariant characteristic of the reach-to-grasp movement. Invariant (unchanging) characteristics of movement are interesting because they help to provide insights into how movement may be organized and controlled (Bate 1997, Charlton 1994).

As recovery occurs (Table 2.2b), movement becomes:

- faster;
- smoother;
- more direct;

Table 2.2b   Change in kinematic characteristics over time.

Reference	Subjects	Task	Measurement schedule	Characteristics
Single joint studies				
Jones et al 1989	8 stroke 36 control	Computer tracking tasks	12 months	Improved movement speed and steadiness, still impaired compared with control subjects
Wing et al 1990	5 stroke	Elbow, attempted movement to and from target	12 months	Increased angular velocity
Reaching				
Lough et al 1984	5 stroke	Moving a handle to a target as fast as possible	2, 6 and 12 months	Increased PV Reduced MT More direct path with fewer deviations
Trombly 1993	5 stroke	Reaching to three targets	2 months	Increased PV Reduced MT Less variable timing of PV Less jerky (fewer velocity peaks)
Turton, 1991 (reported in van Vliet and Turton 2001)	4 stroke	Reaching to target	Up to 65 weeks post stroke	Amount of trunk flexion decreased as shoulder flexion control increased
Broberg 1991	5 stroke 1 control	Moving object between two points	Up to 270 days post stroke	Improved speeds Shoulder–elbow coordination still impaired
Reach and transport				
van Vliet et al 1995b	5 stroke	Reach to pick up, move or drink from cup	3 to 4 weeks	Increased PV Reduced MT Reduced variability in timing of PV Fewer velocity peaks (smoother movement)

MT, movement time; PV, peak velocity.

- better timed;
- with less trunk involvement.

Notwithstanding the criticism that these variables represent only a few of the multitude of variables that could have been measured had the researchers chosen, or been able to do so, we can still identify characteristics of performance that may be important cues for observational assessment. It is probable that these characteristics are important given the fact that they are also nominated and accepted by therapists as cues of movement dysfunction after stroke (Bobath 1990, Carr et al 1987, Charlton 1992, Duncan and Badke 1987, Mulder et al 1995). The next question to ask is whether therapists can observe and rate these characteristics accurately.

Can therapists accurately observe characteristics that differentiate suboptimal from optimal upper limb performance?

In 1998 therapists with a special interest in neurology were asked to watch the videotaped performances of an upper limb transport task performed by a range of neurologically impaired and unimpaired performers and then rate three movement characteristics (Bernhardt et al 1998b):

- speed;
- jerkiness;
- directness.

Visual judgements were recorded on visual analogue scales and these judgements were then compared with the three-dimensional kinematics of the same movements to determine accuracy. Experienced physiotherapists' judgements of speed ($r = 0.79$) and jerkiness ($r = 0.96$) showed good levels of accuracy, and their judgements of path indirectness were moderately accurate ($r > 0.68$). They also showed very high levels of test–retest reliability, suggesting that this skill was stable over time ($r > 0.82$) (Bernhardt et al 1998b). The fact that not all characteristics were judged with equal accuracy raises an important point. It is quite possible that humans may not be able to see all movement characteristics equally well. Therefore, assessment must include those cues that most validly represent the movement disorders of our patients, but we must also determine the movement cues that can be observed most accurately.

A further study examining the accuracy of observation by less experienced therapists and student observers found that observation accuracy was not dependent on years of clinical experience (Bernhardt et al 2002), with all inexperienced observers producing good to excellent levels of accuracy ($r = 0.75$–0.92). This finding suggests that the ability to observe these characteristics of human movement and discriminate between normal and pathological performance represents an intrinsic capacity of the visual system (Pavlova et al 2003). The accuracy of visual judgements of movement timing, associated trunk movements and hand aperture remains untested.

Although the results of these studies are promising, they represent early steps in the process of systematizing observational analysis. Further research is needed to establish the most representative tasks patients should undertake and the most important cues to be observed while undertaking these tasks. We need more detailed studies of patient kinematics during movement performance under a range of environmental influences and over longer time intervals.

These studies will require more complex experimental models to allow derivation of inter-joint coordination and hand function during tasks. Also, given that there are probably a number of critical cues of upper limb performance that must be observed before we are prompted to test hypotheses and design treatment plans, finding out what combination of factors triggers intervention would be a useful undertaking. It is equally possible, however, that a single global cue such as 'effort' is the most influential cue in our decision-making. This too requires further research. Moreover, we have yet to test whether the accuracy found in these studies of videotaped movements can be replicated when observations are undertaken under clinical practice conditions. Work in progress will help answer some of these outstanding questions.

Clinical implications

Therapists identified six characteristics that they used to determine suboptimal upper limb performance (in order of importance):

- abnormal function (essential components);
- speed;
- effort;
- directness;
- smoothness;
- timing.

Three of these – speed, smoothness and directness – have been shown to be characteristics of optimal performance of upper limb tasks, and can be accurately observed. But what of the other three?

First, let's examine abnormal function (or lack of essential components and presence of compensatory strategies). Although characteristics of performance like speed, smoothness and directness seem to be generic to movement, essential components are specific to tasks. It is possible that observation and discrimination of essential components may be dependent on experience and training (Eastlack et al 1991, Jeng et al 1990, Patla and Clouse 1988, Perry 1992, Saleh and Murdoch 1985, Smidt 1974). For example, Perry (1992) states that familiarity with normal function must be developed and imprinted on the observers' memory before what Perry calls an 'organised awareness of normal function' is developed (p. 352). She hypothesizes that this awareness allows therapists to identify deviations from normal (pathological motion). As yet we don't know whether training is necessary before important movement characteristics can be accurately observed (in fact, current data suggest it is not); however, it is likely that training and experience play an important role in the interpretation of what is observed.

Second, let's examine timing. Although the timing of shoulder, elbow and wrist movements during upper limb tasks may be difficult to observe, timing, like speed, probably reflects a more global characteristic of movement that becomes evident as performance deteriorates. Correct timing of hand aperture may be easier to assess using vision, although this remains to be tested. We do know that high levels of accuracy with visual judgements of the temporal asymmetry of gait have been reported (Spencer et al 1992), suggesting that movement timing can be accurately observed under conditions when the movement is repetitive, like walking.

Finally, let's examine the characteristic effort. Effort cannot be directly observed and must be inferred from the observed kinematics of the movement. There is evidence that therapists can accurately infer kinetics from observable kinematics. McGinley and colleagues have found that therapists' visual judgements of the push-off in subjects with hemiplegic gait were strongly correlated with instrumented measurement of ankle joint power (McGinley et al 2003). However, the process of inference allows for many different theoretical considerations to influence the result. For example, when effort in the active limb was noted as a cue for abnormal movement, it was alternatively described as a spastic pattern, an associated reaction, increased tone or as excessive muscle activity. These terms are commonly found in the physiotherapy literature to describe excessive effort but have different meaning to different therapists. For example, spastic patterns are described by Brunnstrom (Sawner and La Vigne 1992), whereas associated reactions and tone are particularly common terms used by Bobath practitioners (Bobath 1990, Davies 1985, Lynch and Grisogono 1991). Within these frameworks, associated reactions indicate the presence of spasticity, the release of abnormal reflex activity, which disrupts the normal postural tone necessary for skilful movement. Treatment within the Bobath or Brunnstrom frameworks emphasizes the inhibition of spasticity in order to facilitate more normal movement. In contrast, excessive muscle activity is a term utilized by Movement Science practitioners (Ada and Canning 1990, Carr et al 1987). Movement Science practitioners view excessive muscle activity leading to 'spastic patterns' as the result of habitual muscle activity in those muscles whose mechanical advantage is greatest, combined with adaptive shortening of soft tissues due to resting postures of the hemiplegic limb adopted by patients. Treatment therefore emphasizes maintenance of soft-tissue extensibility of the limb and training the patient to eliminate unnecessary muscle force during attempts of a motor task (Carr and Shepherd 1987, Carr et al 1995). What is important to note here is that how movement characteristics are labelled reflects the underlying assumptions of therapists about the causes of observed movement abnormality. When therapists observe movements that are 'effortful', they make assumptions about the causes of the abnormality, which are followed by testing of the assumption by, for example, closer examination of the muscles they assume are contributing to effortful movement of the limb for muscle shortening (Movement Science approach) or resistance to passive movement (Bobath approach). Different underlying assumptions for the same observed phenomenon may therefore lead to different hypothesis testing and to a different programme of treatment. It is therefore important that we follow up observation with tests of impairments as well as keeping abreast of new knowledge about the underlying causes of these outward manifestations of dysfunction (see Chapter 5). This will ensure that treatments are directed at the most appropriate contributors to disability.

ASSESSING BALANCE IN NEUROLOGICAL POPULATIONS

There are a large number of measurement instruments used to assess balance dysfunction. This section reviews the rationale for assessing balance, presents a range of measurement instruments and provides a framework to support the choice of appropriate measures and the development of treatment programmes.

Does neurological rehabilitation adequately address balance–related dysfunction?

There is substantial evidence that therapy programmes targeting balance and balance-related function can result in significant improvements in performance in people with a range of neurological disorders (Bernhardt et al 1998c, Dean et al 2000, Duncan et al 1998, Murray et al 2001, Scandalis et al 2001, Yardley et al 1998). However, there are also data indicating that the outcomes achieved are relatively poor if we consider the complex balance demands of independent community mobility. Poor outcomes associated with ongoing balance disturbance include loss of confidence in mobility, reduced physical activity and propensity to stumble or fall. Falls are a clear marker of inadequate recovery of balance, and often result in a vicious cycle triggering further loss of confidence and fear of falling, reduction in activity, deconditioning and subsequent increased falls risk. Falls have been reported to be a major problem for people with neurological dysfunction, for example:

• Up to 47% of patients with stroke experienced one or more falls while in hospital recovering from their stroke (Forster and Young 1995, Langhorne et al 2000, Teasell et al 2002), and up to 73% fell at least once in the 6 months following discharge home (Forster and Young 1995) or later following return home (Hill 1998, Hyndman et al 2002).

• Up to 80% of people with mild to moderate Parkinson's disease have reported falling at least once in a 12-month period

(Ashburn et al 2001, Bloem et al 2001a, Hill 1998, Stack and Ashburn 1999).

- Up to 50% of people with vestibular dysfunction have reported one or more falls (Herdman et al 2000).

- People with polio from the epidemics in the 1950s are now ageing, and many are experiencing exacerbation of symptoms associated with post-polio syndrome. Over 50% of people with polio fall at least once in a 12-month period, and over half of these are multiple fallers (Hill and Stinson 2004, Lord et al 2002).

The examples above demonstrate the magnitude of problems associated with balance and mobility impairment and falls among people with neurological dysfunction. Falls are usually multifactorial in origin and the circumstances surrounding falls indicate that often there may be one or more extrinsic (environmental) and intrinsic (health-related problems affecting the systems involved in balance) factors contributing to falls. Impaired ability to balance effectively when equilibrium is challenged is a major contributor to the risk of falling in people with neurological dysfunction. Strategies effectively to manage people presenting with balance and mobility dysfunction or falls need to be determined based on the judicious selection of assessment procedures that highlight key elements that the retraining programme needs to address. Considerable scope exists for improved outcomes in this area.

Effective balance: the key elements

Before looking more closely at assessment, we first need to define what we mean by balance.

Balance has been defined by Nashner (1993) as 'maintaining the position of the body's Centre of Gravity (COG) vertically over the base of support. When this condition is met, a person can both resist the destabilising influence of gravity, and actively move the COG . . .'. This definition highlights a number of key aspects that need to be integrated into a targeted assessment of balance performance. Withstanding the destabilizing influence of gravity has also been termed static balance. This involves maintaining a steady posture where there is no overt body movement, and it can be assessed using any base of support (e.g. feet together, Sharpened Romberg). Although there is no overt body movement during static balance tasks, a constant interplay between postural muscles occurs to maintain the static posture. This muscle interplay is often not easy to observe; however, it is evident when assessed using force platforms (Boucher et al 1995, Cheng et al 2001, Kantner et al 1991). Most work on static balance relates to standing postures, but the same principles apply to the assessment and training of sitting balance. Achieving effective static balance in the sitting position is significantly correlated with mobility outcomes (Morgan 1994) and can therefore be considered an important early milestone after stroke.

The second component of the balance definition includes moving the centre of gravity, more commonly termed dynamic balance. Active movement of the centre of gravity may involve self-generated movements (perturbations) such as walking, turning or climbing steps, or may involve responses to externally generated forces, such as responding to an uneven surface or a push from behind. Dynamic balance assessment should incorporate evaluation of both self-generated perturbations and externally generated perturbations, although most of the commonly used measures only incorporate self-generated perturbations. Again, dynamic balance can be tested using any base of support. In this chapter, the emphasis will be on standing balance, although the principles are transferable to other positions.

There are several postural synergies commonly observed in response to external perturbations (Allison and Fuller 2001). Although these postural synergies are considered automatic, they are modifiable in response to varying environmental contexts. These postural synergies are:

- Ankle strategy – distal to proximal activation of muscles to achieve small amplitude response to a perturbation in the forwards or backwards direction. Typically occurs when the perturbation is small, slow and near the midline, and when the support surface is broad and stable.

- Hip strategy – proximal to distal muscle activation to achieve moderate amplitude correction of equilibrium, in response to large, fast perturbations. Also evident if small perturbations are applied when the support surface is narrow (e.g. standing on a beam, with the feet perpendicular to the length of the beam).

- Stepping strategy – if the perturbation is excessive to maintain equilibrium, the stepping strategy is adopted to achieve a new, more stable base of support.

While these strategies can be observed in simple clinical and laboratory testing situations, they rarely occur in isolation in everyday activities in which balance is threatened. Instead these strategies may form the basis for more complex balance strategies involved in functional activities (see Carr and Shepherd 1998, p. 162).

The postural alignment of the body also influences an individual's stability. In any base of support, an individual has a specific limit of stability (LOS), which defines the area within which the body's centre of gravity can safely be moved without overbalancing or needing to initiate a protective mechanism such as a stepping strategy (Nashner 1993). In upright standing with the feet 10 cm (4 inches) apart, the LOS have been determined to be approximately 12.5° in the anteroposterior direction and 16° in the side-to-side directions for a person 178 cm (70 inches) tall. In erect upright stance, the body has considerable scope for movement within the LOS without overbalancing. However, if postural alignment is poor (e.g. if there is marked kyphosis associated with osteoporosis/crush fractures), then the body's COG is much closer to the forwards LOS and will require minimal additional perturbation to cause potential overbalancing. Similar association between poor postural alignment in the backwards or lateral direction (e.g. marked asymmetry associated with severe stroke) results in increased risk of overbalancing in the direction of the position of the COG.

Accurate visual, vestibular and somatosensory afferent information, central integration of sensory cues and effective and timely neuromusculoskeletal responses are all necessary for optimal balance. Pathology in any part of the systems involved in balance can lead to impaired balance performance and increased risk of falling.

Balance and mobility tasks are rarely performed in isolation in everyday activities. More commonly, they are undertaken while simultaneously performing at least one other activity such as talking, walking, turning the head or listening. Performance on a task can be quite different when a second task is superimposed (Brauer et al 2001). In general, use of dual tasks has resulted in improved discrimination of mild balance impairments (Condron and Hill 2002, Maylor and Wing 1996). The underlying principles for this are that:

- An individual has a limited attentional capacity, which is usually adequate for single and dual tasks if balance is unimpaired (unless the demands of the task are extremely high).

- When an individual undertakes two or more tasks requiring attention, which is commonly what is experienced in daily activities, then there are fewer available attentional resources for the balance or mobility task. Each of these additional tasks competes with the balance or mobility task for the fixed amount of attentional capacity (Bowen et al 2001).

In summary, effective balance requires efficient and accurate sensory (visual, vestibular and somatosensory) input, central integration and execution of appropriate motor responses to maintain stability during activity. Balance tasks vary in complexity from the relative ease of a static task with a wide base of support, through to dynamic activities such as walking to a seat on a moving bus while putting a wallet in a pocket or balancing on a ladder reaching up to change a high ceiling light globe. Furthermore, we need to be able to perform these functions in both closed (no variability) and open (variable) environments (Gentile 1987), and often during dual or multitask performance. For patients with neurological dysfunction, performance may need to be assessed at all of these levels. The patient's needs, preferences and lifestyle need to be considered as part of the assessment process. The therapist needs to identify the most appropriate tasks to assess to obtain a true indicator of the individual's level and type of dysfunction, and to tailor a training programme to address these factors.

Clinical measures of balance

Observing a patient's responses to tasks that place different demands on the balance system, including what is occurring in the limbs, trunk and head, can be a useful starting point for assessment. The presence of adaptive motor behaviours such as a wide base of support, use of the hands for support, weight shift to the unaffected side, stiffening of the body and avoidance of threats to balance can cue therapists into the presence of balance impairment (see Carr and Shepherd 1998, p. 169). Based on these observations, hypotheses can be generated as to the likely contributory factors to poor performance, and these hypotheses can be tested as part of a more detailed assessment. Although there have been some attempts to define the kinematics of balance dysfunction for patients with stroke (Tyson and DeSouza 2003), this area needs further systematic study similar to that reported for upper limb assessment earlier in this chapter.

More commonly, rating scales or specific performance-based measures (which may or may not rely heavily on observation) are used to assess balance. In some global assessment procedures such as the Motor Assessment Scale, balance is assessed both directly (e.g. balanced sitting) and indirectly as part of the assessment of functional activities that require dynamic standing balance (Carr et al 1985). There are also simple scales that provide a basic framework to support observational assessment, such as the balance component of the Problem Oriented Mobility Assessment (Tinetti 1986) and the Berg Balance Scale (Berg et al 1989), through to more complex performance measures such as the Four Square Step Test (Dite and Temple 2002a, 2002b) or the Functional Obstacle Course (Means et al 1996).

There are a large number of measurement instruments that have been developed to assess balance of both older people generally and those with neurological disorders. Several useful reviews are available that describe many of the assessments, and summarize the research describing the reliability and validity of these measures (Cole et al 1994, Hill et al 2001, Huxham et al 2001). Some of the more commonly reported clinical balance measurement instruments are listed in Table 2.3. Normative scores for healthy older people and scores reported for neurological populations are also presented. Several of the more recently developed measurement procedures such as the Four Square Step Test and the Multiple Task Test have been subjected to little research or clinical application in neurological samples to date. However, the constructs on which they have been derived indicate that they have considerable potential, particularly for the assessment of people with neurological dysfunction with mild levels of balance impairment. Further research is indicated.

The balance performance tasks described in Table 2.3 are a small selection of those that have been reported. The type of tasks assessed can be manipulated across a number of domains to vary the difficulty of the task, as shown in Figure 2.2. Both static and dynamic balance tasks can be modulated by changing:

- the base of support;
- degree of sensory input;
- the environmental demands of the task (open or closed);
- the number of tasks being performed simultaneously (including manipulation); or
- the degree of visual fixation.

Busy therapists are keen to minimize the demands of assessment, while maximizing the information available from the assessment process. The plethora of balance measurement instruments available can be as problematic for the therapist as having too few to choose from. Given that most of the instruments described in Table 2.3 are relatively simple and quick to administer, what other criteria might influence and inform the selection of appropriate tests? Is there one measurement instrument that provides sufficient information to form the basis for determining treatment approaches as well as providing a useful reference for reassessments over time? Or is there a need for a series of measures?

In a study evaluating a number of balance and mobility measurement instruments in patients with stroke undergoing in-patient rehabilitation, factor analysis revealed two factors, or groupings of tests, that accounted for 79% of total variance (Bernhardt et al 1998c). The factors could broadly be considered as static stance balance tasks and dynamic tasks, which also appeared to subgroup into dynamic bilateral stance tasks (reaching tasks) and dynamic single limb stance tasks (including the Step Test and measures of gait). Results of this study suggest that we should include at least one measure from each of these three categories in our assessment battery. Additional data reinforcing the need to consider the use of several selected measures of balance instead of only one, are shown in Figure 2.3 (Hill 1998). Figure 2.3 shows scores on four measures

Table 2.3   Examples of clinical balance assessment tools, and scores reported for healthy older people and people with neurological dysfunction.

Assessment tool	Description of task	Scores reported for neurological samples				Older fallers	Scores reported for healthy older subjects
		Parkinson's disease (PD)	Stroke	Multiple sclerosis (MS)	Polio		
Functional Reach (Duncan et al 1990)	Bilateral stance task, amount of forward reach measured (cm)	PD fallers – 24 cm PD non-fallers – 30 cm Controls – 34cm (Smithson et al 1998)	End rehabilitation – 22 cm (Hill et al 1996)	MS – 31 cm Controls – 39 cm (Frzovic et al 2000)		Single fallers – 26 cm Multiple fallers – 21 cm (Dite and Temple 2002)	Subjects ≥ 70 years Males 33 cm Females 27 cm (Duncan et al 1990)
Timed Up and Go Test (Podsiadlo and Richardson 1991)	Timed task, standing up from a chair, walking 3 m, turning, returning to chair and sitting down (seconds)	17 s (Morris et al 2001)	Average 38 days post stroke, 19.6 s (Salbach et al 2001)			Single fallers – 12.3 s Multiple fallers – 16.7 s (Dite and Temple 2002)	Females ≥ 70 years 9.1 s (Hill et al 1999)
Step Test (Hill et al 1996)	Number of completed steps stepping one foot on then off a 7.5 cm block in 15 s	PD faller – 7 steps/15 s PD non-faller – 12 steps/15 s (Morris et al 2000)	End rehabilitation – 6 steps/15 s (Hill et al 1997)	7 steps/15 s (Frzovic et al 2000)		Single fallers – 11 steps/15 s Multiple fallers – 7 steps/15 s (Dite and and Temple 2002a)	Subjects ≥ 60 years 16 steps/15 s (Hill et al 1996)

table continues

Table 2.3 Examples of clinical balance assessment tools, and scores reported for healthy older people and people with neurological dysfunction—cont'd

Assessment tool	Description of task	Scores reported for neurological samples					Scores reported for healthy older subjects
		Parkinson's disease (PD)	Stroke	Multiple sclerosis (MS)	Polio	Older fallers	
Clinical Test of Sensory Integration of Balance (Shumway-Cook and Horak 1986)	Performance timed up to 30 s on 6 sensory tasks	PD fallers – EO, firm 30 s PD non-fallers – EO, firm 30 s (Morris et al 2000)	Feet 10 cm apart: EO, firm 29 s EC, firm 28 s VC, firm 26 s EO, foam 26 s EC, foam 25 s VC, foam 24 s (Hill et al 1997)		Sway measures recorded: 2 falls: EO, firm 116 mm EC, firm 163 mm 3+ falls: EO, firm 148 mm EC, firm 178 mm (Lord et al 2002)	Feet together Combined score from three foam conditions (max. 30 s/ condition) <81 resulted in age-adjusted odds ratio for falling of 8.7 (Di Fabio and Anacker 1996)	Feet together* EO, firm 30 s EC, firm 30 s VC, firm 30 s EO, foam 29 s EC, foam 17 s VC, foam 19 s (Cohen et al 1993)
Berg Balance Scale (Berg et al 1989)	14 balance-related tasks assessed on a five-point ordinal scale (0–4)		Average 38 days post stroke – mean score 47/56 (Salbach et al 2001) Chronic stroke – mean score 41/56 (Duncan et al 1998)		Mean age 51 years – average score 55/56 (Willen et al 2001)	Cut-off score of less than 45 reported to identify high falls risk (Thorbahn and Newton 1996)	Maximum score of 56

Test	Description	Findings	Sample/normative data
Multi-direction Reach Test (Newton 2001)	Bilateral stance task, amount of forwards, backwards and right and left reach measured (cm)		Sample mean age 74 years (Newton 2001) Forwards – 23 cm Backwards – 12 cm Right side – 17 cm Left side – 17 cm
The Four Square Step Test (FSST) (Dite and Temple 2002a)	A test evaluating the time to complete eight sequential steps around a 2 × 2 grid		Single fallers – 12.0 s Multiple fallers – 24 s (Dite and Temple 2002a) Sample mean age 74 (Dite and Temple 2002a) 8.7 s
The Multiple Tasks Test (Bloem et al 2001)	Eight separate tasks of increasing complexity, administered sequentially (including motor and cognitive dual task)	Patients with PD had significantly more errors than older controls on the motor tasks, increasingly so with increased task complexity (Bloem et al 2001b)	13 older subjects – mean age 62 (Bloem et al 2001b) Assessment involved measurement of errors, defined as hesitations (slowed performance) or blocks (complete cessation). Only 62% performed all motor tasks without any errors. Further research required

EO, eyes open; EC, eyes closed; VC, visual conflict.
*Samples not comprehensively screened, so may underestimate scores for healthy older adults.

Figure 2.2 Domains on which balance assessment and training procedures can be manipulated to grade the level of difficulty for a particular task (darker shading indicates more challenging task conditions for assessment and training).

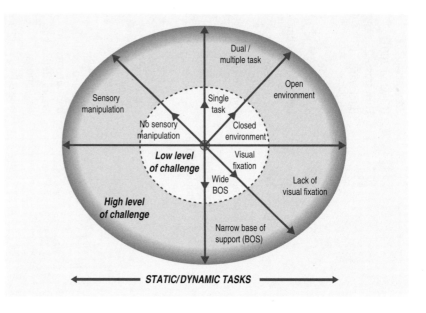

Figure 2.3 Standardized scores for 16 stroke subjects compared with the average for age-matched control subjects. The average score for age-matched control subjects is set at 100%. The scores for subject 1 (dashed line, large circles) indicate the differing performance on different tests for one individual.

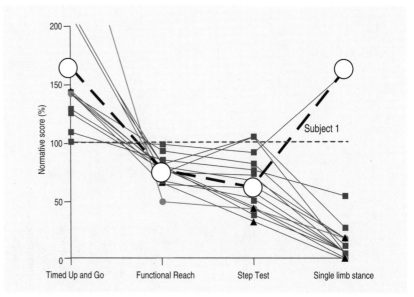

of balance (Timed Up and Go, Functional Reach, Step Test and single limb stance) for 16 female stroke subjects who had returned home following rehabilitation, were independent community ambulators, and were at least 6 months post stroke. Subjects had a mean age of 76.9 (5.1) years, 47% lived at home alone, and the group had experienced a median of one fall in the preceding 12 months. Scores for each test have been standardized to the average scores derived from 16 age-matched healthy community dwelling women who had not fallen in the preceding 12 months, and who were comprehensively screened to exclude any subject with balance dysfunction (Hill et al 1999). Standardization of scores means that 100% represents the mean score for the age-matched sample. The most striking aspect of Figure 2.3 is that level of balance dysfunction varied according to which balance measurement instrument was selected. For example, two of the subjects scored well above the healthy sample mean for single limb stance, although performance for one of these subjects on the Step Test was approximately 65% of the standardized score, Functional Reach was approximately 75% of the standardized score, and Timed Up and Go was approximately 125% of the standardized score. If any one of these measures were used in isolation, different interpretations of balance dysfunction would be derived. These would range from 'no problems with balance' (using the single limb stance score) through to 'moderate impairment of balance performance' (using the Step Test score). A similar profile across tests was identified for a sample of women with Parkinson's disease (Hill 1998). These examples highlight the importance of selecting the most appropriate tests for a particular purpose.

Another factor influencing choice of balance and mobility assessment procedures is the functional level of the patient. Some measurement instruments appear to have ceiling effects, and are therefore more appropriate for patients with moderate levels of dysfunction. A ceiling effect exists if a maximum score is achieved, but there is scope for higher levels of performance to be observed. Figure 2.4 demonstrates performance of patients with stroke on a range of balance and mobility tasks at two time points during inpatient rehabilitation (Bernhardt et al 1998c). Data have been reported relative to performance for healthy older people. From Figure 2.4 it is clear that over 70% of patients with stroke at 16

Figure 2.4 Proportion of stroke subjects achieving normative scores (either maximum score or within 1 standard deviation (SD) of the mean score for healthy older people) at 4 weeks and 16 weeks post stroke on a range of balance and mobility measures. CTSIB, Clinical Test of Sensory Integration of Balance; hemi, hemiplegic. (Based on data from Bernhardt et al 1998c, with the permission of Physiotherapy Research International.)

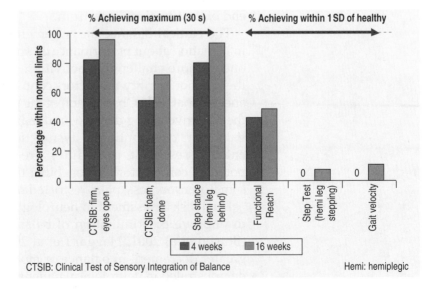

weeks post stroke achieved the maximum score of 30 seconds on the most challenging of the Clinical Test of Sensory Integration of Balance conditions (Shumway-Cook and Horak 1986) (standing on high-density foam with the visual conflict dome), with the feet 10 cm apart. Similarly, another static stance measure (step stance; Goldie et al 1990) also demonstrated limited potential for improved performance at 16 weeks. Other examples of balance measures with potentially limited utility in identifying mild levels of dysfunction (ceiling effects) include the Berg Balance Scale, other components of the Clinical Test of Sensory Integration of Balance, other static stance tests, the Timed Up and Go test and bilateral stance reach tasks such as Functional Reach. Measures that appear to be more sensitive to higher levels of performance are important in identifying early signs of impairment or mild but residual deficits following a neurological event such as stroke. Examples include the Step Test, the Four Square Step Test, the Multiple Tasks Test and other dual task activities. Figure 2.4 shows that at 16 weeks post stroke, less than 10% of patients with stroke were performing within one standard deviation of the mean score for healthy older people on the Step Test.

An equally important issue for patients with marked impairment is the presence of floor effects in measurement. The Step Test, the Four Square Step Test and dual task activities are of limited value for the patient with severe stroke who cannot stand unsupported. Patients at this low functional level will most likely score 0 (unable to do), preventing sensitive identification of change over time. In this instance, static stance tasks and less challenging dynamic tests would be more likely to allow detection of change in performance. Identification of performance change is important for both the patient and the therapist, when patients are at either end of the functional spectrum.

The clinical balance measurements described above provide information about performance on specific task/s that incorporate one or more challenging activities. In most instances, however, they do not identify the factors contributing to impaired performance on that task. Observation of the performance can supplement the objective rating derived, and may identify some of the potential factors contributing to dysfunction. In addition, problem-oriented assessment procedures are required fully to explore potential contributory factors other than balance impairment (e.g. somatosensory loss, pain, restricted range of movement).

Dual task assessment in neurological samples has been shown to improve discrimination of balance or mobility dysfunction (Bowen et al 2001, Haggard et al 2000, Morris et al 2000), and greater decrement in balance or mobility performance has been demonstrated in neurological patients compared with control subjects with addition of the dual task (Morris et al 2000, O'Shea et al 2002). Impairment in balance performance has also been shown to be greater among fallers than non-fallers in neurological samples when dual tasks have been assessed relative to single tasks (Marchese et al 2003, Morris et al 2000). Increased fatigue has also been evident with dual task compared with single task performance (Marshall et al 1997).

Clinical examples of the use of dual tasks in balance and mobility assessment in neurological samples include:

- carrying a tray of different objects while performing the Timed Up and Go test or walking (Bloem et al 2001b, Bond and Morris 2000);

- performance of a cognitive task while performing clinical balance tests such as static stance, Step Test and the arm raise test (Morris et al 2000);

- manipulating an object during gait (O'Shea et al 2002);

- walking and talking (Bowen et al 2001, Lundin-Olsson et al 1997).

Identification of difficulties associated with dual task performance highlights another key area to be targeted in the rehabilitation programme. Giving inadequate consideration to these issues during rehabilitation will result in the patient being unprepared to deal with everyday tasks on their return home.

Interventions based on appropriate assessment

Clearly, people with neurological dysfunction from a range of causes are at high risk of falls. Appropriate assessment will inform treatment options directed at improving functional balance.

Early identification of balance impairment may result in earlier introduction of intervention programmes to improve status, and may prevent potential falls. This is an important goal for older people generally (e.g. an older person who has had a minor fall and is concerned about ongoing risk of falls), in patients with progressive neurological conditions such as Parkinson's disease or multiple sclerosis and in patients with minimal impairment from other neurological dysfunction (e.g. a mild stroke). Measures that do not have ceiling effects will be useful to determine early or minimal balance dysfunction.

A clinical group that is likely to benefit from early assessment of balance dysfunction includes people diagnosed with Parkinson's disease. At the time of diagnosis, and for a number of years afterwards, the main intervention is usually pharmacological. Allied health involvement is often delayed until moderate functional impairments become evident and/or the effectiveness of medications is lessening. Comprehensive balance, mobility and functional assessment of patients early after diagnosis with Parkinson's disease is likely to result in identification of early dysfunction, which may be improved with a targeted treatment programme. This could include advice on postural alignment, balance and other exercises and activities, safety and nutrition. Intermittent reassessments could identify the need for further refinement of the management programme, and have the potential to reduce the magnitude of deterioration in performance longer term.

Exercise training incorporating a balance training component has been shown to be effective in improving performance and reducing falls in older people (Gardner et al 2000, Province et al 1995), in people with moderate neurological dysfunction such as stroke (Chen et al 2002) and in people with Parkinson's disease (Comella et al 1994, de Goede et al 2001). There are a number of important principles that need to be considered in order to maximize potential improvements in balance. Briefly, these include:

- select the appropriate level at which to train balance ensuring that it places moderate demands on the balance system, in a safe manner;

- select a variety of training options that target the specific areas of dysfunction and contributing factors identified from the assessment;

- think about increasing the complexity of the demands on the balance system by changing the base of support, progression to more dynamic tasks, reduction in reliance on visual cues, sensory manipulation and use of dual tasks;

- incorporate balance tasks with a functional element;

- practise tasks in open and variable environments that reflect the demands of functional balance;

- incorporate variability of practice into the functional balance tasks (e.g. vary speed or amplitude of reach or stepping tasks);

- use strategies to maximize both supervised and unsupervised training opportunities;

- regularly reassess with appropriate and sensitive measurement instruments to provide feedback to the patient and to inform ongoing treatment options.

Although rehabilitation programmes often positively influence the balance of patients with a range of neurological conditions, balance dysfunction and falls remain a major problem. There is a need for improved assessment and treatment programmes, as well as complementary research programmes to identify rehabilitation options to address more adequately these ongoing problems.

DISCUSSION

An important task in the development of any systematic approach to assessment is to make sure that therapists know about it, accept it and use it. Maintaining close ties between therapists and researchers is important. There are many examples throughout this book of how information derived from laboratory-based measurement of patients with a range of disabilities has helped inform our clinical practice. There is a need for us to find a common language for describing the movement problems of our patients that is also understood and used by those who undertake movement research. This will ensure that progress can be made not simply in theoretical terms but also in practical ones. Although a large divide exists between our current knowledge about assessment and what we need to know to make our clinical practice truly knowledge (and evidence) based, there are many examples of the successful melding of theory and practice. An excellent example of this lies in the clinical texts of Carr and Shepherd, which successfully integrate up to date science with clinical practice. Ultimately, what we choose to assess is based largely on our background knowledge. And what we treat depends on what we have assessed. For this reason, we must also seek to determine whether training that targets the things we consider important to assess is effective in restoring patient function. Finally, we must remember that the way in which we describe critical elements of assessment is heavily influenced by the theoretical framework we use to explain the disordered movements of our patients. It is therefore essential that therapists keep abreast of research that informs them about contemporary motor control theories together with findings from research that can help us separate critical from non-critical movement characteristics, and important from non-important contributors to motor dysfunction.

References

Ada L, Canning C 1990 Key issues in neurological physiotherapy. Butterworth-Heinemann, Oxford.

Allison L, Fuller K 2001 Balance and vestibular disorders, 4th edn. Mosby, St Louis, MO.

Ashburn A, Stack E, Pickering R M et al 2001 A community-dwelling sample of people with Parkinson's disease: characteristics of fallers and non-fallers. Age and Ageing 30(1):47–52.

Atkinson H W 1992 Principles of assessment. In: Downie P A (ed) Cash's textbook of neurology for physiotherapists, 4th edn. Wolf Publishing, London, pp 104–146.

Bate P 1997 Motor control theories – insights for therapists. Physiotherapy 83(8):397–405.

Berg K, Wood-Dauphinee S, Williams J et al 1989 Measuring balance in the elderly: preliminary development of an instrument. Physiotherapy Canada 41:304–311.

Bernhardt J 1998 Observational kinematic assessment of upper limb movement. PhD thesis, La Trobe University, Bundoora, Australia.

Bernhardt J, Bate P, Matyas T 1998a The scene through our eyes: observation experience doesn't matter. Fifth International Congress of the Australian Physiotherapy Association May;179.

Bernhardt J, Bate P J, Matyas T A 1998b Accuracy of observational kinematic assessment of upper-limb movements. Physical Therapy 78:259–270.

Bernhardt J, Ellis P Denisenko S et al 1998c Changes in balance and locomotion measures during rehabilitation following stroke. Physiotherapy Research International 3:109–122.

Bernhardt J, Matyas T, Bate P 2002 Does experience predict observational kinematic assessment accuracy? Physiotherapy Theory and Practice 18(3):141–149.

Bernhardt J, Bate P, Matyas T et al 2003 Important cues for visual assessment of the hemiplegic upper limb: can physiotherapists agree? 14th International World Confederation of Physical Therapy Congress, Barcelona.

Bloem B R, Grimbergen Y A, Cramer M et al 2001a Prospective assessment of falls in Parkinson's disease. Journal of Neurology 248(11):950–958.

Bloem B R, Valkenburg V V, Slabbekoorn M et al 2001b The multiple tasks test. Strategies in Parkinson's disease. Experimental Brain Research 137(3–4):478–486.

Bloem B R, Valkenburg V V, Slabbekoorn M et al 2001c The Multiple Tasks Test: development and normal strategies. Gait and Posture 14(3):191–202.

Bobath B 1990 Adult hemiplegia: evaluation and treatment, 3rd edn. Heinemann Medical Books, London.

Bond J M, Morris M 2000 Goal-directed secondary motor tasks: their effects on gait in subjects with Parkinson disease. Archives of Physical Medicine and Rehabilitation 81(1):110–116.

Bond M J, Harris R D, Smith D S et al 1992 An examination of the factor structure of the Frenchay Activities Index. Disability and Rehabilitation 14(1):27–29.

Boucher P, Teasdale N, Courtemanche R et al 1995 Postural stability in diabetic polyneuropathy. Diabetes Care 18:638–645.

Bowen A, Wenman R, Mickelborough J et al 2001 Dual-task effects of talking while walking on velocity and balance following a stroke. Age and Ageing 30(4):319–323.

Brauer S G, Woollacott M, Shumway-Cook A 2001 The interacting effects of cognitive demand and recovery of postural stability in balance-impaired elderly persons. Journal of Gerontology 56(8):M489–496.

Broberg, R A 1991 Functional arm movement: the recovery of motor function following stroke. Proceedings of the Eleventh International Congress of the World Confederation for Physical Therapists, London, UK.

Carr J H, Shepherd R B 1987 A motor relearning programme for stroke, 2nd edn. Butterworth Heinemann, Oxford.

Carr J H, Shepherd R B 1998. Neurological rehabilitation: optimizing motor performance. Butterworth-Heinemann, Woburn, MA.

Carr J, Shepherd R 1990a A motor learning model for rehabilitation of the movement-disabled. Heinemann Medical, Oxford.

Carr J H, Shepherd R B 1990b Physiotherapy in disorders of the brain: a clinical guide. Heinemann Medical Books, London.

Carr J H, Shepherd R B, Nordholm L et al 1985 Investigation of a new motor assessment scale for stroke patients. Physical Therapy 65:175–180.

Carr J H, Shepherd R B, Gordon J et al 1987 Movement science: foundations for physical therapy in rehabilitation. Aspen Publishers, Rockville, MD.

Carr J H, Shepherd R B, Ada L 1995 Spasticity: research findings and implications for intervention. Physiotherapy 81:421–429.

Charlton J L 1992 Motor control considerations for assessment and rehabilitation of movement disorders. In: Summers J J (ed) Approaches to the study of motor control and learning. Elsevier Science, Amsterdam, pp 441–467.

Charlton J 1994 Motor control issues and clinical implications. Physiotherapy Theory and Practice 10:185–190.

Chen I C, Cheng P T, Chen C L et al 2002 Effects of balance training on hemiplegic stroke patients. Chang Gung Medical Journal 25(9):583–590.

Cheng P T, Wu S H, Liaw M Y et al 2001 Symmetrical body-weight distribution training in stroke patients and its effect on fall prevention. Archives of Physical Medicine and Rehabilitation 82(12):1650–1654.

Chieffi S, Gentilucci A, Allport A et al 1993 Study of selective reaching and grasping in a patient with unilateral parietal lesion. Brain 116:1119–1137.

Cirstea MC, Levin MF 2000 Compensatory strategies for reaching in stroke. Brain 123:940–953.

Cohen H, Blatchly C, Gombash L A 1993 Study of the Clinical Test of Sensory Interaction and Balance. Physical Therapy 73:346–351.

Cole B, Finch E, Gowland C et al 1994 Physical rehabilitation outcome measures. Canadian Physiotherapy Association, Toronto.

Comella C L, Stebbins G T, Brown-Toms N et al 1994 Physical therapy and Parkinson's disease: a controlled clinical trial. Neurology 44(3 Pt 1): 376–378.

Condron J, Hill K 2002 Reliability and validity of a dual task force platform assessment of balance performance: effect of age, balance impairment and cognitive task. Journal of the American Geriatrics Society 50:157–162.

Craik R L, Oatis C A 1985 Gait assessment in the clinic: issues and approaches. Churchill Livingstone, New York.

Davies P M 1985 Steps to follow: a guide to the treatment of adult hemiplegia. Springer-Verlag, Berlin.

Dean C M, Richards C L, Malouin F 2000 Task-related circuit training improves performance of locomotor tasks in chronic stroke: a randomized, controlled pilot trial. Archives of Physical Medicine and Rehabilitation 81(4):409–417.

Dean C M, Richards C L, Malouin F 2001 Walking speed over 10 metres overestimates locomotor capacity after stroke. Clinical Rehabilitation 15(4):415–421.

Di Fabio R, Anacker S 1996 Identifying fallers in community living elders with a clinical test of sensory integration of balance. European Journal of Physical Medicine and Rehabilitation 6:61–66.

Dite W, Temple V 2002a A clinical test of stepping and change of direction to identify multiple falling older adults. Archives of Physical Medicine and Rehabilitation 83:1566–1571.

Dite W, Temple V 2002b Development of a clinical measure of turning for older adults. American Journal of Physical Medicine and Rehabilitation 81:867–868.

Duncan P, Badke M 1987 Determinants of abnormal motor control. Year Book Medical Publishers, Chicago.

Duncan P, Weiner K, Chandler J et al 1990 Functional Reach: a new clinical measure of balance. Journal of Gerontology 45:M192–197.

Duncan P, Richards L, Wallace D et al 1998 A randomised, controlled pilot study of a home-based exercise program for individuals with mild and moderate stroke. Stroke 29:2055–2060.

Eastlack M, Arvidson J, Snyder-Mackler L et al 1991 Interrater reliability of videotaped observational gait-analysis assessment. Physical Therapy 71:465–472.

Fisk J D, Goodale M A 1988 The effects of unilateral brain damage on visually guided reaching: hemispheric differences in the nature of the deficit. Experimental Brain Research 72:425–435.

Forster A, Young J 1995 Incidence and consequences of falls due to stroke: a systematic inquiry. British Medical Journal 311:83–86.

Friedman P, Richmond D, Baskett J 1988 A prospective trial of serial gait speed as a measure of rehabilitation in the elderly. Age and Ageing 17:227–235.

Frzovic D, Morris M E, Vowels L 2000 Clinical tests of standing balance: performance of persons with multiple sclerosis. Archives of Physical Medicine and Rehabilitation 81(2):215–221.

Gardner M M, Robertson M C, Campbell A J 2000 Exercise in preventing falls and fall related injuries in older people: a review of randomised controlled trials. British Journal of Sports Medicine 34(1):7–17.

Gentile A M 1987 Skill acquisition: action, movement, and neuromotor processes. In: Carr J H, Shepherd R B (eds) Movement science: foundations for physical therapy in rehabilitation. Aspen Publishers, Rockville, MD, pp 93–154.

de Goede C J, Keus S H, Kwakkel G et al 2001 The effects of physical therapy in Parkinson's disease: a research synthesis. Archives of Physical Medicine and Rehabilitation 82(4):509–515.

Goldie P, Matyas T, Spencer K et al 1990 Postural control in standing following stroke: test–retest reliability of some quantitative clinical tests. Physical Therapy 70:234–243.

Goodale M A, Milner A D, Jakobson L S et al 1990 Kinematic analysis of limb movements in neuropsychological research: subtle deficits and recovery of function. Canadian Journal of Psychology 44(2):180–195.

Granger C, Cotter A, Hamilton B et al 1993 Functional assessment scales: a study of persons after stroke. Archives of Physical Medicine and Rehabilitation 74:133–138.

Guyatt G H, Sullivan M J, Thompson P J et al 1985 The 6-minute walk: a new measure of exercise capacity in patients with chronic heart failure. Canadian Medical Association Journal 132(8):919–923.

Haggard P, Cockburn J, Cock J et al 2000 Interference between gait and cognitive tasks in a rehabilitating neurological population. Journal of Neurology, Neurosurgery and Psychiatry 69(4):479–486.

Hamilton B, Granger C 1994 Disability outcomes following inpatient rehabilitation for stroke. Physical Therapy 74:494–503.

Hawthorne G, Richardson J, Osborne R 1999 The Assessment of Quality of Life (AQoL) instrument: a psychometric measure of health-related quality of life. Quality of Life Research 8(3):209–224.

Herbert R, Moore S, Moseley A et al 1993 Making inferences about muscle forces from clinical observations. Australian Journal of Physiotherapy 39:195–201.

Herdman S J, Blatt P, Schubert M C et al 2000 Falls in patients with vestibular deficits. American Journal of Otolaryngology 21(6):847–851.

Higgins J R, Higgins S 1995 The acquisition of locomotor skill. Mosby Year Book, St Louis, MO.

Hill K 1998 Studies of balance in older people. PhD thesis, University of Melbourne.

Hill K, Stinson A A pilot study of falls, fear of falling, activity level and falls prevention actions in older people with polio. Ageing: Clinical and Experimental Gerontology 16:126–131.

Hill K, Bernhardt J, McGann A et al 1996 A new test of dynamic standing balance for stroke patients: reliability, validity and comparisons with healthy elderly. Physiotherapy Canada 48:257–262.

Hill K, Ellis P, Bernhardt J et al 1997 Balance and mobility outcomes for stroke patients: a comprehensive audit. Australian Journal of Physiotherapy 43:173–180.

Hill K, Schwarz J, Flicker L et al 1999 Falls among healthy community dwelling older women: a prospective study of frequency, circumstances, consequences and prediction accuracy. Australian and New Zealand Journal of Public Health 23:41–48.

Hill K, Miller K, Denisenko S et al 2001 Manual for clinical outcome measurement in adult neurological physiotherapy. Australian Physiotherapy Association (Neurology Special Group), Melbourne.

Holden M K, Gill K M, Magliozzi M R 1986 Gait assessment for neurologically impaired patients. Standards for outcome assessment. Physical Therapy 66:1530–1539.

Huxham F, Goldie P, Patla A 2001 Theoretical considerations in balance assessment. Australian Journal of Physiotherapy 47:89–100.

Hyndman D, Ashburn A, Stack E 2002 Fall events among people with stroke living in the community: circumstances of falls and characteristics of fallers. Archives of Physical Medicine and Rehabilitation 83(2):165–170.

Jeng S, Schenkman M, O'Riley P et al 1990 Reliability of a clinical kinematic assessment of the sit-to-stand movement. Physical Therapy 70:512–520.

Jones R G, Donaldson I M, Parkin P J 1989 Impairment and recovery of ipsilateral sensory-motor function following unilateral cerebral infarction. Brain 112:113–132.

Kantner R M, Rubin A M, Armstrong C W et al 1991 Stabilometry in balance assessment of dizzy and normal subjects. American Journal of Otolaryngology 12(4):196–204.

Karnath H, Dick H, Konczak J 1997 Kinematics of goal-directed arm movements in neglect: control of hand in space. Neuropsychologia 35:435–444.

Keshner E A 1991 Commentary. Physical Therapy 71(11):828–829.

Kurtzke J 1983 Rating neurologic impairment in multiple sclerosis: an expanded disability status scale (EDSS). Neurology 33:1444–1452.

Langhorne P, Stott D, Robertson L et al 2000 Medical complications after stroke: a multicenter study. Stroke 31:1223–1229.

Levin M F 1996 Interjoint coordination during pointing movements is disrupted in spastic hemiparesis. Brain 119:281–293.

Lord S R, Allen G M, Williams P et al 2002 Risk of falling: predictors based on reduced strength in persons previously affected by polio. Archives of Physical Medicine and Rehabilitation 83(6):757–763.

Lough S 1987 Visual control of arm movement in the stroke patient. International Journal of Rehabilitation Research 10:113–119.

Lough S, Wing A M, Fraser C et al 1984 Measurement of recovery of function in the hemiplegic upper limb following stroke: A preliminary report. Human Movement Science 3:247–256.

Lundin-Olsson L, Nyberg L, Gustafson Y 1997 'Stops walking when talking' as a predictor of falls in elderly people. Lancet 349:617.

Lynch M, Grisogono V 1991 Strokes and head injuries: a guide for patients, families, friends and carers. John Murray, London.

McGinley J L, Goldie P A, Greenwood K M et al 2003 Accuracy and reliability of observational gait analysis data: judgments of push-off in gait after stroke. Physical Therapy 83(2):146–160.

Malouin F 1995 Observational gait analysis. In: Craik R L, Oatis C A (eds) Gait analysis: theory and applications. Mosby Year Book, St Louis, MO, pp 112–124.

Marchese R, Bove M, Abbruzzese G 2003 Effect of cognitive and motor tasks on postural stability in Parkinson's disease: a posturographic study. Movement Disorders 18(6):652–658.

Marshall S C, Grinnell D, Heisel B et al 1997 Attentional deficits in stroke patients: a visual dual task experiment. Archives of Physical Medicine and Rehabilitation 78(1):7–12.

Maylor E, Wing A 1996 Age differences in postural stability are increased by additional cognitive demands. Journal of Gerontology 51B:P143–154.

Means K, Rodell D, Sullivan P 1996 Use of an obstacle course to assess balance and mobility in the elderly. American Journal of Physical Medicine and Rehabilitation 75:88–95.

Morgan P 1994 The relationship between sitting balance and mobility outcome in stroke. Australian Journal of Physiotherapy 40(2): 91–96.

Morris M, Iansek R, Smithson F et al 2000 Postural instability in Parkinson's disease: a comparison with and without a concurrent task. Gait and Posture 12:205–216.

Morris S, Morris M E, Iansek R 2001 Reliability of measurements obtained with the Timed 'Up and Go' test in people with Parkinson disease. Physical Therapy 81(2):810–818.

Mulder T, Pauwels F, Nienhuis B 1995 Motor recovery following stroke: towards a disability-orientated assessment of motor dysfunction. Churchill Livingstone, Edinburgh.

Murray K, Hill K, Carroll S 2001 Relationship between change in balance and self-reported handicap following a course of vestibular rehabilitation therapy. Physiotherapy Research International 6:251–263.

Nashner L 1993 Practical biomechanics and physiology of balance. In: Jacobson G, Newman C, Kartush J (eds) Handbook of balance function testing. Mosby Year Book, St Louis, MO, pp 61–79.

Newton R A 2001 Validity of the multi-directional reach test: a practical measure for limits of stability in older adults. Journal of Gerontology 56(4):M248–252.

O'Shea S, Morris M E, Iansek R 2002 Dual task interference during gait in people with Parkinson disease: effects of motor versus cognitive secondary tasks. Physical Therapy 82(9): 888–897.

Patla A E, Clouse S D 1988 Visual assessment of human gait: reliability and validity. Rehabilitation Research (October) 87–96.

Pavlova M, Staudt M, Sokolov A et al 2003 Perception and production of biological movement in patients with early periventricular brain lesions. Brain 126:692–701.

Perry J 1992 Gait analysis: normal and pathological function. McGraw-Hill, New York.

Podsiadlo D, Richardson S 1991 The timed 'Up and Go': a test of basic functional mobility for frail elderly persons. Journal of the American Geriatrics Society 39:142–148.

Province M, Hadley E, Hornbrook M et al 1995 The effects of exercise on falls in elderly patients: a preplanned meta-analysis of the FICSIT trials. Journal of the American Medical Association 273:1341–1347.

Richards M, Marder K, Cote L et al 1994 Interrater reliability of the Unified Parkinson's Disease Rating Scale motor examination. Movement Disorders 9:89–91.

Rothstein J M 1985 Measurement and clinical practice: theory and application. Churchill Livingstone, Broadway, NY.

Salbach N M, Mayo N E, Higgins J et al 2001 Responsiveness and predictability of gait speed and other disability measures in acute stroke. Archives of Physical Medicine and Rehabilitation 82(9):1204–1212.

Saleh M, Murdoch G 1985 In defense of gait analysis. Journal of Joint and Bone Surgery 67B(2):237–241.

Sawner K A, La Vigne J M 1992 Brunnstrom's movement therapy in hemiplegia: a neurophysiological approach. J B Lippincott, Philadelphia.

Scandalis T A, Bosak A, Berliner J C et al 2001 Resistance training and gait function in patients with Parkinson's disease. American Journal of Physical Medicine and Rehabilitation 80(1):38–43; quiz 44–46.

Scroggie G 1998 An investigation into the kinematic characteristics of upper limb segments of stroke patients performing an object transport task. Honours thesis, La Trobe University, Bundoora, Australia.

Shumway-Cook A, Horak F 1986 Assessing the influence of sensory interaction on balance: suggestion from the field. Physical Therapy 66:1548–1550.

Simeonsson R J, Lollar D, Hollowell J et al 2000 Revision of the International Classification of Impairments, Disabilities, and Handicaps: developmental issues. Journal of Clinical Epidemiology 53(2):113–124.

Smidt G 1974 Methods of studying gait. Physical Therapy 54:13–17.

Smith A 1990 The measurement of human motor performance. Butterworth-Heinemann, Oxford.

Smithson F, Morris M, Iansek R 1998 Performance on clinical tests of balance in Parkinson's disease. Physical Therapy 78:577–592.

Spencer K, Goldie P, Matyas T 1992 Criterion-related validity of visual assessment of the temporal symmetry of hemiplegic gait. In: Proceedings of the Australian Physiotherapy Association National Congress, p 68.

Stack E, Ashburn A 1999 Fall events described by people with Parkinson's disease: implications for clinical interviewing and the research agenda. Physiotherapy Research International 4(3):190–200.

Teasell R, McRae M, Foley N 2002 The incidence and consequences of falls in stroke patients during inpatient rehabilitation: factors associated with high risk. Archives of Physical Medicine and Rehabilitation 83(3):329–333.

Thomas S A 1989 Clinical decision making. In: King N, Remenyi A G (eds) Psychology for the health sciences. Nelson–Wadsworth, Melbourne, pp 163–170.

Thorbahn L D, Newton R A 1996 Use of the Berg Balance Test to predict falls in elderly persons. Physical Therapy 76(6):576–583; discussion 584–585.

Tinetti M 1986 Performance-oriented assessment of mobility problems in elderly patients. Journal of the American Geriatrics Society 34:119–126.

Trombly C A 1993 Observations of improvement of reaching in five subjects with left hemiparesis. Journal of Neurology, Neurosurgery and Psychiatry 56(1):40–45.

Tyson S, DeSouza L 2003 A clinical model for the assessment of posture and balance in people with stroke. Disability and Rehabilitation 25:120–126.

Vanclay F 1991 Functional outcome measures in stroke rehabilitation. Stroke 22:105–108.

Vertesi A, Darzins P, Lowe S et al 2000 Development of the Handicap Assessment and Resource Tool (HART). Canadian Journal of Occupational Therapy 67(2):120–127.

van Vliet P M, Turton A 2001 Directions in retraining reaching. Criticial Reviews in Physical and Rehabilitation Medicine 13(4):313–338.

van Vliet P, Kerwin D G, Sheridan M R et al 1995a Study of reaching movements in stroke patients. In: Harrsion M (ed) Physiotherapy in stroke management. Churchill Livingstone, Edinburgh, pp 183–191.

van Vliet P, Sheridan M, Kerwin D G et al 1995b The influence of functional goals on the kinematics of reaching following stroke. Neurology Report 19(1):11–16.

Wade D T 1992 Measurement in neurological rehabilitation. Oxford University Press, Oxford.

Willen C, Sunnerhagen K S, Grimby G 2001 Dynamic water exercise in individuals with late poliomyelitis. Archives of Physical Medicine and Rehabilitation 82(1):66–72.

Wing A M, Lough S, Turton A et al 1990 Recovery of elbow function in voluntary positioning of the hand following hemiplegia due to stroke. Journal of Neurology, Neurosurgery and Psychiatry 53:126–134.

Wu C, Trombly C A, Lin K et al 2000 A kinematic study of contextual effects on reaching performance in persons with and without stroke: influences of object availability. Archives of Physical Medicine and Rehabilitation 81: 95–101.

Yardley L, Beech S, Zander L et al 1998 A randomized controlled trial of exercise therapy for dizziness and vertigo in primary care. British Journal of General Practice 48(429):1136–1140.

Chapter 3

The quest for measurement of infant motor performance

Suzann K. Campbell

The difficulty of reliably recognizing the signs of cerebral palsy (CP), even in the presence of evidence of a brain insult from imaging technology, results in long delays in diagnosis and provision of physical therapy for many children. Children with CP are typically diagnosed and treated only at about 9–12 months of age, when they fail to learn to stand and walk (Weindling et al 1996). This situation is akin to allowing adults with traumatic brain injury or a cerebral vascular accident to remain untreated for 9–12 months following the insult. Yet truly these are not even comparable situations because under normal conditions the brain is developing at a rapid rate in early infancy. Given the well-known plasticity of the infant brain, the critical period of time when recovery could be maximally facilitated is being entirely wasted. As a result, we really have no idea what the potential might be to limit impairments and disability in daily life for children with CP.

PLASTICITY, INTERVENTION AND MEASUREMENT

> . . . for rehabilitation (including physiotherapy) to be effective in
> aiding an individual to regain optimal functional recovery, there
> needs to be more emphasis on methods of 'forcing' use of affect-
> ed limbs and providing task-related experience and training.
> There is mounting evidence that neural reorganization reflects
> patterns of use (Carr and Shepherd 1998, p. 3).

Although Carr and Shepherd have written about the plasticity
available for access to recovery primarily in the adult nervous system, I agree wholeheartedly with their observations that successful
treatment of brain damage involves forcing the system to adapt to
task-specific situations along with maintaining the integrity of the
muscular system as rehabilitation begins and progresses. Of course,
in the case of injury to the developing neuromuscular system,
infants must be helped to learn movement patterns and negotiate
the force of gravity in ways they have never before experienced.
Having worked with children with CP and their families for my
entire professional life, and having been trained as a neuroscientist
to appreciate the marvellous potential of neural plasticity, I am constantly aware of the lost opportunities created by late diagnosis and
treatment of CP and have devoted my career to changing this situation. Effecting change requires reliable diagnostic examinations to
(1) identify children with CP at an early date and (2) facilitate production of research to document the efficacy (or lack thereof) of
early versus later intervention. Although, theoretically, early brain
plasticity should provide the opportunity for intervening to shape
the outcome of neonatal brain injury, it is unknown whether a critical period exists during which intervention can reduce the ultimate
level of disability for children with CP.

> Many therapists and physicians set great store by the assessment
> of tone, since they would also believe that spasticity is the major
> impairment following acute lesion such as stroke. These views
> have not, however, resulted in the development of any objective
> measures suitable for use in the clinic (Wade 1992, quoted in Carr
> and Shepherd 1998, p. 55).

Over many years I studied the information available about
pathophysiology and impairments in CP and believed that assessment of reflexes and postural tone held the key to early diagnosis
because these were such salient features of the fully developed syndrome. With the advent of neonatal intensive care units (NICUs), I
examined younger and younger infants at risk for central nervous
system (CNS) dysfunction because of hypoxic–ischaemic or haemorrhagic events. As a result, I realized along with others that abnor-

mal tone and reflexes were unreliably observed during the first year of life and, because of their sometimes transient nature, were less predictive than had been hoped. Of more importance, I also came to believe that abnormal tone was probably not the principal impairment that could be observed in early infancy, but was more likely a developmental adaptation to the primary CNS dysfunction. Other measures of impaired posture and movement were needed to capture the essence of the initial signs of CP.

GENESIS OF A RESPONSIVE MEASURE OF INFANT MOTOR PERFORMANCE

> Measurement carries with it a number of responsibilities. Therapists need to consider carefully, with their medical colleagues and the patients, what questions need answers (Carr and Shepherd 1998, p. 62).

The story in this chapter describes the path to development of a tool called the Test of Infant Motor Performance to provide answers to the following questions:

1. How can one identify delayed development in early infancy and document the presence of specific markers of CNS dysfunction (evaluative or diagnostic measure)?
2. How can one determine goals of treatment to improve functional motor performance and postural control (prescriptive measure)?
3. How can one quantify the effects of physical therapy to improve functional motor performance, regardless of the specific treatment strategy employed (responsive measure)?

As Carr and Shepherd insist, one must have the right tools to measure functional limitations and assess progress in order to test the value of scientifically based theories of intervention.

Physical therapists had long understood that impaired quality of movement was the hallmark of CP but had not succeeded in describing its features in measurable ways. In about 1982, I created a Checklist of Abnormal/Immature Motor Responses containing 36 items to document features of posture and movement in premature infants and others with serious perinatal medical complications I was treating. The observational categories included lists of abnormal behaviours (i.e. positive signs) and behaviours that failed to develop (i.e. negative signs). These included various aspects of head control, oculomotor control, postural tone, poverty of movement or asymmetry, postural abnormalities (e.g. scissoring, hamstring muscle tightness, scapular retraction, opisthotonus), growth, nervous system reactivity (Moro, clonus, asymmetrical tonic neck reflex) and anti-gravity activities (e.g. poor weight-bearing, excessive trunk flexion in supported sitting, absence of the lateral hip abduction reaction). The choice of behaviours to be observed was based on the idea that features such as the ability to centre the head along the midline of the body and perform anti-gravity activities would be lacking and, therefore, diagnostic in infants with developing CP.

At about the same time, a talented physical therapist and neuro-development therapy (NDT) instructor, Gay Girolami, came to work on her master's degree with me at the University of North Carolina at Chapel Hill. Having been trained in treatment of infants with CP in Switzerland by Mary Quinton, she was determined to evaluate the efficacy of NDT in promoting postural control in premature infants at risk for CNS dysfunction as defined by the presence of abnormal reflexes at 34 weeks postconceptional age. A challenge to this work was identification of a reliable outcome assessment tool that would be responsive to the effects of NDT.

As one of the few standardized tests of newborn behavioural organization then available, Girolami chose to use the Brazelton Neonatal Behavioral Assessment Scale (NBAS; Brazelton 1973) as one of the outcome measures in her study, but because she believed that the NBAS was unlikely to be responsive to anticipated improvements in postural control, she developed a Supplemental Motor Test (SMT). Girolami used several of my Checklist's dichotomously scored items of spontaneous posture and movement, added more dichotomous Observed Items to assess activities such as hand function and pelvic lifting, designed a way to quantify the asymmetrical tonic neck reflex (ATNR) and developed new items to assess head and trunk control using 0- to 4-point rating scales. When used as a measure of postural control in high-risk preterm infants at approximately 37 weeks postconceptional age after 7–17 days of twice daily therapy in a small controlled clinical trial, the SMT was incredibly responsive to the effects of NDT and showed, furthermore, that treated preterm infants had postural control more like that of full-term control subjects than like that of infants in the placebo-treated preterm control group (Girolami and Campbell 1994). This work was not only the first to demonstrate that NDT provided in the NICU could improve postural control in high-risk preterm infants, but also suggested that the sensitive test designed by Girolami might not only be useful as a treatment outcome measure, but also held promise as a means of diagnosing delayed development of postural control in early infancy, a prerequisite for initiating therapy. With further development, the SMT evolved into the Test of Infant Motor Performance (TIMP), a functional motor scale for infants under the age of 4 months.

Others began assessing quality of movement in a variety of ways. For example, the Movement Assessment of Infants (MAI) showed promise as a diagnostic measure based on assessment of reflexes, postural tone, spontaneous movement and posture at 4 and 8 months of age; its sensitivity at 4 months was reported to be 83% with a specificity of 78% (Swanson et al 1992). Later, the longitudinal videotaped observations of high-risk infants pioneered by Prechtl and his colleagues led the way to recognition of the unique diagnostic value of a syndrome of cramped synchrony in movement and the failure to develop a qualitative aspect of movement called 'fidgety'. The General Movement (GM) assessment demonstrated sensitivity of 100% and specificity of 92.5–100% depending on age of assessment for diagnosis of CP before 60 weeks postmenstrual age (Ferrari et al 2002). The first piece of the puzzle of early diagnosis and the search for effective treatment appeared to be in place. Although, because of its dichotomous nature (diagnosis of movement as normal versus abnormal), GM assessment is unlikely to be responsive to the effects of intervention or to be helpful in determining treatment goals, the GM assessment can be used to identify individuals as well as groups of infants who are likely to have CP before they would be expected to demonstrate failure to learn to roll over, sit, crawl or walk. Using the GM assessment makes it possible to predict the development of CP with high reliability by 3–4 months of age.

At the same time that Prechtl's group developed the GM assessment as a diagnostic tool for early identification of CP from repeated examinations in early infancy, the renaissance of interest in motor development led by Thelen brought about new insights into infant motor performance in typically developing infants (Thelen et al 1987, Thelen and Smith 1994, Thelen 1995). Using dynamic systems theory to guide exploration of the processes of motor development, Thelen and her colleagues showed through a variety of ingenious experiments that long-held beliefs in maturation of motor behaviour based on inhibition of primitive reflexes, cephalocaudal and proximodistal development and the brain as the unique determinant of motor development were unlikely to be true (Thelen and Fisher 1982, Thelen 1995). Although early development of the TIMP was driven empirically on the basis of clinical knowledge and observations, as test development continued, dynamic systems theory and research results came to inform the process and evolving content of the test.

> . . . good measures exist for evaluating outcome and . . . clinicians must agree on measures, collect data routinely and reliably and act on the results of evaluation. Nevertheless, in the search for the 'perfect' scale clinicians keep developing new functional scales to address their own particular concerns . . . and it may be that more time and money is spent in this endeavour and in the

continuing testing of reliability and validity than in using available tests actually to evaluate patient performance (Carr and Shepherd 1998, p. 63).

Here, I respectfully disagree with this quote from Carr and Shepherd. It is my hope that the remainder of this chapter, which describes the evolution and validation of the Test of Infant Motor Performance from its early incarnation as the Supplemental Motor Test, will demonstrate the value of the more than 15 years and over a million US dollars that I and my colleagues have expended in validating a new diagnostic test of functional motor performance for use in paediatric rehabilitation.

TIMP ITEM DEVELOPMENT: CONTENT AND CONSTRUCT VALIDITY

Ever since the SMT was demonstrated to be responsive to the effects of NDT in the NICU, I had hoped someday to further develop the test as a diagnostic, prescriptive and responsive measure for use in early intervention with infants. In the 1990s, a team consisting of myself, physical therapists Gay Girolami and Thubi Kolobe and occupational therapists Beth Osten and Maureen Lenke came together to work towards this goal. Girolami's SMT was originally designed to assess postural and reflex development at term age, so development first concentrated on expansion of the item content to cover a wider age range as well as item specifications that would reflect postural control in all parts of the body, first and foremost that of head control, the major developmental milestone of the first few months of life, but also arm, leg and trunk control. Based on clinical experience and review of the research literature, each test developer contributed new items, revised previous SMT items or developed rating scales for behaviours on the Checklist of Abnormal/Immature Motor Responses so that the age range of the revised test was from 32 weeks post-conceptional age to 13.5 weeks post term. The SMT originally included 15 dichotomous Observed Items (scored on the basis of infants' spontaneous movements) and 28 Elicited Items (scored with Likert-type scales reflecting the infants' responses to being placed in various positions or stimulated with interesting sights and sounds). Subsequent versions of the test, renamed the Test of Infant Motor Performance (TIMP), had 22 (and then 27) Observed Items and 30 Elicited Items. Additions included Observed Items assessing selective movement of fingers, wrists and ankles, and more Elicited Items assessing lateral righting reactions, neck and trunk rotation, crawling movements, anti-gravity responses in prone suspension and standing and defensive reactions to a cloth placed over the eyes. The items measuring the ATNR were deleted because Girolami's research had demonstrated that they were not reliably rated by independent observers.

Version 2 of the TIMP was used to study content validity based on expert judgement, rater reliability (Osten, unpublished research, 1993), scaling properties of the test and validity for responsiveness to developmental change with age. Rasch psychometric analysis was used to assess:

1. difficulty levels of each item, i.e. how likely babies of different abilities (or ages) were to succeed in performing various activities;
2. construct validity, i.e. how well items reflected a similar construct, that of postural and selective control of movement needed for functional performance in daily life;
3. item misfit, i.e. items that raters scored inconsistently or that babies performed in ways that did not conform to our expectations (Wright et al 1993).

TIMP V.2 Elicited Items were reviewed by 21 experts in paediatric physical therapy, occupational therapy or psychology (Campbell et al 2002a, Conti and Runde, unpublished research, 1990). The results supported the content validity of the TIMP: expert reviewers believed the items to be sensitive to developmental change over time (84% of the items) and to be useful for detecting developmental deviance in young infants (96% of the items).

The sensitivity to developmental change of TIMP V.2 was examined in a cross-sectional sample of 137 infants from three race/ethnicity groups in the Chicago metropolitan area: non-Latino/a white, black (African or African-American) and Latino/a (Mexican or Puerto Rican) (Campbell et al 1993, 1995). TIMP performance correlated with age at $r = 0.83$ (Campbell et al 1995), thus meeting the construct validity requirement that infants' scores must increase linearly with increasing age (or ability). Furthermore, infants with more medical complications did less well than same-age healthier peers.

After study of Rasch analysis results on TIMP V.2 and a review of new literature on typical development and on possible predictors of abnormal outcome, the test developers honed their theoretical understanding of what the TIMP should accomplish and made several more changes to the test. As a result, Version 3 of the TIMP was developed to include 28 Observed Items and 31 Elicited Items, 6 of which were paired items used to test different sides of the body so that asymmetry of movement would be reflected in results.

Although the TIMP was developed for use in clinical settings by paediatric physical therapists and occupational therapists, the test developers believed that TIMP items reflected demands for movement that infants experience during naturalistic handling in daily life interactions with caregivers. This hypothesis was tested in a master's thesis by Murney using V.3 of the TIMP. Murney's study (Murney and Campbell 1998) assessed the demands for movement placed on 22 infants varying in age and ethnicity during bathing, dressing and play interactions with their mother or nurse. These demands for movement placed on infants by caregivers were compared with item administration instructions for the 25 unique TIMP V.3 Elicited Items to quantify how well TIMP items reflect daily life performance demands. The findings indicated that 92% of TIMP item administration instructions were similar in the demands placed on infants to those that occurred naturally in caregiver–infant interactions. The modal infant experienced demands similar to about 37% of the TIMP Elicited Items during a typical caregiving interaction (range = 16–68%). Many demands were experienced by the infant repeatedly during a typical caregiving sequence such that demands related to TIMP items occurred, on average, 1.58 times per minute. This research was used to inform the next revision of the test: no items were considered for removal from the TIMP in Version 4 that were highly related to naturally occurring demands used by caregivers (Campbell et al 2002a).

Some examples of demands on the part of parents or nurses that are similar to TIMP item administration procedures include handling similar to that occurring during nappy changing or diapering (lifting and releasing legs in supine), dressing (rolling the infant to the side by moving the arm or leg; holding the infant in prone suspension while straightening clothing), encouraging the infant to use eyes and head to track moving objects or to look at still objects during playtime and evoking orientation to sounds such as the caregiver's voice or a rattle (Campbell et al 2002a, Murney and Campbell 1998). Caregivers also frequently pull infants up into sitting from supine and place infants in positions that challenge their ability to defy gravity, such as supported sitting or standing with the head unsupported. Parents were not observed to place their infants in prone very often so it was more difficult to find a match up between TIMP prone items and functional demands in natural interactions. Overall, the results of this study provided strong support for the content and construct validity of the TIMP for capturing movement demands in ecologically relevant situations, not just the clinical setting. We believed that a test such as this would be responsive to the effects of task-specific interventions.

The items in TIMP V.3 were further studied with the results of 1723 tests obtained on 159 infants in a longitudinal and test–retest reliability study conducted during 1994–99 (Campbell 1999a, Campbell and Hedeker, 2001, Campbell and Kolobe 2000). Following assessment of item difficulty, item scaling and item misfit based on Rasch psychometric analysis, the 59 items of V.3 were reduced to a 42-item Version 4 (Campbell et al 2002a).

To summarize the results of study of several versions of the TIMP leading to the current V.4, the majority of the changes made have been intended primarily to improve the clarity of scoring for each level of each item to promote reliable scoring among raters. Although a variety of items have been added and subtracted from the test during its development, the major changes that occurred were (1) expansion of item content to cover a larger range of age, and (2) deletion of reflex, that is, ATNR, and some arm/hand items that proved to be unreliably rated or demonstrated by infants. As a result, V.4 of the test is clearly an assessment of gross motor functional performance, primarily head and trunk control in all positions in space and in response to visual and auditory stimulation. The construct underlying the TIMP items is that of postural and selective control of movement needed for function in daily life activities up to 4 months (corrected) age. The infant who performs well on the TIMP at 3–4 months of age has the head and trunk control needed to move on to independent rolling and sitting. An infant who performs better than –0.5 SD from the mean has a 98% chance of having normal gross motor development within the typical range at 12 months (Campbell et al 2002b).

Recently, photographs of infants performing at every level of each of the Elicited Items in V.4 were added to the test form to improve its educational value for parents, thus forming the current illustrated form of the TIMP, V.5.1. A self-instructional CD is available to assist therapists in learning the TIMP (Liao and Campbell 2002). The TIMP V.5.1. is currently being normed on 1200 infants selected to reflect the racial/ethnic and geographic diversity of low-birthweight infants in the USA. The results of this study will allow the test to be used to diagnose delayed functional motor performance with norms for 2-week age intervals from 34 weeks postconceptional age to 16 weeks post term. Furthermore, a subset of 21 items is also under study for development as a screening version of the scale. The full test takes an average of 30 minutes to perform, whereas the screening version will take about 10 minutes. By comparing results of screening tests with performance on the full TIMP, we will be able to provide guidelines for making clinical decisions regarding the need for full TIMP testing given results on the screening test. This development will facilitate use of the TIMP in clinical practice by reducing examination time overall and by allowing more fragile infants to be screened with a shorter version of the test than is currently available.

TIMP PREDICTIVE VALIDITY

The research described thus far has documented that the TIMP is a valid and reliable scale for examining postural and selective control of movement in early infancy, that is, scores change systematically upwards with increasing age or ability. A useful test in infancy would also discriminate among infants with varying risk for developmental disability and predict outcome. Campbell and Hedeker (2001) documented that longitudinal growth curves of performance on the TIMP discriminated among groups with varying degrees of medical complications. Further research by Campbell and colleagues (Campbell et al 2002b) demonstrated that 3-month performance on the TIMP could be used to predict motor development on the Alberta Infant Motor Scale at 12 months of age (corrected for prematurity if necessary) with a high degree of accuracy. Sensitivity for prediction to delayed development at 12 months of age was 0.92 while specificity for prediction to typical development was 0.76. A specificity lower than the sensitivity value indicates that some children who are not performing well on the TIMP at 3 months will, nevertheless, perform within the typical range by 12 months of age, a not unexpected finding in a population with serious medical complications at birth, some of whom require a long period of recovery. Recently, Kolobe et al (2003) assessed developmental outcome of 61 of the 82 infants in the original TIMP predictive validity study at 4–5 years of age to determine the relationship between TIMP scores at 3 months corrected age and motor performance on the Peabody Developmental Motor Scales at 4–5 years of age. Sensitivity of the 3-month TIMP for prediction to gross motor performance was 0.67 and specificity was 0.92. Children who were missed (i.e. had high scores at 3 months but low Peabody scores at 4–5 years) may have had problems like attention deficits that affected their performance on the motor test, rather than serious gross motor problems. Positive and negative predictive validity were excellent (0.73 and 0.89 respectively). The results of this study support the conclusion that high-risk infants who are able to recover by 3 months corrected age have a high probability (0.92) of having normal gross motor performance 4–5 years later.

FURTHER APPLICATION TO CLINICAL PRACTICE

Despite the fact that some children with low TIMP scores in early infancy might recover on their own, Lekskulchai and Cole (2001) demonstrated that using TIMP scores to identify low-scoring premature infants at hospital discharge and to provide them with a home physical therapy programme resulted in significant gains in motor performance over a 4-month period. The average infant who received treatment performed as well as infants who were deemed not to need treatment at discharge because they were scoring well on the TIMP. On the other hand, infants who received the home programme performed significantly better at 4 months of age than other infants scoring poorly at discharge who were randomly assigned to the no-treatment control group. The longitudinal design of this study, using monthly measurement of TIMP performance, revealed the growing gap over time between average performance of treated versus untreated infants, while the gap between high performers at discharge and treated low-scoring infants disappeared. Thus, the TIMP has not only been shown to be useful to diagnose delayed development in preterm infants at hospital discharge, but was also demonstrated to be responsive to the effects of intervention in a large, controlled clinical trial conducted by an independent group of investigators.

With performance standards from a population-based sample of US infants available soon, the test designers will have met their goal of developing an evaluative test to diagnose delayed motor development in the NICU and the developmental follow-up clinic. But can the TIMP also be used to plan treatment goals? We believe that it can because TIMP item content reflects functionally significant movement demands that infants experience frequently in daily life. The results of the studies by Murney and Campbell (1998) and Girolami and Campbell (1994) support the idea that performance on the TIMP could also be used to identify goals for treatment by identifying the next steps in development that infants are lacking and using them to develop both a treatment and an outcome assessment plan (see Campbell 1999b for examples).

Research has not yet revealed specific differences between children with varying diagnoses, but current work by Barbosa documents the early impairment of performance of infants with CP on the TIMP (Barbosa et al 2003) and aims to analyse individual item performance of infants with CP towards the goal of describing a diagnostic profile of motor impairments that characterize this condition as it evolves over the first 4 months of life. Anecdotally, our clinical experiences also suggest that the items capable of reflecting asymmetry are useful in describing the development of children with congenital torticollis, that poor performance on items involving visual or auditory stimulation of head movements can be helpful in discriminating children who should be referred for evaluation of possible vision or hearing deficits, and that items requiring neck and trunk flexion are especially delayed in children with congenital heart conditions who have undergone open-heart surgery as newborns.

TESTING OF SCIENTIFICALLY BASED REHABILITATION THEORIES

Active interaction with the environment is known to be necessary for an animal or human to extract the appropriate information from that environment. It is apparent from studies of animals that the nature of the environment (physical structure, possibilities for social interaction, physical activity and exercise) affect brain organization and reorganization after a lesion (Carr and Shepherd 1998, p. 10).

Of great importance to the goal of testing the efficacy of scientifically based rehabilitation theories, Murney and Campbell (1998) documented the relationship between TIMP items measuring postural control and the typical movement demands of activities (tasks) occurring in naturalistic interactions between infants under 4 months of age and their caregivers. We believe that performance on TIMP items can reflect functional outcomes of task-specific interventions, but can also be used to compare treatment effects based on a variety of theoretical approaches. For infants at risk for CP, we believe that there are at least three existing theoretical approaches that should be tested:

1. NDT, an approach involving significant amounts of physical handling of infants aimed at facilitation of postural and selective control of movement, aspects of motor control that are impaired in CP (Girolami and Campbell 1994);
2. dynamic systems-based Tscharnuter Akademie for Movement Organization (TAMO) therapy, which emphasizes child-initiated movement with minimal hands-on aimed at helping the child to improve body contacts with the support surface so as to optimize the biomechanics of physical activity (Tscharnuter 2002);
3. a task-oriented approach using parent-identified goals and environmental organization to structure movement experiences, which has been successfully tested with older children with CP but requires elaboration and testing in newborns (Ketelaar et al 2001).

These approaches vary in the amount of handling that is prescribed, in how the environment is used in intervention and in how, and by whom, goals of treatment are determined.

Major clinical research emphasis should now be placed, in our view, on studying the effects of different rehabilitation methods upon brain morphology and function as well as on behavior (Carr and Shepherd 1998, p. 4).

The proposed research, if well controlled for effects of maturation and designed to compare various treatment strategies, would allow us to know whether the TIMP is sensitive to the effects of early intervention and how large these effects are for treatment strategies derived from various theoretical points of view. From my perspective, however, the critical question is whether earlier versus later treatment can reduce the ultimate level of disability, implying that the course of brain development has been altered by intervention during the course of recovery from insult. We have previously argued that assessment of outcomes must be multidimensional in order to study the processes by which functional performance and quality of life for people with disabilities are affected by interventions (Almeida et al 1997). The combination of assessment of changes in impairments and functional outcomes with brain imaging to assess changes in morphology or physiology will be especially fruitful in addressing the question of timing effects of intervention.

> It is certain that the brain will reorganize (adapt) after a lesion whatever happens to the individual. However, given the evidence from investigations of the differential and context-dependent effects on reorganization, it is possible to hypothesize that the nature of that reorganization must depend on the inputs received and the outputs demanded post-lesion, and particularly during the rehabilitation process . . . Physiotherapy intervention is typically regarded as enabling the individual to make the most of what is left after the lesion, inferring a static system, rather than actually affecting or driving the recovery (reorganization) process itself. There is, however, increasing support in the neurosciences for the argument that what the person does and experiences in rehabilitation, and the rehabilitation environment itself, affects the recovery process (Carr and Shepherd 1998, p. 9).

An alternative to the currently existing theoretical perspectives would be a highly focused approach based on research on brain organization and plasticity and the effects of training and movement exploration on the nervous system (Black 1998, Sporns and Edelman 1993). If, as I believe, there may be a critical period for altering the course of recovery and the evolution of disability in infants with brain insults, the developing system must be forced to exercise capacities that have been impaired at a much more intense level and earlier in the course of development than is typically offered in early intervention today. As Black (1998) suggests, the damage from pathological experience may be long-lasting and quite difficult to undo so interventions must begin early and be substantial. Furthermore, to test for a critical period for altering outcomes, some children will need to be treated intensively during, say, the first 4 months of life, while others are treated only during the second 4 months of life because critical period tests require that both groups must receive the same amount and intensity of intervention but at different timepoints (Bruer 2001). The idea of beginning intensive intervention early will also present a challenge to the now generally accepted idea that the high-risk infant must be protected from excessive stimulation (Campbell 1999b). This idea is based on the belief that the natural self-organizing tendencies of the human organism (Thelen et al 1987) will promote typical development; however, the ability of children with brain damage to use these mechanisms effectively is doubtful. In fact, we find that such children may even show regressions in motor performance.

Based on Barbosa's analysis of data (Barbosa, unpublished data) on TIMP performance over time of 10 infants with CP, we note the following critical sequence of negative signs during the course of development:

1. inability to maintain a midline position of the head in supine at 3–4 weeks corrected age;
2. poor anti-gravity arm movement and neck flexion when pulled to sit at 5–6 weeks;
3. poor upright head control and inability to inhibit the neonatal neck-righting reaction at 9 weeks;
4. poor prone head control and failure to develop extensor synergies in head, trunk and legs during activities such as turning towards a sound in prone, leg reactions to hip flexion in supine and head righting during facilitated rolling at 12 weeks.

Furthermore, regression may occur in the ability to perform anti-gravity hip flexion, kicking and isolated ankle movements. These findings confirm the general impression that development of head control is the earliest impairment observed in children with CP, and intervention in the first 4 months of life should target this skill aggressively. The regressions in leg movements we recorded also suggest a focused approach that would strengthen leg muscles and exercise the activity of the central pattern generator(s) for production of reciprocal interlimb coordination (Piek 2001, Piek and Gasson 1999). Based on Turvey and Fitzpatrick's (1993) concepts regarding pattern formation during development, shaping behaviour of leg movements using the paradigm of Angulo-Kinzler et al (2002)* to prevent regressions and promote eye–ear–leg perception–action patterns based on the infant's ability to control leg movements to operate a mobile might also be fruitful. How to promote the decoupling of tight intralimb linkages (Vaal et al 2000) that should occur as development progresses, however, would need to be considered.

The studies proposed entail a large degree of ethical challenge. In the USA, infants with defined developmental diagnoses or documented developmental delay have a legal right to early intervention services funded and provided by the states under the aegis of federal laws. Inclusion of an untreated control group in such a situation requires careful thought and justification, but can conceivably be defended in light of the fact that children with CP today are seldom identified and treated before the age of 9 months. Long delays in getting intervention also exist in most state systems even after a child is deemed eligible for treatment. I believe that study of whether a critical period exists for early intervention to reduce the ultimate level of disability in children with CP would involve treatment at a time when most of these children receive either no treatment or very limited treatment. I agree with Carr and Shepherd (1998, p. 3) that intensive treatment to force the production of useful movement will be needed to make a difference so even a control group that is allowed access to 'usual' treatment will receive much less intervention of a relatively unstructured nature than any experimental treatment group in a well-designed study. Despite the challenges of research on scientifically based approaches to early intervention for infants with brain insults, the economic costs of treating such children over a lifetime and the challenges faced by their families demand that this research be done (Campbell 1997).

ACKNOWLEDGEMENTS

The work described in this manuscript was supported by the Foundation for Physical Therapy, the National Center for Medical Rehabilitation Research of the US Public Health Service, National Institutes of Health (HD32567 and HD38867) and the Ministry of Education of Brazil (Barbosa). The TIMP test materials and self-instructional CD are available from Infant Motor Performance Scales, LLC, 1301 W. Madison St #526, Chicago, IL 60607-1953, USA. URL: www.thetimp.com.

---

[*]I would like to acknowledge my debt to Linda Fetters for bringing this work to my attention.

References

Almeida G L, Campbell S K, Girolami G L et al 1997 Multi-dimensional assessment of motor function in a child with cerebral palsy following intrathecal administration of baclofen. Physical Therapy 77:751–764.

Angulo-Kinzler R M, Ulrich B, Thelen E 2002 Three-month-old infants can select specific leg motor solutions. Motor Control 6:52–68.

Barbosa V M, Campbell S K, Sheftel, D et al 2003 Longitudinal performance of infants with cerebral palsy on the Test of Infant Motor Performance and on the Alberta Infant Motor Scale. Physical and Occupational Therapy in Pediatrics 23:7–29.

Black J E 1998 How a child builds its brain: some lessons from animal studies of neural plasticity. Preventive Medicine 27:168–171.

Brazelton T B 1973 The Neonatal Behavioral Assessment Scale. Clinics in Developmental Medicine No. 50. J B Lippincott, Philadelphia.

Bruer J T 2001 A critical and sensitive period primer. In: Bailey D B Jr, Bruer J T, Symons F J et al (eds) Critical thinking about critical periods. Paul H Brookes, Sydney, pp 3–26.

Campbell S K 1997 Therapy programs for children that last a lifetime. Physical and Occupational Therapy in Pediatrics 17(1):1–15.

Campbell S K 1999a Test-retest reliability of the Test of Infant Motor Performance. Pediatric Physical Therapy 11:60–66.

Campbell S K 1999b The infant at risk for developmental disability. In: Campbell S K (ed) Decision making in pediatric neurologic physical therapy. Churchill Livingstone, New York, pp 260–332.

Campbell S K, Osten E, Kolobe T H A et al 1993 Development of the Test of Infant Motor Performance. Physical Medicine and Rehabilitation Clinics of North America 4(3):541–550.

Campbell S K, Kolobe T H A, Osten E T et al 1995 Construct validity of the Test of Infant Motor Performance. Physical Therapy 75:585–596.

Campbell S K, Kolobe T H A 2000 Concurrent validity of the Test of Infant Motor Performance with the Alberta Infant Motor Scale. Pediatric Physical Therapy 12:1–8.

Campbell S K, Hedeker, D 2001 Validity of the Test of Infant Motor Performance for discriminating among infants with varying risk for poor motor outcome. Journal of Pediatrics 139: 546–551.

Campbell S K, Wright B D, Linacre J M 2002a Development of a functional movement scale for infants. Journal of Applied Measurement 3(2): 191–205.

Campbell S K, Kolobe T H A, Wright B D et al 2002b Validity of the Test of Infant Motor Performance for prediction of 6-, 9-, and 12-month scores on the Alberta Infant Motor Scale. Developmental Medicine and Child Neurology 44:263–272.

Carr J, Shepherd R 1998 Neurological rehabilitation: optimizing motor performance. Butterworth-Heinemann, Oxford.

Ferrari F, Cioni G, Einspieler C et al 2002 Cramped synchronized General Movements in preterm infants as an early marker for cerebral palsy. Archives of Pediatrics and Adolescent Medicine 156:460–467.

Girolami G, Campbell S K 1994 Efficacy of a Neuro-Developmental Treatment program to improve motor control of preterm infants. Pediatric Physical Therapy 6(4):175–184.

Ketelaar M, Vermeer A, 't Hart H et al 2001 Effects of a functional therapy program on motor abilities of children with cerebral palsy. Physical Therapy 81:1534–1545.

Kolobe T H A, Bulanda M, Sussman L 2003 Predictive ability of the Test of Infant Motor Performance at preschool age (abstract). Pediatric Physical Therapy 15:68.

Lekskulchai R, Cole J 2001 Effect of a motor development program on motor performance in infants born preterm. Australian Journal of Physiotherapy 47:169–176.

Liao P-J M, Campbell S K 2002 Comparison of two methods for teaching therapists to score the Test of Infant Motor Performance. Pediatric Physical Therapy 14:191–198.

Murney M E, Campbell S K 1998 The ecological relevance of the Test of Infant Motor Performance Elicited Scale items. Physical Therapy 78:479–489.

Piek J P 2001 Is a quantitative approach useful in the comparison of spontaneous movements in fullterm and preterm infants? Human Movement Science 20:717–736.

Piek J P, Gasson N 1999 Spontaneous kicking in fullterm and preterm infants: are there leg asymmetries? Human Movement Science 18:377–395.

Sporns O, Edelman G M 1993 Solving Bernstein's problem: a proposal for the development of coordinated movement by selection. Child Development 64:960–981.

Swanson M W, Bennett F C, Shy K et al 1992 Identification of neuromotor abnormality at 4 and 8 months by the Movement Assessment of Infants. Developmental Medicine and Child Neurology 34:321–337.

Thelen E 1995 Motor development: a new synthesis. American Psychologist 50:79–95.

Thelen E, Fisher D 1982 Newborn stepping: an explanation for a disappearing reflex. Developmental Psychology 18:760–775.

Thelen E, Smith L B 1994 A dynamic systems approach to the development of cognition and action. MIT Press, Cambridge, MA.

Thelen E, Kelso J A S, Fogel A 1987 Self-organizing systems and infant motor development. Developmental Reviews 7:39–65.

Tscharnuter I 2002 Clinical application of dynamic theory concepts according to Tscharnuter Akademie for Movement Organization (TAMO) therapy. Pediatric Physical Therapy 14:29–37.

Turvey M T, Fitzpatrick P 1993 Commentary: development of perception-action systems and general principles of pattern formation. Child Development 64:1175–1190.

Vaal J, van Soest A J, Hopkins B et al 2000 Development of spontaneous leg movements in infants with and without periventricular leukomalacia. Experimental Brain Research 135:94–105.

Wade D T 1992 Measurement in neurological rehabilitation. Oxford University Press, Oxford.

Weindling A M, Hallam P, Gregg J et al 1996 A randomized controlled trial of early physiotherapy for high-risk infants. Acta Paediatrica 85:1107–1111.

Wright B D, Linacre J M, Heinemann A W 1993 Measuring functional status in rehabilitation. Physical Medicine and Rehabilitation Clinics of North America 4(3):475–491.

Chapter 4

Muscle performance after stroke

Di J. Newham

CHAPTER CONTENTS

The pioneering work of Janet Carr and Roberta Shepherd radically changed the approach of physiotherapists to neurological rehabilitation in a number of ways and has made a substantial contribution to this field. In the 1980s, they came to believe that the rehabilitation techniques widely practised were far from optimal on the basis of the ongoing disabilities of many people with neurological conditions. Furthermore, they held that the rehabilitation techniques themselves could actually be contributing to the residual disability (Carr and Shepherd 1980, 1982).

At that time, the major influences on stroke rehabilitation for therapists came from the techniques of Bobath (Bobath 1969, 1970, 1990), Rood (Goff 1969, Rood 1954, Stockmeyer 1967) and proprioceptive neuromuscular facilitation (PNF) (Knott and Kabat 1954, Voss 1967). While they had different approaches, they were based on developmental movement patterns and had in common an emphasis on postural stability, normal movement patterns and muscle tone. The treatment and prevention of spasticity/muscle tone was considered to be of prime importance. It was considered that nothing should be done that might initiate or increase it, and that this excluded making strong or difficult efforts. These schools of thought developed organically and paid little attention to knowledge developing in the neurological sciences, nor did they consider the context-dependent nature of movement.

Carr and Shepherd developed the Motor Relearning Programme (MRP), which considered motor control as a key contributor to function, along with the elimination of unnecessary muscle activity, feedback and practice. They embraced the evolving neurophysiological knowledge that aided the understanding of the changes associated with brain injury and recovery, along with the analysis of normal and abnormal movement in different contexts. Evidence started to emerge at around this time that the brain was not the hard-wired organ previously envisaged, and they incorporated the concept of motor learning as an aid to enhancing plasticity in the brain after stroke. This new approach opened up neurological rehabilitation and enabled active consideration of areas previously not considered, such as the role of muscle strength.

Stroke rehabilitation comprises a complex, multiprofessional package (Young 1996). It is recognized that physiotherapists contribute to many components of this package in ways that are often poorly understood (Pomeroy and Tallis 2002a) and that the interventions vary widely, depending largely on the preferred approach of the individual therapist (Woldag and Hummelsheim 2002). Physical interventions can be broadly categorized into (1) high-level – aimed at preventing the translation of impairments into disability or handicap; and (2) low-level – aimed at reducing impairment (Pomeroy and Tallis 2002b). This may be an oversimplification in cases where strategies have both effects. Generally, high-level interventions help function after stroke, but could be limited by the extent of motor ability available. If this can be improved by low-level strategies, then the potential for recovery of function is even greater (Pomeroy and Tallis 2002a).

This chapter will focus on muscle performance – the effect of stroke and the role of improving muscle performance in rehabilitation. It will start by briefly reviewing current knowledge on cerebral plasticity and the ways that rehabilitation techniques may enhance plasticity in order to optimize function after stroke.

MUSCLE STRENGTH

Muscle strength has only been seriously considered in stroke rehabilitation in relatively recent years. Initial concerns that measurements would be unreliable (e.g. Rothstein et al 1989) and strengthening would exacerbate any tendency for increased tone have not been borne out for most of the muscle groups studied (Bohannon 1989, Eng et al 2002, Gregson et al, 2000, Hsu et al 2002, Levin and Hui-Chan 1994, Pohl et al 2000).

A number of studies have now shown that people affected by stroke are weak during isometric contractions – see review by Ng and Shepherd (2000) and the work of others (Andrews and Bohannon 2000, 2003, Canning et al 1999, Chae et al 2002a, Davies et al 1996, Levin et al 2000, Maeda et al 2001, Newham and Hsiao 2001, Sunnerhagen et al 1999). Distal muscles seem to be more affected than proximal, and flexors more than extensors – a distribution of weakness different from that commonly thought to occur (Andrews and Bohannon 2000).

Weakness is seen when people affected by stroke are compared with age- and sex-matched healthy control subjects. It is present in the quadriceps and hamstring muscle groups soon after mild to moderate stroke and recovers slowly (Figure 4.1) (Newham and Hsiao 2001). Davies et al (1996) found significant weakness in

Figure 4.1   Isometric maximal voluntary torque in the quadriceps (a) and hamstrings (b) for control subjects (diamonds) and the paretic (black squares) and non-paretic (blue squares) legs of stroke subjects in the first 6 months after stroke. For the first 3 months the torque of the paretic limbs was significantly less than control ($P < 0.01$–0.0002). Mean and SEM. (Data redrawn from Newham and Hsiao 2001.)

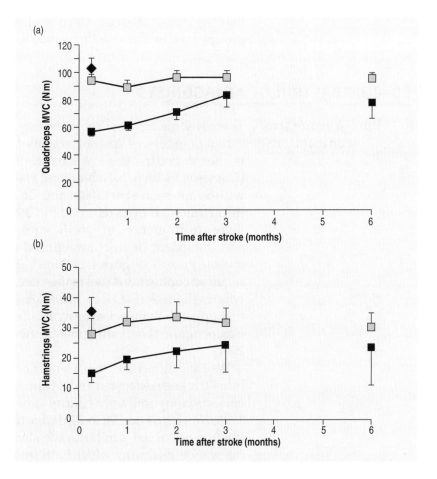

these muscle groups in people affected by stroke up to 42 months previously (range 3–42 months).

From this time course it is clear that the usual rehabilitation package does not restore normal muscle strength. The evidence argues against the widely held belief that any weakness will spontaneously recover with increased activity, and strongly suggests that muscle strength should be directly addressed during rehabilitation.

It is often assumed that any muscle weakness is the result of disuse atrophy caused by inactivity. However, the finding that it occurs so soon after stroke (Andrews and Bohannon 2000, 2003, Newham and Hsiao 1998, 1999, 2001) does not support this. Harris et al (2001) reported reduced force from the externally stimulated quadriceps in the first week after stroke. These changes occur too rapidly to be accounted for by disuse atrophy and suggest that at least some of the muscle weakness seen is a direct and long-lasting consequence of the brain lesion. This is supported by our findings (Hsiao and Newham 1999, 2001) that muscle weakness, even on the 'non-paretic' side, is evident very soon after stroke. Clinically, it is often thought that muscle strength is essentially normal – usually based on the results of subjective, manual muscle testing – but that the effects of excessive co-contraction of antagonistic muscle groups and/or increased tone may reduce it in practice.

CO-CONTRACTION OF ANTAGONISTS

During isometric contractions

There is some controversy in the literature about the presence and extent of excessive co-contraction of antagonist muscles. During isometric contractions we have not found evidence for this (Davies et al 1996, Newham and Hsiao 1998, 2001) in agreement with Svantesson et al (2000) and Gowland et al (1992). However, its presence has been reported by Chae et al (2002a). It may be that there are differences in specific stroke populations in this respect, and the extent of co-contraction does vary between limbs and muscle groups (Figure 4.2) (Newham and Hsiao 2001), speed of required contractions (Basmajian and De Luca 1985) and familiarity with the task (De Luca and Mambrito 1987). There is evidence that upper limb muscles are more affected by excessive co-contraction of agonists and antagonists after stroke (Kamper and Rymer 2001).

We have found that the extent of co-contraction during maximal isometric knee extension and flexion is similar in both legs of stroke subjects compared with control subjects (Figure 4.2) (Davies et al 1996, Newham and Hsiao 2001). Furthermore, the extent of co-contraction remained similar in the stroke subjects over a period of many months during which both strength and function improved.

Figure 4.2   Similar levels of co-activation of antagonist muscle groups are seen during isometric knee extension and flexion efforts of control subjects (dark blue), non-paretic (mid blue) and paretic (pale blue) limbs of stroke patients. Mean and SEM. (Data redrawn from Newham and Hsiao 2001.)

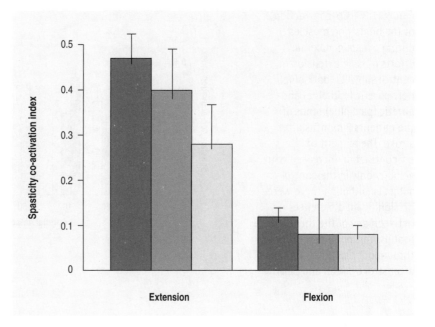

Figure 4.2 shows the amount of co-contraction of antagonists during a maximal voluntary isometric contraction measured by the Spasticity Co-activation Index (Fung and Barbeau 1989), in which antagonist electromyographic activity is expressed as a ratio of the maximum the muscle can produce when it is acting as an agonist.

During dynamic contractions

Spasticity is defined as a velocity-dependent phenomenon. Therefore, if it impairs force generation, a greater effect should be seen during high-velocity contractions. We studied this (Newham and Hsiao 1998, 2001, unpublished data) during maximal isokinetic flexion and extension at angular velocities up to 300°/s using an isokinetic dynamometer. The control subjects showed more co-contraction during dynamic contractions (Figure 4.3) than isometric contractions (Figure 4.2), and this tended to increase with increasing velocity (Figure 4.3). Both legs of the people affected by stroke showed little systematic change in the amount of co-contraction with increasing velocity and there were no significant differences compared with the control subjects during the first 6 months after stroke. These data do not give any indication of the presence of an abnormal velocity-dependent increase in antagonist co-contraction in people affected by stroke, in agreement with the results reported by Bierman and Ralston (1965). In contrast, Knutsson and Martensson (1980) did find antagonist co-contraction that increased with movement velocity; however, there was large individual variation and the extent of clinically

Figure 4.3 Co-contraction of the hamstring muscles during dynamic maximal efforts of knee extension in control subjects (dark blue), non-paretic (mid blue) and paretic (pale blue) limbs of the patients 3 months after stroke. The amount of co-contraction increased with velocity only in the control subjects, although there were no significant differences between any of the three groups. This remained the case throughout the first 6 months after stroke. Mean and SEM.

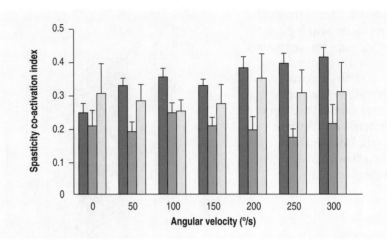

assessed resistance to passive movement was greater than in the subjects we studied.

ABNORMAL TONE

The abnormal tone frequently associated with stroke has long been one of the main focuses of rehabilitation, and for many years the restoration of 'normal' tone was one of the key aims of treatment. Tone may be low immediately after the brain lesion, but in the rehabilitation phase the problem is usually one of increased tone. The prevalence of increased tone has recently been estimated as affecting 38% of people 1 year after stroke, even though several joints were assessed (Watkins et al 2002). This is lower than previous estimates and fits with the clinical impression that abnormal tone is considered to be less of a problem than it used to be. The reason for this is unknown and could be the result of medical management, rehabilitation, or a combination of both.

The phenomenon of increased muscle tone after upper motor neuron lesions is regarded as 'hypertonia', and this term is often used interchangeably with spasticity. The most widely accepted definition of spasticity is 'a motor disorder characterized by a velocity dependent increase in tonic stretch reflexes ("muscle tone" with exaggerated tendon jerks, resulting from hyper-excitability of the stretch reflex as one component of the upper motor neurone syndrome'; Lance 1980). However, the increased resistance to passive movement (hypertonia) is affected not only by the stretch reflex and may contain both neural and non-neural components.

Clinically, spasticity is usually measured by subjective assessments, such as the Modified Ashworth Scale (MAS) (Bohannon and Smith 1987), which rate the resistance to passive movement. One obvious problem with this is that the velocity-dependent nature of spasticity is not taken into account. Scales that rate the resistance to passive movement are unable to distinguish between an increase in tone due to neural factors and that caused by changes in stiffness of the contractile or non-contractile connective tissue (Katz et al 1992). Furthermore, reliability of such assessments has often been reported as poor (e.g. Pomeroy et al 2000).

If increased tone is the result of neural factors, then passive movement would be accompanied by muscle activity that would be detectable by electromyography (EMG). We studied the resistance to passive movement in a group of patients with mild–moderate spasticity on the MAS, and found an increased resistance to passive movement during knee extension in the people affected by stroke without any EMG activity (Davies et al 1996). An increased resistance to passive movement was found bilaterally during passive knee extension but not during passive knee flexion (Figure 4.4). Wilson et al (1999) suggested that muscle spindle activity is normal in people recently affected by stroke and that fusimotor dysfunction has little effect on motor deficit. If increased tone is not the result of neural influences causing either voluntary or reflex muscle activity, then the underlying mechanism must come from non-contractile tissue.

Figure 4.4 The resistance to passive knee extension at an angular velocity of 30°/s. Both the non-paretic (mid blue) and paretic (pale blue) limbs of the stroke patients showed increased resistance compared with the control subjects (dark blue) (P < 0.01). Mean and SEM. (Data from Davies et al 1996.)

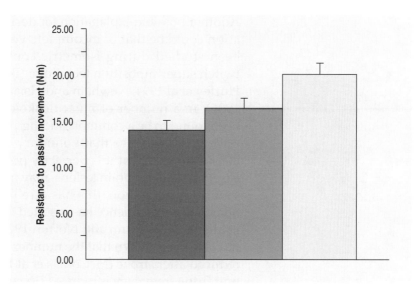

NON-NEURAL COMPONENTS OF INCREASED TONE

There is substantial support for the hypothesis that changes in non-neural stiffness make a major contribution to the increased tone found after stroke. Our findings of increased resistance to passive movement without increased EMG activity (Davies et al 1996; Figure 4.4) support this. Furthermore, the findings of Fowler et al (1998) and Ada et al (1998) suggest that soft-tissue changes, rather than hyperreflexia, result in the increased resistance to passive movement. Svantesson and Stibrant Sunnerhagen (1997) investigated the stretch-shortening cycle and found that prior activity increased the concentric torque output of the paretic legs without any increase in EMG activity. They concluded that this was the result of better utilization of elastic energy due to muscle stiffness. Subsequently, Svantesson et al (2000) reported that muscle stiffness was higher, but tendon stiffness lower, in the triceps surae muscles of the paretic leg. In the same muscle group, passive stiffness of the muscle–tendon complex was found to contribute more to total stiffness during gait in paretic limbs than both non-paretic and control limbs (Lamontagne et al 2000). A review by Singer et al (2001) highlights the importance of non-neural changes after acquired brain injury. These include collagen proliferation and remodelling involving non-contractile material, and also increasing actin-myosin cross-bridge linkages that reduce the rate of cross-bridge detachment. The latter might account for the prolonged activity reported at the end of a contraction of paretic muscle (Riley and Bilodeau 2002).

VOLUNTARY ACTIVATION

Another possible explanation for decreased voluntary force generation could be that of incomplete voluntary activation. This has been studied during isometric contractions, mainly using the twitch superimposition technique (Belanger and McComas 1981, Hurley et al 1994, Newham and Hsiao 1998, 2001, Rutherford et al 1986), in a number of musculoskeletal conditions where it has been found to be a common finding.

There is evidence that voluntary activation failure is present after stroke. Whilst it is perfectly possible that neurological disease, particularly brain lesions, may impair the ability for maximal voluntary activation, this has rarely been directly investigated. Some indirect evidence has resulted from EMG studies (Gowland et al 1992, Sahrmann and Norton 1977, Tang and Rymer 1981). It has also been shown that the number of functioning motor units is reduced after stroke (McComas et al 1973) and also that the motor unit firing frequency is reduced (Rosenfalck and Andreassen 1980,

Tang and Rymer 1981). The twitch speed is also reduced (Newham et al 1996). These factors could all affect voluntary activation.

We have studied voluntary activation failure in the quadriceps during isometric contractions throughout the first 6 months after stroke (Hsiao 1998, Newham and Hsiao 2001). Significant voluntary activation failure, compared with matched control subjects, was found bilaterally. Furthermore, it was greater in the paretic muscle group and remained unchanged over 6 months (Figure 4.5). Similar findings have been reported in the paretic upper limb by Kamper and Rymer (2001) and also Riley and Bilodeau (2002), who found that the extent of activation failure increased during prolonged activity.

The presence of voluntary activation failure supports the theory that the neurological insult has direct effects on skeletal muscle. It could be due to a failure of motor unit recruitment or reduced firing rates in the active units. Furthermore, it is striking that the activation failure in our study was bilateral. While many studies do not investigate the so-called 'unaffected' limbs, there is a growing body of evidence that the consequences of a unilateral cerebrovascular accident are manifested bilaterally (Bohannon and Walsh 1992, Chollett et al 1991, Colebatch and Gandevia 1989, Davies et al 1996, Harris et al 1997).

Voluntary activation failure might also be expected to coexist with excessive activity of antagonist muscles, but this was not the case in our study (Figure 4.2). The failure might also be caused by an interruption of the corticospinal pathways after stroke. If this was the case, then recovery of activation failure would imply that either a reorganization of the central nervous system or collateral

Figure 4.5   Voluntary activation in the quadriceps muscle during isometric contractions. It was reduced in both the non-paretic (mid blue, $P < 0.0002$) and paretic (pale blue, $P < 0.005$) limbs of the stroke subjects compared with control subjects (dark blue). Mean and SEM. (Data from Newham and Hsiao 2001.)

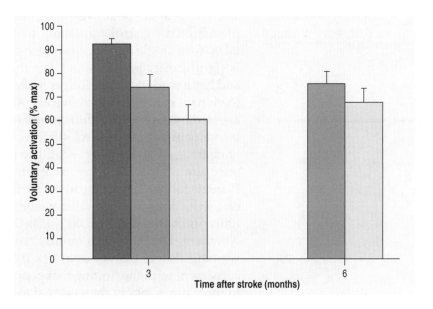

sprouting has occurred. However, we saw no change in the extent of activation failure over a 6-month period.

The frequent occurrence of flaccidity immediately after stroke, at a time too early for any secondary changes in the peripheral neuromuscular system, demonstrates that activation failure is a common feature of brain injury. The finding that significant levels of activation failure persist, and are found bilaterally, may well have important implications for rehabilitation and recovery of function. It remains to be seen whether a period of strength training increases the level of voluntary activation in people affected by stroke.

GENERATION OF POWER

There have been numerous investigations of muscle strength – isometric and dynamic – after stroke, and the clear consensus is that a level of weakness exists that would be expected to adversely affect normal function. Although these studies are valuable, it is important to bear in mind that our main requirement of muscles is to generate power. Because power is the product of force and velocity, the speed at which force can be generated is of crucial importance. There is no functional benefit in having large muscles, capable of generating high forces, if movement can only be performed at velocities below those required for safe function. Therefore, speed and its determinants will now be considered, along with the literature on the generation of power after stroke.

Contribution of
contractile speed

There appears to be universal agreement that the muscles of people affected by stroke are slow to contract and relax. The time taken for a single quadriceps twitch to relax to half of its peak force is significantly longer than normal in the paretic limb ($P < 0.01$) and has a tendency to be longer in the non-paretic limb (Figure 4.6) (Newham et al 1996). We have also shown that people chronically affected by stroke with mild clinical spasticity achieve lower angular velocities than control subjects in both the quadriceps and hamstrings (Davies et al 1996). The paretic limb was also slower, once again indicating the involvement of a central mechanism. Patients followed over the first 6 months after stroke showed bilateral reductions in maximal movement speed that remained essentially unchanged ($P < 0.005$–0.00005) for 3 months (Hsiao and Newham, 2001). After 6 months, movement in the paretic limb was still slower than normal ($P < 0.01$; Figure 4.7). This is also in agreement with the finding that people affected by stroke take two to three times longer than normal to generate force (Canning et al

Figure 4.6 Relaxation speed from a single quadriceps twitch in control subjects (dark blue) and the non-paretic (mid blue) and paretic (pale blue) limbs of chronic stroke patients. There was a tendency for slowed relaxation in the non-paretic muscle group while this was significant in the paretic ($P <$ 0.01). Mean and SEM.

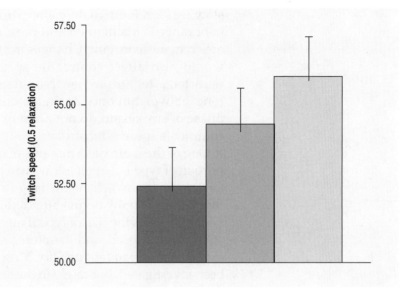

Figure 4.7 The maximal angular velocity that could be achieved during knee extension in control subjects (diamond) and in paretic (pale blue squares) and non-paretic limbs (mid-blue squares) during the first 6 months after stroke. In the stroke patients this was initially reduced bilaterally, showed no change over the first 3 months and was still less than normal in the paretic limb after 6 months. Mean and SEM.

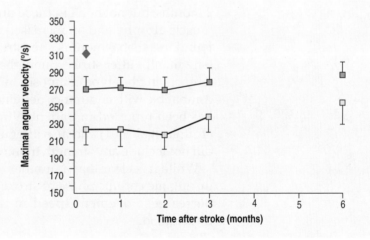

1999). The delayed contraction and relaxation times correlated with physical disability (Chae et al 2002b). Slow movement speeds have also been reported during the activity of standing up (Carr et al 2002).

The number of sarcomeres in series, that is the length of muscle fibre, is proportional to the speed at which a muscle can contract and relax (Jones and Round 1996). Therefore, any loss of joint movement would result in reduced contractile speed if the sarcomere number was reduced. This is a likely scenario in chronic stroke where joint range has been lost, but does not account for the slowing seen immediately after stroke, or in chronic cases where joint range is maintained and presumably the number of sarcomeres remains constant. Changes in stiffness of the muscle/tendon would also affect contractile speed. Such changes have been reported after stroke (see 'Non-neural components of increased tone' above), but once again are unlikely to develop in the acute phase of stroke and do not account for the early changes seen in contractile speed after stroke.

One of the main determinants of contractile function is the proportion of type I (aerobic, slow-twitch, fatigue-resistant) and type II (anaerobic, fast-twitch, highly fatiguable) muscle fibres. It is accepted that disuse atrophy occurs after reduced physical activity and particularly affects the size of type II muscle fibres. This causes reduced strength and speed, and therefore power output, but would not be expected to impair fatiguability. Muscle composition after stroke has been investigated, but rarely in the acute phase. One study reported a transient loss of muscle mass at 7 days after stroke (Jorgensen and Jacobsen 2001). Interestingly, muscle mass had recovered after 1 year only in the non-paretic leg of those who were able to walk after 2 months, but not at all in those unable to walk at this point. Total muscle atrophy and an increased intramuscular fat content were found less than 6 months after stroke (Ryan et al 2002). In patients 6–12 months after stroke, Sunnerhagen et al (1999) reported no differences in fibre type composition but a reduced capillary density, compatible with endurance detraining or inactivity. Type II atrophy has been reported in patients 9 months to 12 years after stroke (Toffola et al 2001) and also after a rehabilitation programme that did not include any strength training (Hachisuka et al 1997).

While it is clear that a number of changes take place in muscle during the chronic phase of stroke recovery, the factors that cause decreased movement speed in the acute phase remain poorly understood.

Power output

The work on isometric strength generation is valuable and informative. Nevertheless it is important to remember that the main functional requirement of skeletal muscle is to generate power and movement. Since power is the product of force and velocity, the isometric studies showing that both of these are reduced after stroke clearly indicate that power is also reduced. However, the reduction in power will be greater than the reduction in either force or velocity alone. Direct studies of power output (the rate of doing work) after stroke are rare.

We studied the power output of the knee flexors and extensors at a range of angular velocities up to 300°/s in the first 6 months after stroke (Hsiao and Newham 2001). Most of the stroke subjects were unable to achieve angular velocities $\geq 250°/s$, and there were insufficient data for analysis. At the remaining movement velocities in the first weeks after stroke the power output in both paretic and non-paretic legs of the stroke subjects was less ($P < 0.01–0.0001$ and $P < 0.045–0.01$, respectively) than that of control subjects. The reduction in the non-paretic limb was less consistent than in the paretic but in both limbs was more pronounced at lower velocities ($\geq 150°/s$). The hamstrings generally showed a greater reduction in power output than the quadriceps. Although there was a slow improvement over time, the power output at 6 months after stroke remained low, particularly in the paretic limb, and this was most obvious at lower movement speeds (Figure 4.8).

Kautz and Brown (1998) studied the power output and EMG of the quadriceps and hamstrings of the hemiplegic leg during moderate intensity cycle ergometry. They found that the external mechanical work output of the plegic leg was significantly less. Abnormal timing of EMG activity in the quadriceps and hamstrings resulted in less positive work (concentric contractions) and more negative work (eccentric contractions) than in the control subjects. The work done at different pedalling speeds and workloads was studied by the same workers (Brown and Kautz, 1999) in people affected by stroke more than 6 months after stroke. This decreased as pedalling speed increased, but as the pattern of EMG activity did not change with velocity they concluded that this was due to mechanical factors.

Dynamometry studies of the plantarflexors after stroke by Nadeau et al (1997) found that although the peak torque was similar in the people affected by stroke, the slow development of torque at the start of movement resulted in reduced power output. Torque, power and rate of torque development were correlated with each other and also with some, but not all, clinical measures.

Figure 4.8 Maximal power output of the quadriceps at three angular velocities in control subjects (dark blue), non-paretic (mid blue) and paretic (pale blue) limbs of stroke subjects. Stroke subjects were tested 0.25, 2 and 6 months after stroke (left to right). Power output was reduced bilaterally (particularly in the paretic limb), and changed little over time. Mean and SEM.

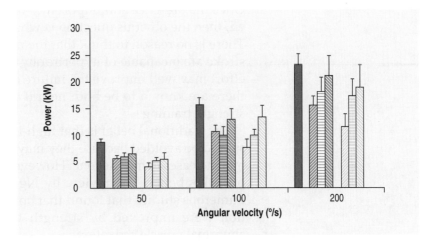

It is clear that the performance of skeletal muscle is impaired by stroke; this is seen too soon afterwards to be simply the result of disuse. Furthermore, it affects both limbs – not just the paretic – and does not fully recover with standard rehabilitation intervention. A key issue is whether these abnormalities are related to function.

RELATIONSHIP BETWEEN MUSCLE PERFORMANCE AND FUNCTION

Ng and Shepherd (2000) reviewed the literature on weakness after stroke and its implications for function and rehabilitation. They concluded that there is good evidence that strength relates directly to function and that both can be improved by intensive strength training without any adverse effects. This is in agreement with our findings that knee muscle strength in the paretic limb in the first few weeks after stroke was significantly correlated with the sit to stand and walking component of the Motor Assessment Scale developed by Carr et al (1985) and the Barthel Index (Mahoney and Barthel 1965) ($P = 0.01–0.002$), but not the 10-m timed walk (Hsiao 1998, Hsaio and Newham 1999). Six months later, all of these measures of disability were significantly correlated ($P = 0.03–0.0002$) with quadriceps strength. At all times, there was a significant relationship between strength and the maximal velocity of movement ($P < 0.0005$). Significant correlations between strength and function have also been reported more recently by other workers (Andrews and Bohannon 2001, Chae et al 2002a, 2002b, Maeda et al 2001, Nadeau et al 1999, Suzuki et al 1999, Teixeira-Salmela et al 1999).

STRENGTH TRAINING

Once the presence and importance of muscle weakness is accepted, then the obvious question is what can be done to improve it. There is no reason to think that the muscles of people affected by stroke are incapable of hypertrophy, and repeated high-intensity effort may well improve the failure of voluntary activation since there are known to be both neural and peripheral responses to strength training.

The traditional belief is that high-intensity muscle contractions should be avoided because they may initiate or exacerbate abnormal increases in muscle tone. However, the evidence does not support this belief. The review by Ng and Shepherd (2000) cited numerous studies that found that both muscle strength and function were improved by strength training without increasing abnormal muscle activation.

Table 4.1   Characteristics of the quadriceps stretch reflex before and after an exercise session consisting of repeated maximal isometric and isokinetic voluntary contractions at angular velocities of 30–300°/s. There was no indication of increased excitability after exercise.

	Non–paretic		Paretic	
	Before	After	Before	After
Amplitude (mV)	0.18 ± 0.03	0.18 ± 0.03	0.13 ± 0.03	0.11 ± 0.02
Onset latency (ms)	19.25 ± 0.67	20.85 ± 1.09	20.05 ± 0.69	19.47 ± 0.78
Peak latency (ms)	24.10 ± 0.64	25.55 ± 0.93	25.68 ± 0.97	25.29 ± 1.09

We have examined the characteristics of the stretch reflex of the quadriceps muscle before and after repeated maximal isometric and isokinetic maximal voluntary contractions, such as would be used during strength training (Hsiao and Newham 1999). No indications were found of an increase in the excitability of the stretch reflex after isokinetic maximal voluntary contractions in the period 6 months after stroke (Table 4.1), and occasionally a decrease was found. It is worth noting that the subjects often spontaneously reported that their muscles felt 'better' and 'looser' after exercise. There was no sign of increased muscle activity or associated reactions.

More recently, a number of authors have similarly reported that high-intensity exercise has a beneficial effect, with no observed adverse effects on muscle tone or function in people affected by stroke (Badics et al 2002, Brown and Kautz 1998, Kim et al 2001, Smith et al, 1999; Teixeira-Salmela et al 1999, 2001, Weiss et al 2000). It is worth noting that a number of these studies involved people affected by stroke in both the acute and chronic phases, and that improvements with strength training were seen in both groups.

CONCLUSION

The work described in this chapter highlights both the novelty and importance of the work of Carr and Shepherd in stroke rehabilitation. They were innovators with an interest in the role of muscle strength in the function of people who have had a stroke. It has since been clearly shown by them and others that muscles are weak after stroke and that muscle weakness is related to function. They do not get stronger during traditional rehabilitation or spontaneously with increased activity. However, high-intensity contractions, once viewed as something to be avoided at all costs, do not generally increase muscle tone and improve both strength and function. The interest of Carr and Shepherd in muscle and stroke initiated studies that revealed voluntary activation failure, implicated a direct action of the brain lesion on muscle performance and found that the effects are not restricted to the paretic limb. To have done this is a remarkable achievement that has consequences in clinical and scientific terms, not least to people affected by stroke themselves. There is still much work to be done to implement these findings into widespread clinical practice and to study further the role of muscle performance and its effect on function after stroke.

References

Ada L, Vattanasilp W, O'Dwyer N J et al 1998 Does spasticity contribute to walking dysfunction after stroke? Journal of Neurology, Neurosurgery and Psychiatry 64:628–635.

Andrews A W, Bohannon R W 2000 Distribution of muscle strength impairments following stroke. Clinical Rehabilitation 14:79–87.

Andrews A W, Bohannon R W 2001 Discharge function and length of stay for patients with stroke are predicted by lower extremity muscle force on admission to rehabilitation. Neurorehabilitation and Neural Repair 15:93–97.

Andrews A W, Bohannon R W 2003 Short-term recovery of limb muscle strength after acute stroke. Archives of Physical Medicine and Rehabilitation 84:125–130.

Badics E, Wittmann A, Rupp M et al 2002 Systematic muscle building exercises in the rehabilitation of stroke patients. Neurorehabilitation 17:211–214.

Basmajian J V, De Luca C J 1985 Muscles alive; their functions revealed by electromyography. Williams & Wilkins, Baltimore.

Belanger A Y, McComas A J 1981 Extent of motor unit activation during effort. Journal of Applied Physiology 51:1131–1135.

Bierman W, Ralston H J 1965 Electromyographic study during passive and active flexion of the normal subject. Archives of Physical Medicine and Rehabilitation 46:71–75.

Bobath B 1969 The treatment of neuromuscular disorders by improving patterns of coordination. Physiotherapy 55:18–22.

Bobath B 1970 Adult hemiplegia: evaluation and treatment. Heinemann Medical Books, London

Bobath B 1990 Adult hemiplegia: evaluation and treatment, 3rd edn. Heinemann Medical Books, London.

Bohannon R W 1989 Is the measurement of muscle strength appropriate in patients with brain lesions? A special communication. Physical Therapy 69:225–236.

Bohannon R W, Smith M B 1987 Interrater reliability of a modified Ashworth scale of muscle spasticity. Physical Therapy 67:206–207.

Bohannon R W, Walsh S 1992 Nature, reliability and predictive value of muscle performance measures in patients with hemiparesis following stroke. Archives of Physical Medicine and Rehabilitation 73:721–725.

Brown D A, Kautz S A 1998 Increased workload enhances force output during pedalling exercise in persons with poststroke hemiplegia. Physician and Sportsmedicine 26:598–606.

Brown D A, Kautz S A 1999 Speed-dependent reductions of force output in people with poststroke hemiparesis. Physical Therapy 79:919–930.

Canning C G, Ada L, O'Dwyer N 1999 Slowness to develop force contributes to weakness after stroke. Archives of Physical Medicine and Rehabilitation 80:66–70.

Carr J H, Shepherd R B 1980 Physiotherapy in disorders of the brain. Heinemann Medical Books, London.

Carr J H, Shepherd R B 1982 A motor learning programme for stroke. Heinemann Medical Books, London.

Carr J H, Shepherd R B, Nordholm L et al 1985 Investigation of a new motor assessment scale for stroke patients. Physical Therapy 65:175–180.

Carr J H, Ow J E G, Shepherd R B 2002 Some biomechanical characteristics of standing up at three different speeds; implications for functional training. Physiotherapy Theory and Practice 18:47–53.

Chae J, Yang G, Kyu Park B et al 2002a Muscle weakness and cocontraction in upper limb hemiparesis: relationship to motor impairment and physical disability. Neurorehabilitation and Neural Repair 16:241–248.

Chae J, Yang G, Park B K et al 2002b Delay in initiation and termination of muscle contraction, motor impairment, and physical disability in upper limb hemiparesis. Muscle and Nerve 25:568–575.

Chollett F, Di Piero V, Wise R J S et al 1991 The functional anatomy of motor recovery after stroke in humans; a study with positron emission tomography. Annals of Neurology 29:63–71.

Colebatch J G, Gandevia S C 1989 The distribution of muscle weakness in upper motor neuron lesions affecting the arm. Brain 112:749–763.

Davies J M, Mayston M J, Newham D J 1996 Electrical and mechanical output of the knee muscles during isometric and isokinetic activity in stroke and healthy adults. Disability and Rehabilitation 18:83–90.

De Luca C J, Mambrito B 1987 Voluntary control of motor units in human antagonist muscles; coactivation and reciprocal activation. Journal of Neurophysiology 58:525–542.

Eng J J, Kim C M, Macintyre D L 2002 Reliability of lower extremity strength measures in persons with chronic stroke Archives of Physical Medicine and Rehabilitation 83:322–328

Fowler V, Canning C G, Carr J H et al 1998 Muscle length effect on the pendulum test. Archives of Physical Medicine and Rehabilitation 79:169–171.

Fung J, Barbeau H 1989 A dynamic EMG profile index to quantify muscular activation disorder in spastic paretic gait. Electroencephalography and Clinical Neurophysiology 73:233–244.

Goff B 1969 Appropriate afferent stimulation. Physiotherapy 51:9–17.

Gowland C, deBruin H, Basmajian J V et al 1992 Agonist and antagonist activity during voluntary upper limb movement in patients with stroke. Physical Therapy 72:624–633.

Gregson J M, Leathley M J, Moore A P et al 2000 Reliability of measurements of muscle tone and muscle power in stroke patients. Age and Ageing 29:223–228.

Hachisuka K, Umezu Y, Ogata H 1997 Disuse muscle atrophy of lower limbs in hemiplegic patients. Archives of Physical Medicine and Rehabilitation 78:13–18.

Harris M L, Polkey M I, Bath P M W et al 1997 Acute hemiplegic ischaemic stroke causes contralateral quadriceps weakness. Journal of Neurology, Neurosurgery and Psychiatry 62:214.

Harris M L, Polkey M I, Bath P M et al 2001 Quadriceps muscle weakness following acute hemiplegic stroke. Clinical Rehabilitation 15:274–81.

Hsiao S-F 1998 Neuromuscular and functional performance in stroke patients; the effect of physiotherapy intervention. PhD thesis, University of London.

Hsaio S-F, Newham D J 1999 The non-paretic side of stroke patients; extent of deficit in mechanical output. Clinical Rehabilitation 13:80–81.

Hsiao S-F, Newham D J 2001 Bilateral deficits of voluntary thigh muscle contraction after recent stroke. In: Gantchev N (ed) From basic motor control to functional recovery. II. Towards an understanding of the role of motor control from simple systems to human performance. Academic Publishing House (Bulgarian Academy of Science), Sofia, pp 376–384.

Hsu A L, Tang P F, Jan M H 2002 Test-retest reliability of isokinetic muscle strength of the lower extremities in patients with stroke. Archives of Physical Medicine and Rehabilitation 83:1130–1137.

Hurley M V, Jones D W, Newham D J 1994 Arthrogenic quadriceps inhibition and rehabilitation of patients with extensive traumatic knee injuries. Clinical Science 86:305–310.

Jones D A, Round J M 1996 Skeletal muscle in health and disease; a textbook of muscle physiology. Manchester University Press, Manchester.

Jorgensen L, Jacobsen B K 2001 Changes in muscle mass, fat mass, and bone mineral content in the legs after stroke: a 1 year prospective study. Bone 28:655–659.

Kamper D G, Rymer W Z 2001 Impairment of voluntary control of finger motion following stroke: role of inappropriate muscle coactivation. Muscle and Nerve 24 673–681.

Katz R T, Rovai G P, Brait C 1992 Objective quantitation of spastic hypertonia; correlation with clinical findings. Archives of Physical Medicine and Rehabilitation 73:339–347

Kautz S A, Brown D A 1998 Relationships between timing of muscle excitation and impaired motor performance during cyclical lower extremity movement in post-stroke hemiplegia. Brain 121:515–526.

Kim C M, Eng J J, MacIntyre D L et al 2001 Effects of isokinetic strength training on walking in persons with stroke: a double-blind controlled pilot study. Journal of Stroke and Cerebrovascular Diseases 10:265–273.

Knott M, Kabat H 1954 Proprioceptive facilitation therapy for paralysis. Physiotherapy 40:171–176.

Knutsson E, Martensson A 1980 Dynamic motor capacity in spastic paresis and its relation to prime mover dysfunction; spastic reflexes and antagonist co-activation. Scandinavian Journal of Rehabilitation Medicine 12:93–106.

Lamontagne A, Malouin F, Richards C L 2000 Contribution of passive stiffness to ankle plantarflexor moment during gait after stroke.

Archives of Physical Medicine and Rehabilitation 81:351–358.

Lance J W 1980 Symposium synopsis. In: Feldman R G, Toung R R, Koella W P (eds) Spasticity: disordered motor control. Year Book Medical Publishers, Chicago, pp 485–494

Levin M F, Hui-Chan C 1994 Ankle spasticity is inversely correlated with antagonist voluntary contraction in hemiparetic subjects. Electromyography and Clinical Neurophysiology 34:415–425.

Levin M F, Selles R W, Verheul M H et al 2000 Deficits in the coordination of agonist and antagonist muscles in stroke patients: implications for normal motor control. Brain Research 853:352–369.

McComas A J, Sica R E P, Upton A R M et al 1973 Functional changes in motoneurones of hemiparetic patients. Journal of Neurology, Neurosurgery and Psychiatry 36:183–193.

Maeda T, Oowatashi A, Kiyama R et al 2001 Discrimination of walking ability using knee joint extension muscle strength in stroke patients. Journal of Physical Therapy Science 13:87–91.

Mahoney F I, Barthel D W 1965 Functional evaluation: the Barthel Index. Maryland State Medical Journal 14:61–65.

Nadeau S, Gravel D, Arsenault A B et al 1997 Dynamometric assessment of the plantarflexors in hemiparetic subjects: relations between muscular, gait and clinical parameters. Scandinavian Journal of Rehabilitation Medicine 29:137–46.

Nadeau S, Arsenault A B, Gravel D et al 1999 Analysis of the clinical factors determining natural and maximal gait speeds in adults with a stroke. American Journal of Physical Medicine and Rehabilitation 78:123–130.

Newham D J, Hsiao S-F 1998 Muscle performance of patients with recent stroke: weakness or antagonist restraint? Clinical Rehabilitation 12:163–164.

Newham D J, Hsiao S-F 1999 Voluntary strength and activation of quadriceps after stroke; the first six months. Clinical Rehabilitation 13:92.

Newham D J, Hsiao S-F 2001 Knee muscle isometric strength, voluntary activation and antagonist co-contraction in the first six months after stroke. Disability and Rehabilitation 23:379–386.

Newham D J, Mayston M J, Davies J M 1996 Quadriceps isometric force, voluntary activation and relaxation speed in stroke. Muscle and Nerve Suppl 4:S53.

Ng S S, Shepherd R B 2000 Weakness in patients with stroke: implications for strength training in neurorehabilitation. Physical Therapy Reviews 5:227–238.

Pohl P S, Startzell J K, Duncan P W et al 2000 Reliability of lower extremity isokinetic strength testing in adults with stroke. Clinical Rehabilitation 14:601–607.

Pomeroy V M, Tallis R C 2002a Restoring movement and functional ability after stroke: now and the future. Physiotherapy 88:3–17.

Pomeroy V M, Tallis R C 2002b Neurological rehabilitation; a science struggling to come of age. Physiotherapy Research International 7:76–89.

Pomeroy V M, Dean D, Sykes L et al 2000 The unreliability of clinical measures of muscle tone: implications for stroke therapy. Age and Ageing 29:229–233.

Riley N A, Bilodeau M 2002 Changes in upper limb joint torque patterns and EMG signals with fatigue following a stroke. Disability and Rehabilitation 24:961–969.

Rood M S 1954 Neurophysiologic reactions: a basis for physical therapy. Physical Therapy Review 34:444–449.

Rosenfalck A, Andreassen S 1980 Impaired regulation of force and firing pattern of single motor units in patients with spasticity. Journal of Neurology, Neurosurgery and Psychiatry 43:907–916.

Rothstein J M, Riddle D I, Finucane S D 1989 Commentary. Physical Therapy 69:230–235.

Rutherford O M, Jones D A, Newham D J 1986 Clinical and experimental application of the percutaneous twitch superimposition technique for the study of human muscle activation. Journal of Neurology, Neurosurgery and Psychiatry 49:1288–1291.

Ryan A S, Dobrovolny C L, Smith G V et al 2002 Hemiparetic muscle atrophy and increased intramuscular fat in stroke patients. Archives of Physical Medicine and Rehabilitation 83:1703–1707.

Sahrmann S A, Norton B S 1977 The relationship of voluntary movement to spasticity in the upper motor neurone syndrome. Annals of Neurology 2:460–465.

Singer B, Dunne J, Allison G 2001 Reflex and non-reflex elements of hypertonia in triceps surae muscles following acquired brain injury; implications for rehabilitation. Disability and Rehabilitation 23:749–757.

Smith G V, Silver K H C, Goldberg A P et al 1999 Task oriented exercise improves hamstring strength and spastic reflexes in chronic stroke patients. Stroke 39:2112–2118.

Stockmeyer S A 1967 An interpretation of the approach of Rood to the treatment of neuromuscular dysfunction. American Journal of Physical Medicine 46:900–955.

Sunnerhagen K S, Svantesson U, Lonn L et al 1999 Upper motor neuron lesions: their effect on muscle performance and appearance in stroke patients with minor motor impairment. Archives of Physical Medicine and Rehabilitation 80:155–1561.

Suzuki K, Imada G, Iwaya T et al 1999 Determinants and predictors of the maximum walking speed during computer-assisted gait training in hemiparetic stroke patients. Archives of Physical Medicine and Rehabilitation 80:179–182.

Svantesson U, Stibrant Sunnerhagen K 1997 Stretch-shortening cycle in patients with upper motor neuron lesions due to stroke. European Journal of Applied Physiology and Occupational Physiology 75:312–318.

Svantesson U, Takahashi H, Carlsson U et al 2000 Muscle and tendon stiffness in patients with upper motor neuron lesion following a stroke. European Journal of Applied Physiology and Occupational Physiology 82:275–279.

Tang A, Rymer W Z 1981 Abnormal force-EMG relations in paretic limbs of hemiparetic human subjects. Journal of Neurology, Neurosurgery and Psychiatry 44:690–698.

Teixeira-Salmela L F, Olney S J, Nadeau S et al 1999 Muscle strengthening and physical conditioning to reduce impairment and disability in chronic stroke survivors. Archives of Physical Medicine and Rehabilitation 80:1211–1218.

Teixeira-Salmela L F, Nadeau S, McBride I et al 2001 Effects of muscle strengthening and physical conditioning training on temporal, kinematic and kinetic variables during gait in chronic stroke survivors. Journal of Rehabilitation Medicine 33:53–60.

Toffola E D, Sparpaglione D, Pistorio A et al 2001 Myoelectric manifestations of muscle changes in stroke patients. Archives of Physical Medicine and Rehabilitation 82:661–665.

Voss D E 1967 Proprioceptive neuromuscular facilitation. American Journal of Physical Medicine 46:838–898.

Watkins C L, Leathley M J, Gregson J M et al 2002 Prevalence of spasticity post stroke. Clinical Rehabilitation 16:515–522.

Weiss A, Suzuki T, Bean J et al 2000 High intensity strength training improves strength and functional performance after stroke. American Journal of Physical Medicine and Rehabilitation 79:369–376.

Wilson L R, Gandevia S C, Inglis J T et al 1999 Muscle spindle activity in the affected upper limb after a unilateral stroke. Brain 122:2079–2088.

Woldag H, Hummelsheim H 2002 Evidence based physiotherapeutic concepts for improving arm and hand function in stroke patients: a review. Journal of Neurology 249:518–528.

Young J 1996 Rehabilitation and older people. British Medical Journal 313:677–681.

Chapter **5**

Changing the way we view the contribution of motor impairments to physical disability after stroke

Louise Ada and Colleen Canning

The neurologist Hughlings Jackson, in the late 19th century, observed that the motor problems resulting from lesions of the central nervous system (CNS) could be categorized as either positive or negative. Negative impairments are those that represent a loss of pre-existing function, such as loss of strength and dexterity, whereas positive impairments are additional, such as abnormal postures, increased proprioceptive reflexes (i.e. spasticity) and increased cutaneous reflexes. Furthermore, because brain damage usually results in impairments that take time to resolve, secondary impairments (such as contracture and reduced cardiovascular fitness) arise as adaptations to the primary impairments. A major concern of neurological physiotherapists is understanding the relative contribution of the positive versus negative, and primary versus secondary impairments to disability (Figure 5.1). This chapter presents the contribution to this understanding made by studies examining brain damage caused by stroke, carried out in the School of Physiotherapy at the University of Sydney.

POSITIVE IMPAIRMENTS

Before the 1970s, the positive impairments, particularly spasticity, were seen as the major contributors to disability by neurologists and therapists alike. In 1974, Landau published a landmark paper questioning this view (Landau 1974). Over the next decade, there were a number of investigations into the contribution of spasticity to disordered voluntary movement. One method of investigation examined muscle activity during voluntary movement and came to the conclusion that excessive antagonist activity could not have caused the observed movement abnormality (e.g. Dietz et al 1981, Norton and Sahrmann 1978, Sahrmann and Norton 1977). Another method of investigation reduced spasticity, using either drugs (McLellan 1977) or training (Neilson and McCaughey 1982), and found that function

Figure 5.1   Schematic showing the relation of primary motor impairments to secondary motor impairments and the relation of these impairments to disability after stroke.

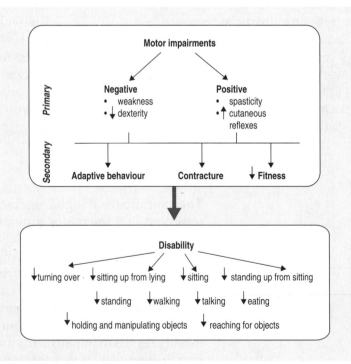

was not improved. Around this time, Carr and Shepherd were observing in the clinic that, while it was possible to reduce spasticity temporarily, this did not necessarily improve function. By the publication of their landmark book in 1982, *A Motor Relearning Programme for Stroke* (Carr and Shepherd 1982), they were already placing more emphasis on treating the negative impairments, especially training motor control, rather than reducing spasticity. This position was a reflection of their clinical observations and synthesis of this early scientific literature. As the emphasis shifted towards the negative impairments, new questions about spasticity, such as its relation with contracture, were being raised (Dietz et al 1981, Perry 1980). It was this context that provided the background for the following studies investigating positive impairments.

Characteristics of spasticity

Spasticity has often been used to describe a wide range of motor impairments (both negative and positive) and this in itself has made understanding its contribution to disability difficult. However, in the early 1980s, a conference of leading neurologists and neurophysiologists agreed upon a consensus definition that described spasticity as: 'a motor disorder characterised by a velocity-dependent increase in tonic stretch reflexes ("muscle tone") with exaggerated tendon jerks resulting from hyperexcitability of the stretch reflex' (Lance 1980, 1990).

The existence of this widely accepted definition of spasticity has produced investigations of spasticity with a consistent theoretical view. The definition asserts that spasticity is an abnormality of the stretch reflex, and this has meant that it is necessary to measure muscle activity to be sure that the increase in muscle tone referred to in the definition is the result of hyperreflexia.

Appropriate methods of describing and examining spasticity in line with this definition enable close scrutiny of its characteristics. For example, the relationship between spasticity and associated reactions was investigated (Ada and O'Dwyer 2001). Associated movements (or synkineses) are unintentional movements that accompany, but are not necessary for, volitional movement (Zülch and Müller 1969). It is common to observe associated movements during the performance of tasks in neurological conditions and when underlying pathology is present; these movements have been called associated reactions (Walshe 1923). Associated reactions have been assumed to be a manifestation of spasticity, that is, they have been seen as a part of the spastic syndrome (Walshe 1923) and are believed to occur only in the presence of spasticity (Bobath 1990, Cornall 1991, Stephenson et al 1998). The question of whether the presence of spasticity is essential for the expression of associated reactions was investigated in people after stroke (Ada and O'Dwyer 2001). Associated reactions were identified by the presence of muscle activity in the affected muscle and quantified as the amount of torque produced during a moderate contraction of contralateral muscles. Spasticity was measured, according to Lance's definition, as the presence of abnormal stretch-related activity (Figure 5.2). Associated reactions were present in 29% of subjects, which is much the same as previously reported. Although the incidence of associated reactions was about the same as that of spasticity (21%), the two were not related, suggesting that these phenomena are separate impairments. Indeed, it has been shown that hemiparetic subjects can be trained to reduce their associated reactions without any reduction in spasticity (Dvir and Penturin 1993). It may be more logical to think of associated reactions as a negative impairment, that is, the result of a problem of coordination of muscles. Either way, the associated reactions found in this study were not large, suggesting that they are not usually a major problem for everyday function after stroke.

Characteristics of contracture and its relation to spasticity

By the mid-1980s, it was becoming recognized that factors other than reflex hyperexcitability (i.e. spasticity) may produce an increase in resistance to passive movement (i.e. hypertonia). It had been found in animal studies that a decrease in joint range (i.e. contracture) was accompanied not only by a decrease in numbers of sarcomeres, but also by an increase in stiffness. Human studies unable to account for movement abnormality by an increase in

Figure 5.2   Response to passive stretch for (a) a stroke subject with normal reflexes and (b) a stroke subject with hyperactive reflexes. The top trace is the angle through which the joint is moved, where the downwards section represents stretch of the muscle. The middle trace is the muscle response. In the normal response, the integrated electromyogram (IEMG) in the bottom trace illustrates no muscle response to stretch whereas the IEMG of the stroke subject illustrates the similarity and timing of the abnormal muscle response to the stretch.

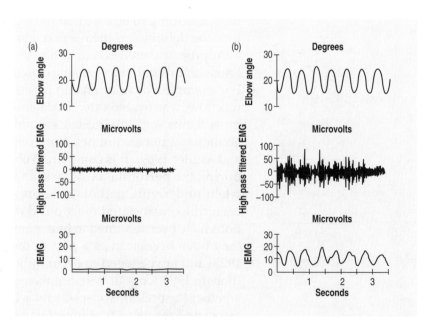

antagonist activity hypothesized that contracture could be the cause of hypertonia rather than, or in addition to, spasticity (e.g. Dietz et al 1981).

In order to address this issue, it is important that hypertonia can be clearly distinguished from spasticity. Spasticity is most commonly measured in the laboratory by slowly moving the joint (mechanically or manually) and (1) quantifying the resistance to stretch or (2) quantifying the electromyographic (EMG) activity in response to stretch. However, the first method is a measure of hypertonia whereas the second is a measure of reflex hyperexcitability (i.e. spasticity). These laboratory measures were collected in two groups of stroke subjects (Vattanasilp and Ada 1999) and their relationship examined. There was a relation between the two measures only in one group, illustrating that other impairments can contribute to hypertonia. Unless stretch-evoked muscle activity can be demonstrated by electromyography, increased resistance to passive movement (i.e. hypertonia) cannot be unconditionally attributed to reflex hyperexcitability (i.e. spasticity).

In order to determine whether contracture could be a cause of hypertonia, hemiparetic subjects who were within 1 year of their first stroke were assessed for the presence of hypertonia, spasticity and contracture (O'Dwyer et al 1996). Hypertonia was measured as stretch-related resistance to movement. Spasticity was measured as the presence of abnormal stretch-related muscle activity. Contracture was measured as passive range of motion using a standardized force. Interestingly, in this group of subjects, contracture was more prevalent than spasticity. Hypertonia was associated with contracture but not with reflex hyperexcitability. Increased reflexes were observed only in a subgroup of those with contracture and, where present, could usually be elicited only at the end of muscle range. This study was the first to show that in humans contracture produced an increase in stiffness. This finding was replicated in another group of stroke subjects. Subjects whose muscles felt clinically stiff after stroke were assessed for the presence of thixotropy, spasticity and contracture (Vattanasilp et al 2000). Hypertonia was measured at two speeds – slow and fast. In this group of subjects, most exhibited spasticity and only about one-third displayed contracture. However, only contracture contributed to the measure of stiffness when tested at the slow speed. Spasticity only contributed to stiffness when tested at the fast speed, presumably because the stretch reflex is velocity dependent. So, it appears that the presence of hypertonia after stroke is as likely to be the result of contracture as it is spasticity.

In order to investigate the causal relation between spasticity and contracture, it is necessary to show time precedence. Therefore, the development of spasticity and contracture was followed from

2 weeks to 1 year after stroke (Ada et al, unpublished work). Spasticity developed early and remained at the same low level over the year. Contracture was generally more prevalent than spasticity and worsened up to 4 months then resolved to some extent. At no time was spasticity directly correlated with contracture. However, early spasticity was correlated with later contracture, at least up to 4 months when contracture was developing. The finding that moderate spasticity correlates with the development of contracture strengthens the case for the aggressive prevention of contracture, especially in patients early after stroke who show signs of spasticity.

Contribution of spasticity versus contracture to disability

It is difficult to measure spasticity during the performance of movement in order to assess its contribution to disability. One reason for this is that the presence of a voluntary contraction changes the response of the stretch reflex. When a muscle is stretched passively, there is normally no electrical response if the stretch is within the physiological speed of movement. After stroke, however, there may be an abnormal response as a result of hyperactive reflexes (i.e. spasticity). On the other hand, when a normal active muscle is stretched, the muscle activity is modulated by the stretch. During the stance phase of walking, the gastrocnemius muscle is active, first eccentrically to decelerate the rotation of the shank forwards and then concentrically to achieve plantarflexion before toes off. Therefore, in order to assess the contribution of spasticity to walking after stroke, stretch-related activity of the gastrocnemius muscle was measured in ambulant stroke subjects and compared with control subjects under conditions that mimicked the stance phase of walking (Ada et al 1998). In long sitting, with the gastrocnemius muscle contracting, the ankle was dorsiflexed through 20° of range thereby stretching the muscle at the same time as it was actively contracting. Only the stroke subjects exhibited a response under passive conditions. Both groups exhibited responses under active conditions, however, and the reflexes of the stroke subjects were of similar magnitude, rather than exaggerated, to those of the control subjects. Furthermore, there was no evidence that these reflexes contributed a higher resistance to stretch than in the control subjects. Hence, in people ambulant after stroke, when the ankle is dorsiflexing during stance phase, it is unlikely that an increase in resistance to dorsiflexion is solely due to exaggerated reflex activity.

The picture that has emerged from this study and other investigations (e.g. Berger et al 1984, Ibrahim et al 1993) is that, after stroke, the stretch reflex cannot be modulated to respond differently under passive versus active conditions. In order to see if this would improve as a result of rehabilitation, the stretch reflex of the gastrocnemius muscle was examined as walking recovered after stroke (Vattanasilp 1998). The ability of the stretch reflex to modulate was investigated by examining the difference between the reflex under passive and active conditions. On the whole, the magnitude of the reflexes did not change from pre-ambulation to post-ambulation. In addition, the modulation of the reflex did not increase – it either stayed the same or decreased. It appears that the inability to modulate the stretch reflex, which is a characteristic of spastic muscles, does not prevent the recovery of function.

The question remains of the relative contribution of negative versus positive and primary versus secondary impairments to disability. In order to determine this, the evolution of spasticity (a primary positive impairment), contracture (a secondary impairment) and weakness (a primary negative impairment) was measured in stroke subjects over a year and compared with disability (Ada et al, unpublished work). Spasticity was only a contributing factor at 4 months and early contracture predicted function at 2 months, the period where contracture is worsening. However, strength always made a significant contribution to function. This study reinforces the now widely accepted view that the major contribution to disability after stroke is not the result of the positive impairments but rather the negative impairments.

Assessment of spasticity and contracture

Valid clinical procedures for the assessment of spasticity and contracture are necessary in order that the two impairments are accurately differentiated from each other. Only in this way will appropriate intervention be provided. In order to assess contracture, it is necessary to passively move the joint to the end of range without neural input influencing the endpoint. The easiest way to achieve this is to passively move the joint to the end of range as slowly as possible, because the stretch reflex, which is velocity dependent, is unlikely to be elicited under these conditions.

In order to assess spasticity accurately, its contribution to hypertonia needs to be clearly demonstrated. In a study comparing the clinical measure of spasticity using the Ashworth scale with the gold-standard laboratory method of stretch-related muscle activity and stretch-related resistance to movement (Vattanasilp and Ada 1999), the Ashworth scale was only related to the stretch-related resistance to movement (i.e. hypertonia). Unless stretch-evoked muscle activity can be demonstrated by electromyography, increased resistance to passive movement cannot be assumed to be due to reflex hyperexcitability. However, measuring stretch-related muscle activity is not feasible in everyday clinical practice. Many years ago Tardieu (Tardieu et al 1954, Held and Pierrot-

Deseilligny 1969) designed a scale that is very similar to the Ashworth scale but differs in two important ways. First, it assesses hypertonia at different speeds of limb movement and, second, the quality of the muscle response is more likely to reflect abnormal neural input. For example, Grade 3 of the Ashworth scale is 'considerable increase in tone – passive movement difficult' whereas Grade 3 on the Tardieu scale is 'fatiguable clonus appearing at a precise angle'. Therefore, it was hypothesized that the Tardieu scale would be better able to distinguish spasticity from contracture. To test this hypothesis, stroke subjects with a mixture of spasticity and contracture were assessed clinically using the Ashworth and the Tardieu scales (Patrick 2002). Their contracture and spasticity were also assessed using gold-standard laboratory tests. The percentage exact agreement between the presence of spasticity as determined by the Tardieu scale and the presence of stretch-related EMG was 100% compared with 63% for the Ashworth scale. The percentage exact agreement between the presence of contracture as determined by the Tardieu scale and the presence of loss of range of motion measured using a standardized force was 97% whereas the Ashworth scale does not address contracture. The Tardieu scale, therefore, provides a more accurate assessment of spasticity than the Ashworth scale, and its use should allow clinicians to differentiate between spasticity and contracture in order to focus on the impairment(s) that need(s) attention.

Decreasing spasticity and contracture after stroke

The findings from these studies add to our understanding of the contribution of spasticity and contracture to disability. On the whole, contracture is more prevalent than spasticity. Even when spasticity is present in people after stroke, it is generally only mild to moderate. Because mild to moderate spasticity has been shown not to be related to, or to interfere with, function, in most situations it can probably be ignored. In those situations where spasticity requires intervention, it has been shown that it is possible for people with brain damage to learn to modulate the stretch reflex using EMG biofeedback (Neilson and McCaughey 1982). However, having reduced the hyperreflexia, attention should then be turned towards the negative impairments.

The finding that moderate spasticity correlates with the development of contracture suggests that prevention of contracture, especially in patients who begin to show signs of spasticity, should be a routine part of rehabilitation. Early after stroke, whenever patients are not being assisted to move, they tend to spend their time sitting in a chair. In this position, the hips are flexed and externally rotated, the ankles are usually slightly plantarflexed, the arm rests with the shoulder in internal rotation, the elbow, wrist and fingers in flexion, the forearm in pronation and the thumb in adduction (Figure 5.3a). The muscles resting in a shortened part of their range are at risk of shortening. Animal studies suggest that 15 minutes of stretch at maximum range every 2 days only partially prevents muscle shortening, whereas 30 minutes every day prevents it entirely (Williams 1990). After stroke, in patients who spent most of their day with the arm in internal rotation, positioning the shoulder in external rotation for 30 minutes reduced loss of external rotation range (Ada et al, unpublished work). Currently, a reasonable clinical guideline seems to be that joints at risk of developing disabling contractures should spend at least 20–30 minutes in outer range. An efficient way of achieving this can be to make passive positioning part of routine ward protocols. For example, providing seating where the affected foot is back behind the knee should help maintain dorsiflexion range. Similarly, positioning the arm in neutral on a lap tray when in sitting should assist in maintaining shoulder external rotation range (Figure 5.3b).

NEGATIVE IMPAIRMENTS

The studies presented above reinforce the view that regardless of the presence of spasticity, the negative impairments always contribute to disability. There has been a shift in focus, both in the laboratory and in the clinic, towards the negative impairments, that is, loss of strength and dexterity. In the first and second editions of *A Motor Relearning Programme for Stroke*, Carr and Shepherd (1982, 1987) emphasized the treatment of the negative impairments by outlining strategies for training motor control. By the dawn of the new century, a focus on strengthening muscles in neurological conditions is included in their texts (Carr and Shepherd 1998, 2003). Because therapy now includes both increasing strength and improving dexterity after stroke, it is important that therapists understand as much as possible about the nature of these impairments as well as their relative contribution to disability in order that rehabilitation has a sound scientific basis. In an effort to contribute to this comparatively unexplored area, the following studies investigating negative impairments were carried out.

Characteristics of loss of dexterity

Loss of dexterity refers to a loss of coordination of voluntary muscle activity to meet environmental demands and is not restricted to manual dexterity (Bernstein 1991). Along with the reduction of spasticity, training dexterity (motor control) has been the main focus of rehabilitation. It is difficult to measure loss of dexterity because measures of dexterity (which are typically measures of

(a) (b)

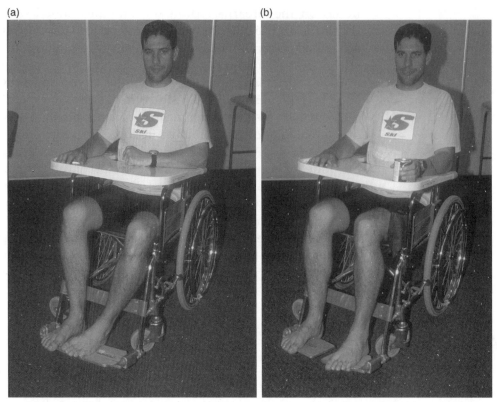

Figure 5.3   (a) Typical sitting position of a person with paralysed muscles after stroke. Although the arm is supported on a lap tray in order to prevent subluxation, its natural resting position will predispose to contracture of the shoulder internal rotators and adductors, forearm pronators and the web space. The resting position of the leg will predispose to contracture of the hip internal rotators and ankle invertors. (b) Modified sitting position of a person with paralysed muscles after stroke. The hand placed around a cylinder at the front of the lap tray positions the shoulder in some external rotation, the forearm in midposition, the wrist in some extension and the thumb in some abduction. A sandbag placed laterally to the knee positions the hip in neutral. The footplates adjusted to the correct height position the ankles in neutral.

function) are usually confounded by weakness, because they rely upon a prerequisite amount of strength to perform the test. To overcome this problem, the measure of dexterity that was used in the following studies is a specialized task in which precise coordination, but minimal strength, is required. Subjects perform a joint position tracking task requiring skilled interaction of agonists and antagonists to track a pseudo-random target, and dexterity is measured as the similarity between target motion and joint position (Figure 5.4). The first study using this method of testing dexterity demonstrated that, after stroke, dexterity and strength were not correlated, that is, they are separate motor impairments (Ada et al 1996).

It is important to differentiate the characteristics of loss of dexterity from weakness per se. Loss of dexterity is a loss of both the spatial and temporal accuracy needed to make movement meet environmental demands whereas weakness is an inability to achieve high levels of torque regardless of accuracy. In a study investigating the muscle activation characteristics associated with loss of dexterity after stroke (Canning et al 2000), low dexterity performance was characterized by excessive biceps muscle activation and decreased coupling of muscle activation to target motion. In particular, loss of dexterity was distinguishable from weakness. Furthermore, the abnormalities associated with loss of dexterity could not be attributed to the presence of positive impairments such as spasticity and excessive co-contraction. The muscle activation abnormalities reflect a loss of skill in generating appropriate spatial and temporal muscle activation patterns that conform to environmental demands. The findings of this study would suggest that, in therapy, opportunities be provided to practise tasks that demand processing of information to produce movements that are consistent with the spatial and temporal demands of the task. Simultaneously, attention should be paid to decreasing excessive, inappropriate muscle activity during task performance. In clinical practice, however, dexterity can only be trained once some strength is present.

Figure 5.4 Five-second excerpts of tracking traces for (a) a stroke subject with normal dexterity and (b) a stroke subject with low dexterity. The target is the black line and the subject's response the blue line. In the normal response, the subject reproduces the target well but with a time delay; in contrast, the stroke subject reproduces very little of the target, tending to freeze or move with very little amplitude and a prolonged time delay.

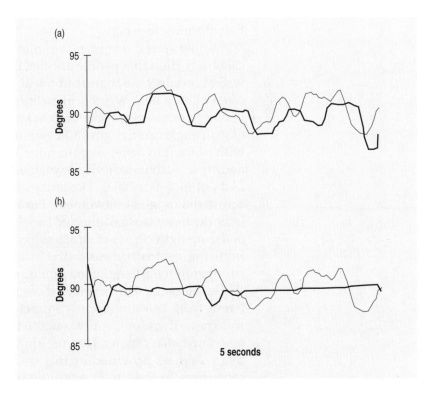

Characteristics of weakness

Weakness, or loss of strength, is an inability to generate high levels of torque. Unlike many musculoskeletal conditions, where weakness is the result of atrophy, weakness immediately after stroke is the result of loss of descending excitation to spinal segments reducing the number of motor units activated. Some authors take exception to the use of the word 'weakness' to describe the lack of ability to activate muscles after stroke (e.g. Bobath 1990, Landau and Sahrmann 2002). However, on clinical testing, there is a decrease in the maximum voluntary torque compared with normal values, which is consistent with the definition of weakness. Clinical observation suggests that, in addition to a reduction in maximum torque, other aspects of torque production are disordered after stroke. Therefore, a series of studies investigating the characteristics of torque production after stroke was carried out.

In order to investigate rate of torque production, the torque generation profile during maximum isometric contractions of elbow flexors and extensors was analysed in a group of stroke subjects undergoing rehabilitation (Canning et al 1999). In addition to reduced peak torque, these subjects were slow to generate peak torque. Furthermore, there was no consistent relationship between level of peak torque and rate of torque development suggesting some independence between these two characteristics of weakness after stroke. This would suggest, therefore, that once a reasonable level of force has been achieved in rehabilitation following stroke, there is a need to focus on increasing the speed of contraction of a muscle group.

Another series of studies was motivated by the common clinical observation that people affected by stroke are able to function well at certain joint angles but not at others; for example, they are often able to bear weight on a slightly flexed knee while being unable to bear weight on a straight knee. In these studies, the effect of joint angle on strength and dexterity after stroke was compared with normal in order to determine whether selective weakness and/or selective dexterity explained this clinical phenomenon (Ada et al 2000, 2003). Dexterity and strength were measured across the range of movement. For both stroke and control subjects, dexterity was not affected by joint angle. However, the shape of the strength curves of stroke subjects was significantly different from the control subjects. The stroke subjects were relatively stronger in their lengthened range and relatively weaker in their shortened range. Furthermore, those with contracture were no different from those without contracture. The origin of selective weakness, therefore, appears not to be attributable to the length-associated adaptations. The confirmation of the existence of selective weakness provided by this study suggests that, as soon as some muscle activity is present, strengthening should include exercises that focus on the shortened range.

In order to examine the neural contribution to weakness, muscle activation during strength measurements was measured throughout range in late stroke subjects and compared with control subjects (Doumit 2001). Although the stroke subjects were weaker, muscle activation was not abnormal, that is, the stroke subjects were able to activate their available motor units as successfully as the control subjects. This suggests that, long term, the weakness is not due to a lack of ability to activate motor units. Several studies (Hara et al 2000, McComas et al 1973) have found that functioning motor units are halved within the first 6 months after stroke, and this is the most likely mechanism underlying this finding. It appears, therefore, that it is important to stimulate maximum excitation of motor units early after stroke (if necesssary by electrical stimulation), not only in order to promote recovery, but also to prevent loss of motor units as recovery takes place.

Contribution of loss of dexterity versus weakness to disability

It is clear that both loss of strength and loss of dexterity contribute to disability after stroke. However, the relative contribution of each impairment to the physical disability experienced during recovery after stroke is not so clear. Therefore, a longitudinal study was carried out to determine the relative contributions of strength and dexterity to function during the first 6 months of recovery after stroke (Canning et al 2004). Not surprisingly, strength and dexterity together contributed significantly to function at all times. However, strength made a significant additional contribution to function at all times. These findings suggest that, in a typical population of people affected by stroke undergoing rehabilitation, loss of strength is a more significant contributor to physical disability than loss of dexterity. Therefore, where significant weakness is present, exercises designed to increase strength will be required to decrease disability. This represents a paradigm shift in stroke rehabilitation and requires that therapists identify the most effective ways of strengthening very weak muscles after stroke.

Assessment of weakness and loss of dexterity

The findings discussed above show that loss of strength and dexterity are major contributors to disability. However, clinically it is necessary to determine the contribution of each to disability in order to intervene effectively. First, it is essential to establish the level of disability, by observing the patient's attempts at performing everyday tasks. Then, the severity of individual impairments needs to be determined in order to analyse their individual contribution.

Strength is the maximum torque produced by muscles, and early after stroke this output can be seen as a reflection of neural drive. Assessing strength after stroke is difficult because of the nature of the condition. Not only may other impairments, such as aphasia, make following instructions difficult, but the fact that many muscles are affected means that it is not feasible for patients to change position frequently. Therefore, it is important to be as efficient as possible. Determining strength in a way that does not necessitate a change in position for each muscle group will assist in this endeavour. Additionally, it is probably only necessary to determine the degree of weakness in broad terms in order to decide on appropriate intervention. For example, it is helpful to differentiate whether muscles are paralysed or very weak (such that anti-gravity movement is not possible) versus whether they are just weak (such that anti-gravity movement is possible but not with normal strength), because methods of strengthening will differ accordingly.

Dexterity is the ability to coordinate muscle activity and is usually tested under conditions where some temporal and spatial accuracy are required, for example, fast opposition of the thumb and fingers. However, the easiest way to determine the severity of loss of dexterity may be to test alternating movements as fast as possible (e.g. alternating supination and pronation required in the test for dysdiadochokinesia). Assessing dexterity early after stroke can be difficult because it can only reasonably be tested when some strength is present. Obviously, distal limb movements can be tested with less requirements for strength since there is less mass being moved; for example, toe tapping only requires the ability to move the relatively light foot segment.

Increasing strength and dexterity after stroke

Traditionally, strengthening has not been a significant component of stroke rehabilitation. This is because of the commonly held assumptions that spasticity is the most important contributor to disability after stroke, and that resisted exercise will increase spasticity. However, several studies have shown that strength can be increased after stroke without increasing spasticity (Badics et al 2002, Bütefisch et al 1995, Sharp and Brouwer 1997, Smith et al 1999, Teixeira-Salmela et al 1999). Furthermore, there are now a number of studies examining the efficacy of strengthening after stroke, although not many of them are randomized controlled trials. The clinical trials that have examined intensive efforts directed towards regaining muscle activation and strength early after stroke (Bütefisch et al 1995, Chae et al 1998, Feys et al 1998, Francisco et al 1998, Hummelsheim et al 1996) or strengthening exercises later after stroke (Badics et al 2002, Engardt et al 1995, Sharp and Brouwer 1997, Teixeira-Salmela et al 1999, Weiss et al 2000) are associated with an increase in strength and often with a decrease in disability. Most of these clinical trials have been carried out on subjects who have already regained some strength.

The challenge for therapists is not only to implement strengthening exercises but also to balance the emphasis between strengthening and dexterity training. Table 5.1 is an attempt to provide a conceptual framework for implementing strengthening and dexterity training dependent upon level of strength. Initially after stroke, where there is severe weakness due to a lack of motor unit activation, the principles of strengthening need to be modified. For example, it is important that strengthening exercises are set up so that minimal muscle activity will result in movement (Figure 5.5a,b). This can be achieved by:

● focusing on the mid-range of muscle length where it is usually the strongest;
● decreasing the effect of gravity (e.g. by changing body positions to eliminate the resistance due to gravity);

Table 5.1   Interaction between strength and dexterity training after stroke.

	Group 1 Paralysed (torque = 0)	Group 2 Very weak (torque < gravity)	Group 3 Weak (torque > gravity < normal)	Group 4 Strong (torque ≥ normal)
Strength training	Eliciting muscle activity: Mid-range Gravity-eliminated position ↓Friction (suspension, skateboard, powder, towel) Shorten lever Mental practice EMG biofeedback Electrical stimulation EMG-triggered electrical stimulation	Exercises: Full range Inner range Sustained contraction ↑Speed Add resistance to mid-range	Resisted exercises: Weight machines Free weights Body weight (e.g. standing up, heel lifts, step ups) Theraband Grip dynamometer	Not essential
Dexterity training	Not practical	Task-related training (part or modified): Hip extension over the side of the bed Shoulders forward for standing up Walking with partial body weight support Grasp and release with forearms supported	Task training (whole task): Sitting Standing up Standing Walking (treadmill, overground) Reaching and manipulation	Task training (↑flexibility of performance): ↑Cognitive demand ↑Physical demand

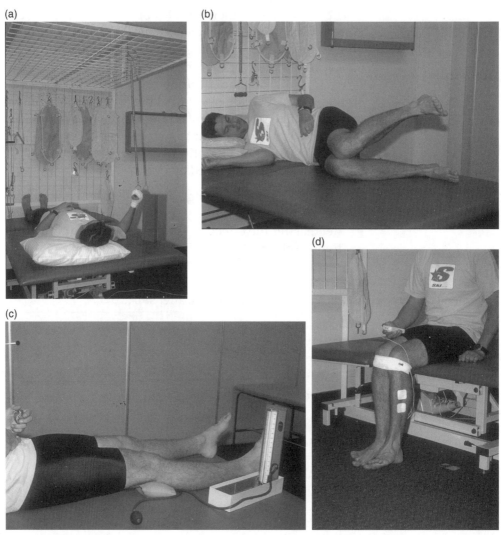

Figure 5.5   (a) Position for strengthening the rotators of the shoulder. The paralysed hand can be bandaged onto the handle, which is connected to a low-tension spring providing some suspension of the forearm. The subject practises external rotation in mid-range by attempting to move the hand towards the target (rectangular box). (b) Position for strengthening the internal rotators of the hip. The subject aims to raise the foot while keeping the knees together, so that the internal rotators rather than the abductors are targeted. (c) Position for strengthening the knee extensors in shortened range. An inflated blood pressure cuff is placed under the knee and as the subject pushes down, he or she gets feedback from the increase in mercury level in the sphygmomanometer. (d) Position for strengthening ankle evertors. The knees are together (held there if necessary) and the feet are 4–5 cm apart. The subject aims to squeeze the ankles together. EMG-triggered electrical stimulation as illustrated can be used when muscles are very weak. A small block of dense foam placed between the ankles can provide resistance as strength improves.

- decreasing friction (e.g. by using suspension or a skateboard);
- decreasing the lever arm of the limb.

In addition, effort can be enhanced by following the principles of mental practice (Van Leeuwen and Inglis 1998), which suggest that practice in situations where movement does not result should include goals, the provision of feedback (via EMG biofeedback, Figure 5.5d) and counters to record a preset number of repetitions. As soon as muscles have some ability to contract, but are still very weak, then the exercises should focus on full range of motion (in particular, shortened range, Figure 5.5c), sustaining contractions, increasing speed and beginning to add resistance to mid-range. When muscles can contract against gravity, but are still weak, resisted exercises can be implemented using methods of resistance such as weight machines, free weights, Theraband and body weight.

Once some strength has been regained, therapy should be directed towards dexterity as well as strength because both are necessary for optimal function. However, the dexterity training should be appropriate to the level of strength available (Table 5.1). For example, when muscles are not strong enough to move against gravity, then practice of the whole task should be modified. This can be achieved by practising part of the task where muscles are working in a similar manner to full task performance (e.g. hip extension over the side of the bed in order to practise loading the affected leg in preparation for standing) (Carr and Shepherd 1982, 1987, 1998, 2003). The task can also be modified by reducing the strength requirements during performance of the whole task (e.g. providing partial body weight support using a harness while walking). When muscles are strong enough to move against gravity, the whole task can be practised with less likelihood of learning compensatory strategies. Then, to train flexibility of whole task performance, cognitive and/or physical demands can be added (e.g. walking while carrying on a conversation and/or carrying a glass of water).

In clinical practice, progress needs to be monitored. The most appropriate way of monitoring progress is to quantify the change in disability over time using efficient measurement tools such as disability scales (e.g. the Motor Assessment Scale for stroke, the Berg Balance Scale) or standardized tests of motor performance (e.g. the timed 10-m walk, the 6-minute walk test, the nine-hole peg test). On the other hand, although it is important to assess the severity of all impairments in order to determine their contribution to disability, it is only necessary to measure those impairments that are the focus of intervention.

CONCLUSION

We have found that classifying impairments after brain damage as negative or positive, originally proposed more than a century ago, is a useful framework for investigating the underlying causes of disability after stroke. Carr and Shepherd's challenge of the assumption that spasticity was the major contributor to disability was influential in the direction of our investigations by stimulating us to ask pertinent questions. Our findings have reinforced the now current view that the positive impairment of spasticity is usually only of moderate intensity and has little effect on function after stroke. In addition, the prevailing view that the negative impairments of weakness and loss of dexterity are the major contributing factors to disability has also been supported by our findings. As such, an in-depth understanding of the nature of both weakness and loss of dexterity as well as their interaction should enable accurate assessment tools and effective intervention strategies to be developed and tested.

References

Ada L, O'Dwyer N 2001 Do associated reactions in the upper limb after stroke contribute to contracture formation? Clinical Rehabilitation 15:186–194.

Ada L, O'Dwyer N J, Green J et al 1996 The nature of loss of strength and dexterity in the upper limb following stroke. Human Movement Sciences 15:671–687.

Ada L, Vattanasilp W, O'Dwyer N et al 1998 Does spasticity contribute to walking dysfunction following stroke? Journal of Neurology, Neurosurgery, and Psychiatry 64:628–635.

Ada L, Canning C, Dwyer T 2000 Effect of muscle length on strength and dexterity after stroke. Clinical Rehabilitation 14:55–61.

Ada L, Canning C, Low S-L 2003 Muscle length has a selective effect on strength after stroke. Brain 126:724–731.

Ada L, Goddard E, McCully J et al 2004 30 minutes of positioning reduces the development of shoulder external rotation contracture after stroke: a randomized controlled trial. Archives of Physical Medicine and Rehabilitation in press.

Badics E, Wittmann A, Rupp M et al 2002 Systematic muscle building exercises in the rehabilitation of stroke patients. Neurorehabilitation 17:211–214.

Berger W, Horstmann G, Dietz V (1984) Tension development and muscle activation in the leg during gait in spastic hemiparesis: independence of muscle hypertonia and exaggerated stretch reflexes. Journal of Neurology, Neurosurgery, and Psychiatry 47(9):1029–1033.

Bernstein N A (1991) On dexterity and its development. Physical Culture and Sport Press, Moscow (in Russian); cited in Latash L P, Latash M K 1994 A new book by Bernstein: 'On dexterity and its development'. Journal of Motor Behavior 26:56–62.

Bobath B (1990) Adult hemiplegia evaluation and treatment, 3rd edn. Butterworth-Heinemann, London.

Bütefisch C, Hummelsheim H, Denzler P et al 1995 Repetitive training of isolated movements improves the outcome of motor rehabilitation of the centrally paretic hand. Journal of the Neurological Sciences 130:59–68.

Canning C G, Ada L, O'Dwyer N 1999 Slowness to develop force contributes to weakness after stroke. Archives of Physical Medicine and Rehabilitation. 80:66–70.

Canning C G, Ada L, O'Dwyer N J 2000 Abnormal muscle activation characteristics associated with loss of dexterity after stroke. Journal of the Neurological Sciences 176:45–56.

Canning C, Ada L, Adams R et al 2004 Loss of strength contributes more to disability after stroke than loss of dexterity. Clinical Rehabilitation 18:300–308.

Carr J H, Shepherd R B 1982 A motor relearning programme for stroke. Heinemann Medical, London.

Carr J H, Shepherd R B 1987 A motor relearning programme for stroke, 2nd edn. Heinemann Medical, Oxford.

Carr J H, Shepherd R B 1998 Neurological rehabilitation: optimizing motor performance. Butterworth-Heinemann, Oxford

Carr J H, Shepherd R B 2003 Stroke rehabilitation: guidelines for exercise and training to optimize motor skill. Butterworth-Heinemann, Oxford.

Chae J, Bethoux F, Bohine T et al 1998 Neuromuscular stimulation for upper extremity motor and functional recovery in acute hemiplegia. Stroke 29:975–979.

Cornall C 1991 Self-propelling wheelchairs: the effect on spasticity in hemiplegic patients. Physiotherapy Theory and Practice 7:13–21.

Dietz V, Quintern J, Berger W 1981 Electrophysiological studies of gait in spasticity and rigidity. Brain 104:431–449.

Doumit M A 2001 Mechanisms of chronic weakness following stroke. Honours thesis, University of Sydney.

Dvir Z, Penturin E 1993 Measurement of spasticity and associated reactions in stroke patients before and after training. Clinical Rehabilitation 7:15–21.

Engardt M, Knutsson E, Jonsson M et al 1995 Dynamic muscle strength training in stroke patients: effects on knee extension torque, electromyographic activity and motor function. Archives of Physical Medicine and Rehabilitation 76:419–425.

Feys H, De Weerdt W J, Selz B E et al 1998 Effect of a therapeutic intervention for the hemiplegic upper limb in the acute phase after stroke: a single-blind, randomized, controlled multicenter trial. Stroke 29:785–792.

Francisco G, Chae J, Chawla H et al 1998 Electromyogram-triggered neuromuscular stimulation for improving the arm function of acute stroke survivors: a randomised pilot study. Archives of Physical Medicine and Rehabilitation 79:570–575.

Hara Y, Akaboshi K, Masakado Y et al 2000 Physiologic decrease of single thenar motor units in the F-response in stroke patients. Archives of Physical Medicine and Rehabilitation 81:418–423.

Held J P, Pierrot-Deseilligny E 1969 Reeducation motrice des affections neurologiques. J B Bailliere, Paris, pp 31–42.

Hummelsheim H, Amberger S, Mauritz K H 1996 The influence of EMG-initiated electrical muscle stimulation on motor recovery of the centrally paretic hand. European Journal of Neurology 3:245–254.

Ibrahim I K, Berger W, Trippel M et al 1993 Stretch-induced electromyographic activity and torque in spastic elbow muscles. Differential modulation of reflex activity in passive and active motor tasks. Brain 116:971–989.

Lance J W 1980 Symposium synopsis. In: Feldman R G, Young R R, Koella W P (eds) Spasticity: disordered motor control. Symposia Specialists, Miami, pp 485–494.

Lance J W 1990 What is spasticity? Lancet 335:606.

Landau W M 1974 Spasticity: the fable of a neurological demon and the emperor's new therapy [editorial]. Archives of Neurology 31:217–219.

Landau W M, Sahrmann S A 2002 Preservation of directly stimulated muscle strength in hemiplegia due to stroke. Archives of Neurology 59:1453–1457.

McComas A J, Sica R E, Upton A R et al 1973 Functional changes in motoneurones of hemiparetic patients. Journal of Neurology, Neurosurgery and Psychiatry. 36:183–193.

McLellan D L 1977 Co-contraction and stretch reflexes in spasticity during treatment with baclofen. Journal of Neurology, Neurosurgery and Psychiatry 40:30–38.

Neilson P D, McCaughey J 1982 Self-regulation of spasm and spasticity in cerebral palsy. Journal of Neurology, Neurosurgery and Psychiatry 45:320–330.

Norton B J, Sahrmann S A 1978 Reflex and voluntary electromyographic activity in patients with hemiparesis. Physical Therapy 58(8):951–955.

O'Dwyer N J, Ada L, Neilson P D 1996 Spasticity and muscle contracture following stroke. Brain 119:1737–1749.

Patrick E 2002 Is the Tardieu scale better at differentiating the presence of contracture from spasticity than the Ashworth Scale? Honours thesis, University of Sydney.

Perry J 1980 Rehabilitation of spasticity. In: Feldman R G, Young R R, Koella W P (eds) Spasticity: disordered motor control. Symposia Specialists, Miami, pp 87–100.

Sahrmann S A, Norton B J 1977 The relationship of voluntary movement to spasticity in the upper motor neurone syndrome. Annals of Neurology 2:460–465.

Sharp S A, Brouwer B J 1997 Isokinetic strength training of the hemiparetic knee: effects on function and spasticity. Archives of Physical Medicine and Rehabilitation 78:1231–1236.

Smith G V, Silver K H C, Goldberg A P et al 1999 'Task-oriented' exercise improves hamstring strength and spastic reflexes in chronic stroke patients. Stroke 30:2112–2118.

Stephenson R, Edwards S, Freeman J 1998 Associated reactions: their value in clinical practice? Physiotherapy Research International 3:151–152.

Tardieu G, Shentoub S, Delarue R 1954 A la recherche d'une technique de mesure de la spasticite. Revue Neurologique 91(2):143–144.

Teixeira-Salmela L F, Olney S J, Nadeau S et al 1999 Muscle strengthening and physical conditioning to reduce impairment and disability in chronic stroke survivors. Archives of Physical Medicine and Rehabilitation 80:1211–1218.

Van Leeuwen R, Inglis J T 1998 Mental practice and imagery: a potential role in stroke rehabilitation. Physical Therapy Reviews 3:47–54.

Vattanasilp W 1998 Factors contributing to muscle stiffness and function following stroke. PhD thesis, University of Sydney.

Vattanasilp W, Ada L 1999 Relation between clinical and laboratory measures of spasticity. Australian Journal of Physiotherapy 45:135–139.

Vattanasilp W, Ada L, Crosbie J 2000 Contribution of thixotropy, spasticity and contracture to ankle stiffness after stroke. Journal of Neurology, Neurosurgery and Psychiatry 69:34–39

Walshe F M R 1923 On certain tonic or postural reflexes in hemiplegia, with special reference to the so-called 'associated movements'. Brain 46:1–37.

Weiss A, Suzuki T, Bean J et al 2000 High intensity strength training improves strength and functional performance after stroke. American Journal of Physical Medicine and Rehabilitation 79:369–376.

Williams P E 1990 Use of intermittent stretch in the prevention of serial sarcomere loss in immobilised muscle. Annals of the Rheumatic Diseases 49:316–317.

Zülch K J, Müller N 1969 Associated movements in man. In: Vinken P J, Bruyn G W (eds) Disturbances of nervous function: handbook of clinical neurology, vol 1. North Holland Publishing, Amsterdam, pp 404–426.

Chapter **6**

How muscles respond to stretch

Robert Herbert

In the 1970s, neurological physiotherapy practice was based almost exclusively on neurophysiology. Roberta Shepherd and Janet Carr changed that. They showed how other disciplines, particularly biomechanics, psychology and muscle biology, could influence physiotherapy practice. As a physiotherapy student at the University of Sydney in the early 1980s, I was inspired by Carr and Shepherd's pioneering work, and I set out to research questions in muscle biology that had implications for physiotherapy practice. This chapter describes a line of research in muscle biology that I have contributed to over the intervening years.

During the execution of motor tasks, joints move in response to forces produced by muscles, gravity and the accelerations of distant body segments. The extent of this movement is constrained by tissues that span joints, particularly muscles and ligaments.

Constraints to joint motion are of interest because they provide limits within which the motor control system must operate. Abnormal constraints to joint movement ('contracture' or 'loss of

joint range of motion' or 'inflexibility') can impair motor performance, so physiotherapists often attempt to reduce constraints to
joint motion to improve motor performance. Information about
the nature of constraints to joint motion potentially provides
insights into the way we control movement and might suggest
ways to prevent and treat movement dysfunction.

Different tissues constrain movement at different joints. For
example, extension of the knee is constrained primarily by ligaments, whereas ankle dorsiflexion is constrained primarily by
muscles. Importantly, muscles can constrain the movement available at joints even when completely relaxed (or 'passive'). This
chapter is concerned with how relaxed muscles constrain joint
movement.

The chapter is divided into four parts. The first part discusses
elastic properties of resting muscles: its focus is on the instantaneous relationship between the tension in a muscle and its length.
The second part considers viscous or time-dependent responses
that occur when muscles are stretched for seconds, minutes or
hours. The third section considers adaptive responses (growth and
contracture) that manifest when muscles are exposed to or
deprived of stretch that is sustained or repeated over days or
months. The chapter concludes by describing some clinical studies
of the effects of muscle stretching.

ELASTIC RESPONSES

Relaxed muscles behave very much like elastic bands or springs.
At short lengths they fall slack and develop no tension, but when
lengthened beyond some threshold length (sometimes called the
'slack length') they develop tension and resist further lengthening.
As the muscle is further lengthened, passive tension progressively
increases.

The spring-like properties of muscles can be measured relatively easily in animal muscles. The muscle is isolated and
fixed between two clamps. Then muscle length and tension are
measured as the muscle is lengthened. The relationship between
muscle length and tension can be illustrated with a passive
length–tension curve (Figure 6.1).

Passive length–tension curves of muscles are highly curvilinear.
Below slack length, tension is zero. Immediately above slack length,
large changes in length are accompanied by only small increases in
tension – the muscle is highly compliant. At greater lengths,
changes in length are accompanied by relatively large increases in
tension – the muscle becomes relatively stiff. Compliance decreases
and stiffness increases with increasing muscle length.

Figure 6.1   Passive
length–tension curve of a
rabbit soleus muscle–tendon
unit. The arrow indicates slack
length.

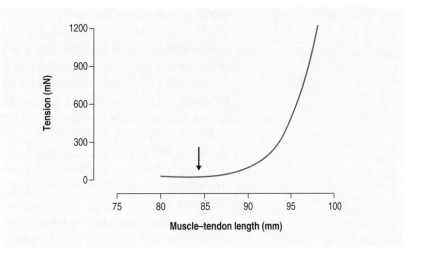

An interesting question concerns whether, at the extreme of available joint motion, muscles become sufficiently short to fall slack. One pertinent observation was made by Refshauge et al (1998). An incision was made in the skin overlying the extensor hallucus longus tendon of an anaesthetized human subject. When the ankle was dorsiflexed passively and the toe was flexed passively there was buckling of the tendon, suggesting that the tendon had fallen slack within the physiological range of joint motion. More quantitative evidence of slack in animal muscles comes from the study that produced the length–tension curve of rabbit soleus muscle in Figure 6.1 (Herbert and Balnave 1993). In that experiment, measurements were also taken of the distance between the soleus muscle's origin and insertion over the full range of physiological ankle positions, so it was possible to relate muscle length to joint angle. At the very short muscle lengths attained when the ankle was fully plantarflexed there was no passive tension in the soleus, indicating that the rabbit soleus muscle falls slack in full plantarflexion. These observations and others (Herbert and Gandevia 1995, Jahnke et al 1989, Wei et al 1986) suggest that some muscles do fall slack at their shortest physiological lengths.

Muscle–tendon units

In some muscles the fibres extend the full distance from proximal to distal tendons. Other muscles contain fibres arranged end to end or in overlapping configurations, so that each fibre extends only part of the distance between tendons (Loeb and Richmond 1994). Regardless of the arrangement, fibres are bundled together in groups called fascicles. Although the anatomy of most muscles is complex, the mechanical properties of whole muscles (muscle–tendon units) can be understood by thinking of them in relatively simple terms. Mechanically, muscle–tendon units can be considered to consist of muscle fascicles connected in series with tendons.

Typically muscle fascicles are short. In most human muscles the fascicles are less than about 7 cm in length (Yamaguchi et al 1990). This is possible, even in muscles with long muscle bellies, because tendons do not usually terminate at the ends of the muscle belly. Instead the tendons blend into the muscle belly in broad intramuscular sheets, variously called intramuscular tendons, tendon plates or intramuscular aponeuroses. Short muscle fascicles need only traverse the small distances between proximal and distal intramuscular tendons, not the entire length of the muscle belly (Figure 6.2a).

In long muscles, short muscle fascicles lie in series with long tendons. An example is the adult human rectus femoris muscle, which has muscle fascicles of approximately 7 cm long (Yamaguchi et al 1990) lying in series with tendons that are about 33 cm long. In this muscle the ratio of tendon length to muscle fascicle length is nearly 5:1. Ratios of more than 10:1 can be observed in other human muscles, such as the gastrocnemius (Herbert et al 2002).

The source of muscle compliance

When joints move, muscle lengths increase and decrease. Theoretically, the changes in muscle length that occur with joint movement could occur in muscle fascicles or tendons, or both. Where do the length changes occur? Is muscle extensibility dominated by the extensibility of muscle fascicles or tendons?

It has usually been assumed that relaxed muscle fibres are much more compliant than tendon, and therefore that most of the length changes occur in the muscle fascicles. However, there is little direct evidence to support that view. Recent evidence suggests

Figure 6.2 Contribution of muscle fascicles and tendons to length changes in resting rabbit soleus muscle. (a) Schematic diagram showing the architecture of the rabbit soleus muscle. Circles indicate the location of markers on the proximal and distal ends of the proximal and distal intramuscular tendons used in the experiment described in the text. Note that muscle fibres do not extend the full length of the muscle belly but instead traverse the relatively short distance between intramuscular tendons. (b) Passive length–tension curve of the whole rabbit soleus muscle–tendon unit and tendons. Pairs of lines envelop the mean (five muscles) ± SE.

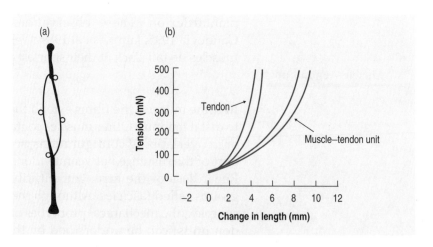

that, in some muscles at least, a large part of the total change in muscle length occurs in tendons.

In 1997 Jack Crosbie and I directly assessed the contributions of muscle fascicles and tendons to changes in length imposed on relaxed rabbit soleus muscle (Herbert and Crosbie 1997). We isolated the muscle and placed small reflective markers on the proximal and distal ends of the proximal and distal muscle fibres (Figure 6.2a). The whole muscle–tendon unit was mounted in a testing jig that could lengthen the muscle at a controlled velocity from less than the muscle's slack length to lengths equivalent to the maximum lengths attained in vivo. As the muscle was lengthened, whole muscle–tendon length was measured with a potentiometer and the muscle was filmed with three video cameras. Subsequently we were able to reconstruct the three-dimensional locations of the markers and determine the change in length of the muscle–tendon unit and of the proximal and distal muscle fascicles. Tendon length was calculated as the difference between change in whole muscle length and change in muscle fascicle length. These data were used to assess the contribution of tendon to the total change in muscle length. The findings were surprising: about half of the total change in length occurs in the muscle fascicles and half in the tendons (Figure 6.2b). That is, the extensibility of the rabbit soleus muscle is determined by the extensibility of both muscle fascicles and tendons in approximately equal degree.

Why do the tendons of the rabbit soleus contribute such a large part to the extensibility of the whole muscle? The answer is not that tendon is intrinsically compliant. In fact, length for length, the tendon of the rabbit soleus deforms only about a quarter as much as the muscle fascicles. The explanation lies in the fact that the tendons of rabbit soleus are about four times longer than its muscle fascicles. Even though the tendon is intrinsically stiffer than the muscle fascicles, there is lots of it. So even proportionately small increases in tendon length produce relatively large increases in the total length of the tendon. Tendon contributes approximately half of the total change in muscle length, even though it is a relatively inextensible material, because there is so much more tendon than muscle fascicles to be lengthened.

Subsequently, we were able to replicate these findings on human muscles using a very different experimental paradigm (Herbert et al 2002). In human muscles it is possible to use diagnostic ultrasonography to visualize muscle fascicles: with ultrasonography, muscle fascicles appear as distinct stripes in the muscle belly (Figure 6.3a). It is a simple matter to measure the distance between the proximal and distal insertions of muscle fascicles. This made it possible to examine the contribution of muscle fascicles and tendon to changes in length of relaxed human muscles. Measurements of gastrocnemius and tibialis anterior fascicle lengths were made with the knee and ankle in a range of positions. We compared measured changes in muscle fascicle lengths with changes in whole muscle length calculated from joint angles. Changes in muscle fascicle length were much smaller than changes in whole muscle length (Figure 6.3b,c). On average, change in length of muscle fascicles contributed only 27% of the total change in length of the gastrocnemius and 55% of the total change in length of the tibialis anterior. Almost all of the rest of the change in length occurred in tendons. Only a small part of the change in length could be attributed to changes in the pennation of muscle fibres. These data confirmed our earlier finding

Figure 6.3   Relationship between muscle fascicle length and change in muscle–tendon length. (a) Ultrasonographic image of the human gastrocnemius muscle. Striations indicate the course of muscle fascicles. (b) Human medial gastrocnemius muscle. (c) Human tibialis anterior muscle. In (b) and (c), each line is the regression for a single subject. The mean slope of the regressions, which indicates the average contribution of change in muscle fascicle length to change in whole muscle length, was 27% for the gastrocnemius muscle and 55% for the tibialis anterior muscle.

(a)

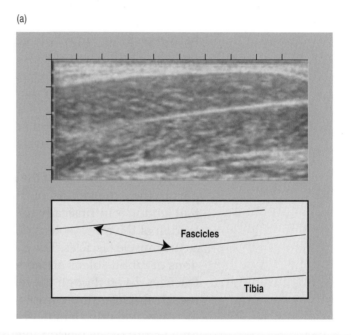

(b)

(c)

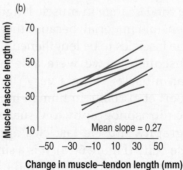

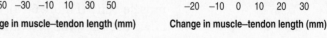

that, in some muscles at least, a large part of the total change in length was due to elongation of the tendon.

Taken together, these studies provide strong evidence that tendons of relaxed muscles undergo considerable changes in length and can contribute a large part of the total changes in muscle length. That is, the extensibility of at least some muscles is attributable in large part to the extensibility of tendons. How well does this finding extrapolate to other muscles? Comparative data are not available, but theoretical considerations suggest the contribution of tendon to whole muscle compliance is probably determined largely by the ratio of muscle fascicle and tendon slack lengths.

Generally, the cross-sectional areas of tendons scale with the physiological cross-sectional areas of their muscle fibres (although the scaling, at least across species, is not proportional; Pollock and Shadwick 1994), but there is enormous variation across muscles in the ratio of muscle fascicle length and tendon length (e.g. Lieber et al 1992). Zajac (1989) has argued that the ratio of muscle fascicle length and tendon length is the major determinant of the contribution of tendon to mechanical properties of contracting muscles. Those arguments apply equally well to the case in which the muscle is relaxed. It is reasonable to expect the contribution of tendon to whole muscle extensibility will be greatest in muscles with long tendons such as the hamstrings, calf muscles, quadriceps, biceps brachii and triceps brachii and the extrinsic hand muscles. The contribution of tendon to whole muscle extensibility will be relatively small in muscles such as the intrinsic muscles of the hand and foot because these muscles have relatively short tendons.

Structural determinants of the elastic properties of tendons and muscle fascicles

What part of tendons and muscle fibres determines their extensibility? This question has been the subject of sporadic research for at least 70 years, but complete answers are only now beginning to appear.

The elastic properties of tendon are conferred primarily by collagen. Collagen fibrils are aggregated in fibres into a Z-like 'crimp' pattern, and the degree of crimping is distributed across fibrils (Rowe 1985a, 1985b, Stolinski 1995). When tension is applied to tendon, some of the fibres are straightened out and lose their crimp. Further increases in tension produce progressive uncrimping until, at forces greater than those usually experienced in resting muscle, all fibres are straightened out. It has been hypothesized that, once straightened, fibrils become able to bear tension. According to this hypothesis it is the sequential uncrimping of collagen fibres that produces the non-linear 'toe' region characteristic of the length–tension properties of tendon (Fratzl et al 1997, Hurschler et al 1997, Kastelic et al 1980, Liao and Belkoff 1999, Maes et al 1989, Stromberg and Wiederhielm 1969). At higher tensions, possibly greater than those experienced by relaxed muscles, other mechanisms come into play. These include the straightening out of random 'kinks' in collagen fibrils and the gliding, relative to each other, of the molecules within a fibril (Fratzl et al 1997).

There is more uncertainty about the origins of the passive mechanical properties of muscle fibres. Over the past six decades the mechanical properties of resting muscle have variously been ascribed to the intramuscular connective tissue (endomysium, perimysium and epimysium; Banus and Zetlin 1938, Borg and Caulfield 1980, Rowe 1981, Williams and Goldspink 1978; cf. Hill 1952, Purslow 1989), the sarcolemma (Fields and Faber 1970, Ramsey and Street 1940; cf. Casella 1950, Podolsky 1964, Rapaport 1972, 1973, Street 1983) or mysterious 'S' ('superfine'!) filaments (Hanson and Huxley 1955). A major breakthrough was the finding, by Magid and Law (1985), that whole muscle, muscle fibres and skinned muscle fibres all had similar stiffness. This strongly suggests that the resting properties of muscles are conferred by structures inside muscle fibres (see also Purslow 1989). The view most consistent with current evidence appears to be that two sets of intracellular structures, weakly bound cross-bridges (Hill 1968) and titin (Wang 1984), determine the mechanical properties of resting muscles at low and high tensions respectively.

D K Hill (1968) showed that muscles exhibited complex behaviours at low forces (see also Alexander and Johnson 1965, Hill 1950, McCarter et al 1971). Subsequently Proske and colleagues have shown that such behaviours can be demonstrated in human muscles and can explain a range of phenomena, including history dependence of proprioception (Proske et al 1993).

Hill observed that when very small stretches were delivered to resting muscles the muscles exhibited linear increases in tension with length changes of up to about 0.2% of muscle optimum length (tensions of ~1.5% of maximal isometric tension at optimal length), above which yielding was evident. He called the component responsible for this behaviour the 'short range elastic component'. Hill noted that both the resting tension and the short-range elastic component increased in hypertonic solutions; this he presumed was because the hypertonic solutions reduced interfilamentary spacing (although this now appears unlikely; see Campbell and Lakie 1998). Consequently, he suggested that a part of the resting tension was also attributable to the formation of resting cross-bridges between the contractile filaments. Hill called this the 'filamentary resting tension', and attributed latency relaxation (a momentary fall in muscle tension that precedes a muscle twitch) to a fall in filamentary resting tension. Claflin and colleagues (1990) later showed that latency relaxation was very closely coincident with an increase in stiffness, confirming that the filamentary resting tension and short-range elastic component were due to similar mechanisms. They and others have hypothesized that such behaviours could be explained if cross-bridges existed in one of three states: a resting state (low tension, low stiffness), an intermediate state (no tension or negative tension and high stiffness) and a force-generating state. The resting state confers the filamentary resting tension, and the intermediate state confers the short-range elastic component and latency relaxation.

An alternative hypothesis was provided by Campbell and Lakie (1998), who developed a 'cross-bridge population displacement mechanism' model. Their model simulates the complex muscle responses to low-force stretch. The model produced behaviours that are qualitatively similar to those observed experimentally. The primary assumption of the model is that actin and myosin filaments of resting muscles are linked by a small number of slowly cycling cross-bridges. According to this hypothesis, the short-range elastic component is attributable to a change in the cross-bridge length distribution produced by relative motion of the contractile filaments.

Currently, it is not clear which of the existing models best describes the mechanisms underlying muscle responses to low-force stretch. Nonetheless, it appears very likely that part of the resting tension and the short-range stiffness of resting muscle is due to an interaction between contractile filaments.

It is difficult to establish the contribution of filamentary resting tension to tension in relaxed muscles at stretched lengths so it is not certain to what degree, if any, the filamentary resting tension accounts for the elastic properties of resting muscles in response to large-amplitude stretches. Granzier and Wang (1993) investigated this by abolishing interactions between contractile filaments in skinned muscle fibres of rabbit psoas and semitendinosus. At physiological temperatures and ionic strengths, and at sarcomere lengths of 2.0–3.0 μm (stresses of up to 3 N/cm^2), abolishing filament interactions had little effect on passive length–tension curves, suggesting that weak cross-bridges contributed relatively little to the total passive tension over this large range of lengths (see also Proske and Morgan 1999).

There is now quite strong evidence to suggest that the mechanical properties of resting muscle fibres are largely determined by a protein called titin. Titin (previously called connectin) has structural and mechanical properties that make it ideally suited to bear resting tension in skeletal muscles (Horowits 1992, Linke et al 1996, Maruyama et al 1977, Wang et al 1991). Immunohistochemical studies show that titin wraps around myosin filaments and extends to the Z line (Linke et al 1996, Wang et al 1991). It is thought that, when the muscle is stretched to physiological lengths, a region of the molecule progressively unfolds, and when the muscle is shortened it progressively refolds (Linke et al 1996, Tskhovrebova et al 1997). Thus, titin forms a molecular spring that constrains the travel of sarcomeres.

Some remarkable experiments have described the mechanical properties of single titin molecules. In these experiments a single molecule is trapped between a microscope slide and a tiny bead that is gripped with atomic tweezers. The bead is displaced in tiny steps, stretching the molecule, and the tension generated in the stretched molecule is determined from the bead's resistance to displacement. Single titin molecules exhibit just the right length–tension properties to account for the length–tension properties observed when large stretches are delivered to muscle fibres or whole muscles (Kellermayer et al 1997, Rief et al 1997, Tskhovrebova et al 1997). Titin also displays viscous properties such as stress relaxation (Tskhovrebova et al 1997) and hysteresis (Kellermayer et al 1997), which could account for part or all of the viscous behaviours seen in whole muscles at high forces. These properties of resting muscles are described in the next section.

To summarize, the available evidence indicates that the extensibility of tendon is due to the crimped morphology of collagen fibres. Muscle fibres exhibit complex responses to low-force stretch, probably reflecting the behaviour of cross-bridges formed between contractile filaments. The response of muscle tissue to large-amplitude stretch is probably determined largely by titin.

VISCOUS RESPONSES

By definition, the elastic properties of muscles determine the instantaneous response to stretch. But muscles do not behave simply as purely elastic structures. The response of muscle to lengthening evolves with time; that is, muscles behave 'viscously'. Viscosity manifests as a range of phenomena, the two most important of which are 'stress relaxation' and 'creep'.

If a muscle is stretched to a fixed length, muscle tension does not remain constant; instead it progressively declines. The decline in tension is initially rapid but becomes progressively slower. This phenomenon is called stress relaxation. Stress relaxation can easily be observed in humans. If a joint is stretched to a fixed angle and held at that angle for some time, the torque required to maintain the angle will gradually decline.

How much does stress decline with sustained stretch, and what is the time course of stress relaxation? Duong et al (2001) examined stress relaxation in human ankles by measuring the decay of ankle torque that occurred in response to a sustained stretch into dorsiflexion (42 minutes of 14 Nm stretch). Figure 6.4a shows the time course of the response. Ankle torque, which reflects tension in ankle plantarflexor muscle and other structures on the plantarflexor aspect of the ankle, declines approximately exponentially with time. (Actually, the decay is bi-exponential, meaning that tension declines as the sum of two exponential processes.) Half of the maximal eventual decline in torque is achieved within the first 5 minutes of the stretch. Ultimately torque declines to 58% of its initial value.

A closely related phenomenon is called creep. Creep occurs when sustained tension is applied to muscle. Under these conditions muscle length gradually increases. As with stress relaxation, the effect is initially quite rapid but it becomes progressively slower. Creep can easily be observed in humans. If a constant torque is applied to the joint of a relaxed subject, the joint angle will slowly increase over time.

The effects of creep and stress relaxation are entirely reversible. If they were not, muscles would gradually accumulate viscous

Figure 6.4 Viscous deformation in relaxed muscle. Data show stress relaxation when a 'strong but not painful' stretch is applied to human ankles. (a) Stress relaxation of eight ankles. Each line is the regression line from one subject. The thick line is the median of all subjects' data. (b) Recovery from stress relaxation when the stretch is released for 2 minutes ('recovery period') after the first 20 minutes of stretch. Curves are drawn from the median regression coefficients for all eight subjects. The average recovery over the 2 minutes was 42%. (c) Time course of recovery from stress relaxation after a 20–minute stretch. Subjects were randomly allocated to recovery times of between 0 and 20 minutes. Each data point indicates the degree of recovery for one subject. Recovery is plotted against the duration of the recovery time.

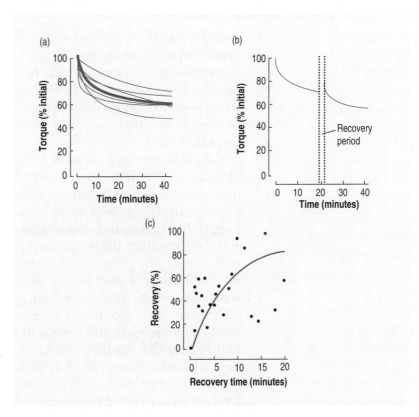

deformation to the point where all possible viscous deformation was exhausted. What is the time course of this recovery? This was examined by applying a sustained dorsiflexion stretch to the ankle and then, after 20 minutes, interrupting the stretch by plantarflexing the ankle (Duong et al 2001). When the muscle is subsequently returned to the initial stretch position, tension is found to have recovered – there is recovery from stress relaxation (Figure 6.4b). To determine the effect of recovery time on the extent of recovery from stress relaxation, subjects were allocated recovery times of up to 20 minutes. Although the degree of recovery was highly variable between subjects it appeared that the time course of recovery was similar to the time course of the viscous deformation (Figure 6.4c). The magnitude of the recovery did not appear to depend on whether muscles rested or actively contracted during the recovery period.

Importantly, reversible viscous deformation occurs without any change in the composition of the muscle. More lasting changes in the properties of muscles are brought about by muscle adaptations that involve changes in muscle composition. These adaptive changes are the topic of the next section.

ADAPTIVE RESPONSES

The growing body is faced with a difficult problem. When bones grow, supporting structures such as ligaments and muscles must grow in synchrony. Asynchronous growth might be problematic because it could cause ligaments and muscles to constrain joint motion inadequately or excessively, or cause muscles to become unable to produce force in the parts of range where force is needed.

The evolutionary solution is a clever one. Longitudinal growth of muscles is regulated by stretch. Muscles are able to sense the degree of stretch that they experience and adjust their growth accordingly. If a muscle experiences a high degree of stretch its longitudinal growth is accelerated, the muscle becomes longer, and the amount of stretch placed on the muscle is reduced. If the muscle is deprived of stretch it shortens until it experiences the requisite levels of stretch. In this way coordination of growth is achieved by homeostasis of stretch.

One way to explore the mechanisms regulating growth in muscles is to immobilize an animal's limb in a cast. Cast immobilization fixes joints at a constant angle. Depending on the angle of immobilization the muscle may be exposed to constant high levels of stretch (when the muscle is immobilized long) or constant low levels of stretch (when the muscle is immobilized short).

Ron Balnave and I investigated the effects of immobilization at a range of joint positions on the passive properties of whole muscles (muscle–tendon units; Herbert and Balnave 1993). One ankle of each of 23 rabbits was immobilized somewhere between full plantarflexion and full dorsiflexion for 10 days. After the immobilization period the length–tension properties of the soleus muscles were tested. We found that muscles immobilized at short lengths had slack lengths that were less than normal and less than those of muscles immobilized at stretched lengths (Figure 6.5a). Muscles immobilized at the most stretched lengths had slack lengths that were normal, or perhaps even greater than normal. However, immobilized muscles were stiffer than normal muscles, regardless of the position of immobilization (Figure 6.5b). One interpretation of these data is that the slack length of muscles is regulated by the degree of muscle stretch (i.e. position of immobilization) but the stiffness of muscles is determined by the amount of joint motion.

How important are these adaptations of muscle slack length? A simple index to assess the effect of a particular reduction in muscle slack length can be obtained by expressing the reduction in muscle slack length as a percentage of the moment arm of the muscle – let's call this the 'shortening index'. Some elementary biomechanics shows that the joint angle at which a muscle falls slack is reduced by 0.6° for every per cent reduction in the shortening index. For example, the reduction in slack length of muscle immobilized at short lengths for 10 days is about 7 mm and the moment arm of the rabbit soleus is about 10 mm (calculated from data in Herbert and Balnave 1993 and Herbert and Crosbie 1997) so the shortening index is about 70%. This means the effect of immobilization is to shift the joint angle at which slack length occurs by about 42°. The same reasoning can be used to estimate

Figure 6.5   Effects of position of immobilization on rest length and stiffness of rabbit soleus muscle. (a) Effect of position of immobilization on muscle rest length. (b) Effect of position of immobilization on muscle stiffness. Stiffness is given by the coefficient in the regression equation: extension = $20 \times e^{\text{stiffness} \times (\text{length} - \text{slack length})}$. Each data point represents one muscle immobilized for 10 days. The shaded bar represents the mean value ± 95% CI for muscles from animals that had not been immobilized.

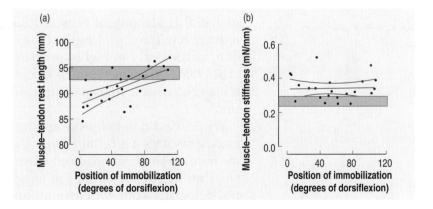

the effects of a given amount of muscle shortening in human muscles. A 10% reduction in the length of the human gastrocnemius muscle (which has a slack length of the order of 30 cm and a moment arm at the ankle of the order of 5 cm) would shift the torque–angle curve of the muscle by about 36°.

The reductions in muscle–tendon length that occur when muscles are immobilized at short lengths are of great interest to physiotherapists because it is these adaptations that underlie the ubiquitous clinical problem of 'contracture', or loss of joint range of motion. Is contracture due to adaptations of muscle fibres or tendons?

Jack Crosbie and I investigated this issue by immobilizing one hindlimb of each of five rabbits in the fully plantarflexed position for 14 days (Herbert and Crosbie 1997). After the period of immobilization we tested the length–tension properties of muscle fascicles and tendons as described above. The slack lengths of rabbit soleus muscles immobilized at short lengths were 8.8% shorter than non-immobilized muscles from the contralateral limb. We showed that most of the reduction in slack length was due to a reduction in the slack length of the tendon and that there was no reduction in the slack length of muscle fascicles. Thus, in the rabbit soleus, immobilization-induced contracture is due primarily to a reduction in tendon slack length. These findings extended earlier observations by Heslinga and Huijing (1992), who observed that immobilization of rat gastrocnemius at short lengths reduced the length of the intramuscular tendon. Together these studies suggest that contracture may be due as much to changes in tendon as to changes in muscle fibres.

What makes tendons become shorter following a period of immobilization at short lengths? There are at least two very different explanations. It could be that there are adaptive changes to the tendon that are in the opposite direction to those that occur during growth. Alternatively, it could be that the tendon does not adapt, but reductions in tendon slack length occur because the tendon plates adhere to muscle tissue, which atrophies in response to immobilization at short lengths. Heslinga and Huijing (1992) speculated that atrophy of muscle fibres could cause an apparent reduction in the slack length of the intramuscular part of the tendon, particularly in highly pennate muscles (see also Heslinga et al 1995). This explanation is fascinating because it suggests that it may be possible to treat contracture by inducing muscle hypertrophy.

While we did not observe any reduction in the slack length of muscle fascicles it is certain that important length changes occur in the fibres of some immobilized muscles. In fact the most important work on length adaptations of muscles, conducted by the British physiologist, Geoffrey Goldspink, and a group of French workers,

Tabary, Tabary, Tardieu and Tardieu, has demonstrated profound adaptations in muscle fibres immobilized at short lengths. In their pioneering work these researchers showed that when the soleus muscle of the adult cat is immobilized at short lengths for short periods (3 weeks) the average number of sarcomeres in series is reduced by about 40% (Tabary et al 1972). The muscle 'recognizes' deprivation of stretch caused by immobilization at short lengths and responds by removal of sarcomeres. In contrast, immobilization at stretched lengths causes an increase in the number of sarcomeres.

Sarcomere number adaptations such as those described by Goldspink and colleagues (see also Williams and Goldspink 1978, Witzmann et al 1982) are likely to contribute to the changes in the passive properties that have been observed in some muscles. The reduction in sarcomere number that occurs when muscles are immobilized at short lengths means that there are fewer sarcomeres end on end at slack length, and fewer sarcomeres to be lengthened (each sarcomere's lengthening limited, presumably, by its own titin springs). It is expected that this would cause muscle fibres to become shorter and less extensible.

Why do some studies of immobilization show important structural changes in muscle fibres (changes in sarcomere number) when others find little change in muscle fascicle length? There may be important differences between muscles that influence their susceptibility to structural and mechanical adaptations but it is difficult to identify what those differences are. Architectural characteristics such as the ratio of muscle fascicle and tendon lengths or the degree of fibre pennation may be important.

Sarcomere number adaptations also influence the contractile properties of muscles. The tension that a muscle can actively generate is a function of the degree of overlap of myosin and actin filaments. Loss of sarcomeres increases sarcomere length at any joint angle, and increases in sarcomere number decrease sarcomere length at any joint angle. Williams and Goldspink (1978) noted that the extent of the increase or loss of sarcomeres appears to be that which maintains the length at which the muscle is best able to produce tension close to the position of immobilization.

Quite different adaptations are observed in the muscles of juvenile animals immobilized at stretched lengths. Tardieu and colleagues (1977) observed that, in the soleus muscles of kittens, immobilization at stretched lengths produces a decrease in sarcomere number, the opposite to the effect observed in adult muscle. They interpreted their data as indicating that the tendons of growing muscle respond to chronic stretch by longitudinal growth. Tendon growth reduces stretch on muscle fibres, inducing a reduction in sarcomere number. This observation is of particular interest to paediatric therapists who use serial casting at stretched lengths to treat contractures in children with cerebral palsy and other conditions. Serial casting could increase the length of tendon and reduce the length of muscle fibres, which might impair function. However, cast-induced lengthening of tendon has not been directly demonstrated in humans.

There have been a few attempts to elucidate the 'critical mechanical stimulus' (Herbert 1993) that regulates muscle length. One clue about the nature of this stimulus comes from the observation that the effect of immobilization is similar (though not identical) in innervated and denervated muscle (Goldspink et al 1974, but see also McLachlan and Chua 1983). This suggests that the homeostatic mechanism is sensitive to imposed changes in length but not to patterns of muscle contraction. An important first step in developing a coherent theory of muscle length adaptations was recently made by Wren (2003). Wren described a simple model that predicts adaptations of muscle belly and tendon length by making assumptions about the critical mechanical stimulus that drives adaptation. The model assumed that tendons grow when under sustained strain (i.e. while even the minimum strain is positive), and that the rate of tendon growth increases linearly with increasing minimum strains. The muscle belly, on the other hand, was assumed to grow at a rate proportional to the average extension of the muscle belly. Wren showed that these simple rules closely predicted changes in muscle belly and tendon length that accompany growth, bone lengthening procedures, immobilization and retinacular release. If the model proves more generally capable of predicting muscle length adaptations it could be very important for clinical practice. It will be interesting to see if the model proves capable of predicting growth of muscle and tendon length in response to therapeutic application of muscle stretch.

CLINICAL STUDIES

Physiotherapists stretch muscles to deal with quite different clinical problems in two quite different populations. Sports people are often advised to stretch before or after exercise. In hospital and rehabilitation environments physiotherapists use muscle stretch to prevent or treat contracture. The following section presents some clinical research that has investigated these applications of muscle stretching.

Stretching before or after exercise

It is widely believed that stretching before exercise prevents the subsequent development of muscle soreness, or reduces risk of injury or enhances performance. What evidence is there that stretching provides these benefits?

Michael Gabriel and I conducted a systematic review of the literature on the effects of stretching before or after activity on development of muscle soreness, risk of injury or athletic performance (Herbert and Gabriel 2002). We searched major medical databases (Medline, Embase, CINAHL, SPORTDiscus and PEDro) for randomized studies that investigated the effects of any stretching technique administered before or after activity on muscle soreness, risk of injury or athletic or sporting performance.

The search identified five studies of the effects of stretching on muscle soreness. Three studies evaluated stretching after exercising, and two evaluated stretching before exercising. Total stretch time per session varied from 300 to 600 s, with the exception of one study in which total stretch time was only 80 s. As there was no evidence of heterogeneity in the outcomes of the studies we combined studies of stretch before and after exercise in a meta-analysis. Figure 6.6 shows the findings of individual studies, as well as pooled estimates obtained by combining the findings of all studies. The pooled estimate of the mean effect of stretching on muscle soreness 48 hours after exercising was just 0.3 mm (95% CI –4.0 to 4.5 mm) on a 100 mm scale, where negative values indicate a beneficial effect of stretching (Figure 6.6a). These data clearly indicate that stretching before or after exercise does not produce worthwhile reductions in muscle soreness.

We found only two randomized trials that had investigated the effects of stretching before exercising on the risk of injury. These studies, conducted by Rod Pope and colleagues, involved military recruits undergoing 12 weeks of initial training (Pope et al 1998, 2000). The first study investigated the effects of supervised stretching of calf muscles before exercising (two stretches of soleus and gastrocnemius muscles for 20 s on each limb, total stretch time 160 s) on the risk of six specific leg injuries (lesions of the Achilles tendon, lateral ankle sprains, stress fractures to the foot and tibia, periostitis or anterior tibial compartment syndrome). The second study investigated the effects of supervised stretching of six muscle

Figure 6.6   Effects of stretching on muscle soreness and injury risk. (a) Meta-analysis of the effects of stretching on muscle soreness 48 hours after exercise. Five studies (squares) provided estimates of the effects of stretching on muscle soreness (mm on a 100-mm visual analogue scale). The names of the authors of the individual studies are given at the left. The pooled estimate of the effect of stretching (diamond) was 0.3 mm (95% CI –4 to 4.5 mm). (b) Survival curves from two trials (Pope et al 1998, 2000) investigating the effects of stretching on injury risk. S and C indicate stretch and control groups respectively. The pooled estimate of the hazard ratio was 0.9 (95% CI 0.78 to 1.16).

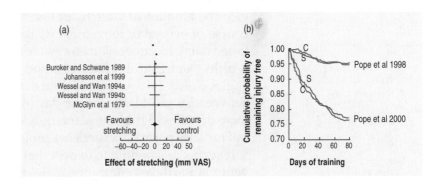

groups in the lower limbs before exercising (one 20 s stretch to each muscle group on each limb, total stretch time 240 s) on risk of soft-tissue injury, bone injury and all injuries. Recruits were considered to have sustained an injury if they were unable to return to full duties without signs or symptoms in 3 days. In both studies, subjects in both stretch and control groups also performed gentle warm-up exercises. The two studies yielded similar estimates of risk reduction: hazard ratios 0.92 (95% CI 0.52 to 1.61) and 0.95 (95% CI 0.77 to 1.18). Time-to-injury data from the two studies (total 2630 subjects) were combined. A total of 181 injuries occurred in stretch groups and 200 injuries in control groups. The pooled estimate of the hazard ratio for the stretch factor was 0.95 (95% CI 0.78 to 1.16), meaning that the best estimate is that stretching reduced risk of injury by 5% of the risk in the control group. This corresponds to the prevention, on average, of one injury for every 23 years of stretching (Pope et al 2000). Such an effect is, by most people's reckoning, too small to be worthwhile. It was concluded that the best available evidence suggests stretching before exercise does not appreciably reduce injury risk. However, as only two trials on army recruits have rigorously investigated this issue, the generality of this conclusion needs to be tested.

We found only one small randomized study that investigated the effects of stretching on sporting performance. This study provided inconclusive results. Therefore, it was concluded that there are not yet sufficient data with which to determine the effects of muscle stretching on sporting performance.

Stretching to prevent or reduce contracture

Animal studies indicate that muscles become shorter when immobilized at short lengths. Muscles that are not immobilized do not get short. This suggests that the stretches normally applied to muscles in the course of everyday movement are sufficient to maintain muscle slack length. How much stretch do muscles receive in the course of everyday movement, and how much stretch is necessary to prevent adaptive shortening?

Claudine Barrett and I conducted a descriptive study to investigate the amount of stretch applied to human calf muscles in the course of everyday movement (C Barrett and R Herbert, unpublished data). Electrogoniometers were attached to the ankles of seven healthy young adult volunteers and a data logger sampled ankle angles over a 24-hour period. The data showed that subjects spent between 5.6 and 14.9 hours per day (mean 9.6 hours) with the ankle more dorsiflexed than the plantargrade position. This shows that the calf muscles normally experience prolonged stretch during a day.

It seems reasonable to expect that physiotherapists could prevent plantarflexor contractures developing in at-risk patients by ensuring that the ankle was stretched by this amount every day. In practice, however, it would be difficult to administer such sustained stretching to muscles at risk of contracture. Instead, physiotherapists usually apply smaller numbers of stretches for a shorter total stretch duration than would normally be experienced in the course of everyday movement.

How effective are these less intensive stretching programmes at preventing or reversing the development of contracture? Only a small number of properly controlled clinical trials have investigated the effects of stretching programmes on the prevention or treatment of contracture, and these studies have mixed findings. Ada et al (2004) randomized patients with upper limb weakness after stroke to either receive a shoulder positioning programme or not. On 5 days each week, the affected shoulders of subjects in the experimental group were positioned in 90° of flexion for 30 minutes and 'maximum comfortable' external rotation for a further 30 minutes. After 4 weeks the mean effect of the positioning programme on shoulder flexion range of motion was less than 3°, but the effect on shoulder external rotation range of motion was about 12°, arguably a clinically worthwhile effect.

One small trial compared the effects of low-load prolonged stretch to high-load brief stretch in treatment of knee flexion contractures in nursing home residents (Light et al 1984). This study found that 4 weeks of twice-daily low-load stretch (each stretch of 1 hour, applied with traction) produced an average of 16° more knee extension than short-duration (3×1 minute) high-load manual stretching (mean effect 16°, 95% CI 10 to 22°). However, another trial with a very similar sample and methodology found that 6 months of daily 3-hour stretches had no greater effect than twice-weekly passive motion and manual stretching (difference of 0°, 95% CI −3 to 4°; Steffen and Mollinger 1995).

Lisa Harvey and her co-workers have examined the effects of sustained stretch on prevention and treatment of contractures in paraplegics and quadriplegics. In the first of two trials, subjects' left and right legs were randomly allocated to treatment and control groups. One leg received 30-minute stretches (ankle stretched into dorsiflexion with the knee straight) daily for 4 weeks, whereas the other leg was not stretched (Harvey et al 2000). Surprisingly, there was no effect of stretching (mean treatment effect of 0°, 95% CI −3 to 3°). The authors surmised that the negative results could have been due to the inclusion of some subjects with normal ankle mobility. Subjects with normal ankle mobility were included to simulate clinical practice where stretches are routinely administered to prevent ankle contractures. However, there was no evidence that the effect of stretching was any greater in subjects with contracture.

A second trial (Harvey et al 2003) examined the effect of stretching the hamstring muscles. In this trial an inclusion criterion was that subjects had to have insufficient hamstring and lower back extensibility to enable unsupported long sitting. Again, subjects' legs were randomly allocated to experimental and control groups. The hamstring muscles of the experimental leg of each subject were stretched for 30 minutes each weekday for 4 weeks. Stretching did not change the extensibility of the hamstring muscles. The mean effect of stretching was 2° (95% CI –1 to 6°). It was concluded that 4 weeks of 30-minute stretches each weekday does not affect the extensibility of the hamstring muscle in people with spinal cord injuries.

An alternative way of applying therapeutic stretch to muscles is with serial casts. This involves casting the joint in a stretched position. Every few days the cast is removed and the joint is recast in a progressively more stretched position. Animal studies such as those by Goldspink and colleagues would suggest that casting is likely to be an effective therapy. The first randomized trial of the effects of serial casting on humans was conducted on head-injured patients with plantarflexor contractures (Moseley 1997). This important study showed that a week of serial casting increased ankle dorsiflexion range of motion by a mean of 12°. The effect of casting was assessed at the time the cast was removed so it is not known if the beneficial effects of casting were sustained for any period of time.

In neurological physiotherapy and in hand therapy, the hand is often splinted to prevent contracture of the wrist and extrinsic finger flexor muscles. Often the wrist is splinted in the 'position of function', with the extrinsic finger flexors at an intermediate length (neither fully stretched nor fully shortened). The findings of animal studies suggest that muscles immobilized at intermediate lengths still undergo adaptive shortening (Herbert and Balnave 1993), so it is not obvious why splinting in the position of function would prevent contracture. Recently, Lannin et al (2003) conducted a randomized controlled trial that demonstrates that splinting the hand in the neutral position following stroke is not helpful (nor, for that matter, is it harmful): patients whose wrists were splinted in the neutral position experienced very similar outcomes in terms of extrinsic finger flexor length, pain and function. If splinting is to prevent contracture it may be necessary to splint at-risk muscles at stretched lengths. This is the focus of a clinical trial that is currently under way.

SUMMARY

The response of relaxed muscles to stretch is characterized by elastic, viscous and adaptive properties. Elastic properties of whole muscles are conferred by both muscle fascicles and tendons. Stretch sustained for seconds, minutes or hours produces reversible viscous responses such as stress relaxation and creep. Deprivation of stretch for days, weeks or months can induce contractures, which may be due to adaptations of muscle or tendon.

Many people stretch before exercise with the aim of preventing muscle soreness, reducing risk of injury or enhancing performance. The best available evidence suggests stretching before or after exercise does not prevent soreness, and probably does not reduce risk of injury. Therapists often stretch muscles to prevent or reverse muscle contracture. Some studies have shown that sustained stretching produces small but possibly worthwhile effects on joint range of motion, but other studies have found no worthwhile effect.

References

Ada L, Goddard E, McCully J et al 2004 30 minutes of positioning reduces the development of external rotation after stroke: a randomised controlled trial. Archives of Physical Medicine and Rehabilitation (in press).

Alexander R S, Johnson P D 1965 Muscle stretch and theories of contraction. American Journal of Physiology 208:412–416.

Banus M G, Zetlin A M 1938 The relation of isometric tension to length in skeletal muscle. Journal of Cellular and Comparative Physiology 12:403–420.

Borg T K, Caulfield J B 1980 Morphology of connective tissue in skeletal muscle. Tissue and Cell 12:197–207.

Buroker KC, Schwane JA 1989 Does postexercise static stretching alleviate delayed muscle soreness? Physician Sports Medicine 17:65–83.

Campbell K S, Lakie M 1998 A cross-bridge mechanism can explain the thixotropic short-range elastic component of relaxed frog skeletal muscle. Journal of Physiology 510:941–962.

Casella C 1950 Tensile force in total striated muscle, isolated fibre and sarcolemma. Acta Physiologica Scandinavica 21:380–401.

Claflin D R, Morgan D L, Julian F J 1990 Earliest mechanical evidence of cross-bridge activity after stimulation of single skeletal muscle fibres. Biophysical Journal 57:425–432

Duong B, Low M, Moseley A et al 2001 Time course of stress relaxation and recovery in human ankles. Clinical Biomechanics 16:601–607.

Fields R W, Faber J J 1970 Biophysical analysis of the mechanical properties of the sarcolemma.

Canadian Journal of Physiology and Pharmacology 48:394–404.

Fratzl P, Misof K, Zizak I et al 1997 Fibrillar structure and mechanical properties of collagen. Journal of Structural Biology 122:119–122.

Goldspink G, Tabary C, Tabary J C et al 1974 Effect of denervation on the adaptation of sarcomere number and muscle extensibility to the functional length of the muscle. Journal of Physiology 236:733–742.

Granzier H L M, Wang K 1993 Passive tension and stiffness of vertebrate skeletal and insect flight muscles: the contribution of weak cross-bridges and elastic filaments. Biophysical Journal 65:2141–2159.

Hanson J, Huxley H E 1955 The structural basis of contraction in striated muscle. Symposia of the Royal Society for Experimental Biology 9:228–264.

Harvey L A, Batty J, Crosbie J et al 2000 Effects of 4 weeks of daily stretching on ankle flexibility in recently injured spinal cord injured patients. Archives of Physical Medicine and Rehabilitation 81:1340–1347.

Harvey L A, Byak A J, Ostrovskaya M et al 2003 Randomised trial of the effects of four weeks of daily stretch on extensibility of hamstring muscles in people with spinal cord injuries. Australian Journal of Physiotherapy 49:176–181.

Herbert R D 1993 The prevention and treatment of stiff joints. In: Crosbie W J, McConnell J (eds) Key issues in musculoskeletal physiotherapy. Butterworth-Heinemann, London, pp 114–141.

Herbert R D, Balnave R J 1993 The effect of position of immobilisation on the resting length, resting stiffness and weight of rabbit soleus muscle. Journal of Orthopaedic Research 11:358–366.

Herbert R D, Crosbie J 1997 Rest length and compliance of non-immobilised and immobilised rabbit soleus muscle and tendon. European Journal of Applied Physiology 76:472–479.

Herbert R D, Gabriel M 2002 Effects of pre- and post-exercise stretching on muscle soreness, risk of injury and athletic performance: a systematic review. British Medical Journal 325:468–472.

Herbert R D, Gandevia S C 1995 Changes in pennation with joint angle and muscle torque: in vivo measurements in human brachialis muscle. Journal of Physiology 484:523–532.

Herbert R D, Moseley A M, Butler J E et al 2002 Change in length of relaxed muscle fascicles and tendons with knee and ankle movement in humans. Journal of Physiology 539:637–645.

Heslinga J W, Huijing P A 1992 Effects of short length immobilization of medial gastrocnemius muscle of growing young adult rats. European Journal of Morphology 30:257–273.

Heslinga J W, te Kronnie G, Huijing P A 1995 Growth and immobilization effects on sarcomeres: a comparison between gastrocnemius and soleus muscles of the adult rat. European Journal of Applied Physiology 70:49–57.

Hill A V 1950 Is relaxation an active process? Proceedings of the Royal Society (Series B) 136:420–435.

Hill A V 1952 The thermodynamics of elasticity in resting striated muscle. Proceedings of the Royal Society (Series B) 139:464–497.

Hill D K 1968 Tension due to interaction between the sliding filaments in resting muscle. The effect of stimulation. Journal of Physiology 208:725–739.

Horowits R 1992 Passive force generation and titin isoforms in mammalian skeletal muscle. Biophysical Journal 61:392–398.

Hurschler C, Loitz-Ramage B, Vanderby R 1997 A structurally based stress–stretch relationship for tendon and ligament. Journal of Biomechanical Engineering 119:392–399.

Jahnke M T, Proske U, Struppler A 1989 Measurements of muscle stiffness, the electromyogram and activity in single muscle spindles of human flexor muscles following conditioning by passive stretch or contraction. Brain Research 493:103–112.

Johansson P H, Lindstrom L, Sundelin G et al 1999 The effects of pre-exercise stretching on muscular soreness, tenderness and force loss following heavy eccentric exercise. Scandinavian Journal of Medical Science in Sports. 9:219–225.

Kastelic J, Palley I, Baer E 1980 A structural mechanical model for tendon crimping. Journal of Biomechanics 13:887–893.

Kellermayer M S Z, Smith S B, Granzier H L et al 1997 Folding-unfolding transitions in single titin molecules characterised with laser tweezers. Science 276:1112–1116.

Lannin N, McCluskey A, Herbert R D et al 2003 Hand splinting in the functional position after brain impairment: a randomized controlled trial. Archives of Physical Medicine and Rehabilitation 84:297–302.

Liao H, Belkoff S M 1999 A failure model for ligaments. Journal of Biomechanics 32:183–188

Lieber R L, Jacobson M D, Fazeli B M et al 1992 Architecture of selected muscles of the arm and forearm: anatomy and implications for tendon transfer. Journal of Hand Surgery (American volume) 17:787–798.

Light K E, Nuzik S, Personius W et al 1984 Low-load prolonged stretch vs high-load brief stretch in treating knee contractures. Physical Therapy 64:330–333.

Linke W A, Ivemayer M, Olivieri N et al 1996 Towards a molecular understanding of the elasticity of titin. Journal of Molecular Biology 261:62–71.

Loeb G E, Richmond F J R 1994 Architectural features of multiarticular muscles. Human Movement Sciences 13:545–556.

McCarter R J M, Nabarro F R N, Wyndham C H 1971 Reversibility of the passive length-tension relation in mammalian skeletal muscle. Archives Internationales Physiologie Biochimie 79: 469–479.

McGlynn G H, Laughlin N T, Rowe V 1979 Effect of electromyographic feedback and static stretching on artificially induced muscle soreness. American Journal of Physical Medicine 58:139–148.

McLachlan E M, Chua M 1983 Rapid adjustment of sarcomere length in tenotomized muscle depends on an intact innervation. Neuroscience Letters 35:127–133.

Maes M, Vanhuyse V J, Decraemer W F et al 1989 A thermodynamically consistent constitutive equation for the elastic force-length relation of soft biological materials. Journal of Biomechanics 22:1203–1208.

Magid A, Law D J 1985 Myofibrils bear most of the resting tension in frog skeletal muscle. Science 230:1280–1282.

Maruyama K, Matsubara S, Natori R et al 1977 Connectin, an elastic protein, of muscle: characterization and function. Journal of Biochemistry 82:317–337.

Moseley A M 1997 The effect of casting combined with stretching on passive ankle dorsiflexion in adults with traumatic head injuries. Physical Therapy 77:240–247.

Podolsky R J 1964 The maximum sarcomere length for contraction of isolated myofibrils. Journal of Physiology 170:110–123.

Pollock C M, Shadwick R E 1994 Allometry of muscle, tendon, and elastic energy storage capacity in mammals. American Journal of Physiology 266:R1022–1031.

Pope R, Herbert R D, Kirwan J 1998 Effects of flexibility and stretching on risk of injury in army recruits. Australian Journal of Physiotherapy 44:165–177.

Pope R, Herbert R D, Kirwan J 2000 Effects of pre-exercise stretching on risk of injury in army recruits: a randomized trial. Medicine and Science in Sports and Exercise 32:271–277.

Proske U, Morgan D L 1999 Do cross-bridges contribute to the tension during stretch of passive muscle? Journal of Muscle Research and Cell Motility 20:433–442.

Proske U, Morgan D L, Gregory J E 1993 Thixotropy in skeletal muscle and in muscle spindles: a review. Progress in Neurobiology 41:705–721.

Purslow P P 1989 Strain-induced reorientation of an intramuscular connective tissue network: implications for passive muscle elasticity. Journal of Biomechanics 22:21–31.

Ramsey R W, Street S F 1940 The isometric length-tension diagram of isolated skeletal muscle fibres of the frog. Journal of Cellular and Comparative Physiology 15:11–34.

Rapaport S I 1972 Mechanical properties of the sarcolemma and myoplasm in frog muscle as a function of sarcomere length. Journal of General Physiology 59:559–585.

Rapaport S I 1973 The anisotropic elastic properties of the frog semitendinosus muscle fiber. Biophysical Journal 13:14–36.

Refshauge K M, Taylor J L, McCloskey D I et al 1998 Movement detection at the human big toe. Journal of Physiology 513:307–314.

Rief M, Gautel M, Oesterhelt F et al 1997 Reversible unfolding of individual titin immunoglobulin domains by AFM. Science 276:1109–1112.

Rowe R W D 1981 Morphology of perimysial and endomysial connective tissue in skeletal muscle. Tissue and Cell 13:681–690.

Rowe R W D 1985a The structure of rat tail tendon. Connective Tissue Research 14:9–20.

Rowe R W D 1985b The structure of rat tail tendon fascicles. Connective Tissue Research 14:21–30.

Steffen T M, Mollinger L A 1995 Low-load, prolonged stretch in the treatment of knee flexion contractures in nursing home residents. Physical Therapy 75:886–897.

Stolinski C 1995 Disposition of collagen fibrils in human tendons. Journal of Anatomy 186:577–583.

Street S F 1983 Lateral transmission of tension in frog myofibers: a myofibrillar network and transverse cytoskeletal connections are possible transmitters. Journal of Cell Physiology 114:346–364.

Stromberg D D, Wiederhielm C A 1969 Viscoelastic description of a collagenous tissue in simple elongation. Journal of Applied Physiology 26:857–862.

Tabary J C, Tabary C, Tardieu C et al 1972 Physiological and structural changes in the cat's soleus muscle due to immobilization at different lengths by plaster casts. Journal of Physiology 224:231–244.

Tardieu C, Tabary J C, Tabary C et al 1977 Comparison of the sarcomere number adaptation in young and adult animals. Influence of tendon adaptation. Journale de Physiologie 73:1045–1055.

Tskhovrebova L, Trinick J, Sleep J A et al 1997 Elasticity and unfolding of single molecules of the giant muscle protein titin. Nature 387: 308–312.

Wang K 1984 Cytoskeletal matrix in striated muscle: the role of titin, nebulin and intermediate filaments. In: Pollock G H, Sugi H (eds) Contractile mechanisms in muscle. Plenum, New York, pp 285–305.

Wang K, McCarter R, Wright J et al 1991 Regulation of skeletal muscle stiffness and elasticity by titin isoforms: a test of the segmental extension model of resting tension. Proceedings of the National Academy of Sciences of the USA 88, 7101–7105.

Wei J Y, Simon J, Randic M et al 1986 Joint angle signaling by muscle spindle receptors. Brain Research 370:108–118.

Wessel J, Wan A 1994 Effect of stretching on the intensity of delayed onset muscle soreness. Clinical Journal of Sports Medicine. 4:83–87.

Williams P E, Goldspink G 1978 Changes in sarcomere length and physiological properties in immobilised muscle. Journal of Anatomy 127:459–468.

Witzmann F A, Kim D H, Fitts R H 1982 Hindlimb immobilisation: length–tension and contractile properties of skeletal muscle. Journal of Applied Physiology 53:335–345.

Wren T A 2003 A computational model for the adaptation of muscle and tendon length to average muscle length and minimum tendon strain. Journal of Biomechanics 36:1117–1124.

Yamaguchi G T, Sawa A G-U, Moran M J et al 1990 A survey of human musculotendon actuator parameters. In: Winters J M, Woo S L-Y (eds) Multiple muscle systems: biomechanics and movement organisation. Springer-Verlag, New York, pp 717–773.

Zajac F E 1989 Muscle and tendon: properties, models, scaling, and application to biomechanics and motor control. Critical Reviews in Biomedical Engineering 17:359–411.

Chapter **7**

Cardiorespiratory fitness after stroke

Sharon L. Kilbreath and Glen M. Davis

Historically, deficits of cardiorespiratory fitness (i.e. aerobic fitness) have not been recognized as an impairment that warranted primary treatment by physiotherapists, or have been considered less important to functional rehabilitation for patients recovering from cerebrovascular accident ('stroke'). The neurodevelopmental paradigms of physiotherapy assumed that the primary sequelae after stroke were spasticity and impaired balance (Gordon 1987). Strengthening of 'weak' muscles using progressive resistance exercises or cardiorespiratory training was discouraged, since it was believed that loading the muscle would lead inter alia to greater spasticity. Thus, it is unsurprising that cardiorespiratory fitness was not considered to be an important component of stroke rehabilitation. Patients were not required to exert themselves and so there was little demand placed upon their cardiorespiratory system to confer improved fitness.

In the 1980s, Carr and Shepherd challenged physiotherapists to examine scientific literature outside of traditional areas referred to by the profession, and they exhorted 'best-practice' models of therapy that were multidisciplinary in nature. In particular, one discipline in which their theoretical basis for the movement sciences paradigm was grounded was motor control (Carr and Shepherd 1982), and one of the abiding principles within the motor learning scientific literature is the importance of practice. For the first time, there was an expectation that patients not only would practise within the physiotherapy session, but would also be expected to practise independently. However, for patients to practise repetitive gross motor activities involving lower limb musculature required a reasonable cardiorespiratory fitness. Hence, recent textbooks on stroke rehabilitation (Carr and Shepherd 1998, 2003) have recognized the importance of adequate levels of cardiorespiratory fitness for training as a component of rehabilitation for people affected by stroke.

FACTORS THAT CONTRIBUTE TO REDUCED CARDIORESPIRATORY FITNESS

The impairment of cardiorespiratory fitness after stroke is probably related to a combination of pathological, physiological and environmental factors. Furthermore, these factors are often interdependent, and by modifying one, the physiotherapist may elicit consequential outcomes upon the others.

Exercise capacity may be compromised after stroke by comorbid cardiovascular disease. In a thorough review of epidemiological evidence, Roth (1993) suggested that up to 75% of people affected by stroke might have clinical or asymptomatic coronary artery disease (CAD). In one study of 200 people with transient ischaemic attack or stroke, 40% demonstrated advanced or severe CAD, and an additional 46% had mild to moderate CAD (Hertzer et al 1985). In other reports (reviewed in Potempa et al 1996, Roth 1993), between 28% and 70% of people with stroke or transient ischaemic attack demonstrated myocardial perfusion defects without a history of CAD.

This comorbid cardiovascular disease is coupled with age-related declines in cardiorespiratory fitness approximating 10% or greater per decade (Bouchard et al 1990). In addition, following stroke, physiological factors, including loss of muscle strength and poor coordination (Burke 1988), result in a reduction in the number of recruitable motor units (Jakobsson et al 1992, Ragnarsson 1988), a diminished capacity for oxidative metabolism in paretic muscle tissue (Landin et al 1977) and 'blunted' cardiovascular responses that are not conducive to performing exercise. Thus, while the primary cause of disability in acute stroke is of neuromuscular aetiology, fitness status includes a constellation of cardiorespiratory impairments and frequent comorbid coronary artery disease.

Finally, environmental factors that contribute to impairment of cardiorespiratory fitness include bed rest and physical inactivity experienced following the stroke. Two Australian studies have reported similar results regarding the small amount of time people affected by stroke spend in physical activities (Esmonde et al 1997, Mackey et al 1996). They spent less than 20% of their day engaged in activities that potentially contributed to their recovery (Mackey et al 1996). Four per cent of their day (i.e. 28 minutes) was spent performing specific 'exercises' with the upper and lower affected limb, and the remaining 16% was spent in the performance of tasks such as walking, sit-to-stand, balanced sitting and standing and using the affected upper limb (Mackey et al 1996). Furthermore, the motor activity performed while in physical and/or occupational therapy is unlikely to be of sufficient potency to confer any cardiorespiratory training effect (Mackay-Lyons and Makrides 2002b).

CURRENT LEVELS OF CARDIORESPIRATORY FITNESS FOLLOWING STROKE

Subacute stroke   In a recent study from our laboratory (Kelly et al 2003), assessment of cardiorespiratory fitness in people affected mild-to-moderately by stroke revealed that aerobic fitness was significantly reduced within 7 weeks of their initial hospitalization. Using assessment criteria and testing strategies based on American College of Sports Medicine guidelines (Franklin 2000), 17 subjects aged between 24 and 84 years undertook both an incremental maximal effort test and a multistage submaximal assessment using cycle ergometer to derive their peak cardiorespiratory fitness. Aerobic fitness estimated from symptom-limited maximal exercise performance and predicted peak oxygen uptake (VO_{2peak}) from the submaximal test both demonstrated a significantly blunted exercise response (Figure 7.1). The median VO_{2peak} from the symptom-limited test was 14.0 ml/kg/min [interquartile range (IQR) 11.8–18.3 ml/kg/min], only 47% of the

Vo_{2peak} estimated for an age-matched sample. When submaximal exercise data were used to extrapolate aerobic fitness to age-predicted maximal heart rate, their median predicted Vo_{2peak} was higher – 79% (IQR 62–90%) of the expected value. This disparity between directly measured and predicted cardiorespiratory fitness highlights the pernicious effects of muscle paresis and cardiovascular deconditioning against achieving a 'true' maximal exercise response in acute stroke. The disparity also demonstrates that directly measured Vo_{2peak} will likely under-predict the 'true' aerobic fitness of patients, whereas an age-predicted maximal heart rate estimate will nearly always over-predict 'true' cardiorespiratory fitness. Unsurprisingly, the younger subjects achieved higher fitness levels compared with their older cohorts, both for the symptom-limited and heart rate-predicted Vo_{2peak} values; but when these were expressed relative to age- and gender-matched normative values their aerobic fitness was no better or worse than the older subjects.

The cardiorespiratory fitness in subacute stroke has also been assessed during treadmill walking (Mackay-Lyons and Makrides 2001). People within 1 month of their first stroke ($n = 29$) underwent a stress test protocol involving increments of both treadmill speed and gradient with 15% body mass support. Measures of cardiorespiratory fitness were uniformly low, with symptom-limited Vo_{2peak} and peak heart rate of 14.4 ± 5.1 ml/kg/min and 123 ± 18.9 beats/min respectively. The authors noted that their patients' cardiorespiratory fitness was only 60% of age- and gender-related normative values for sedentary healthy adults (Figure 7.1). Interestingly, patients in this study were similar in age and time since stroke to those in the investigation of Kelly et al (2003), and achieved similar values for Vo_{2peak} during treadmill walking to

Figure 7.1 Peak cardiorespiratory fitness in people early after stroke. Peak oxygen uptake (Vo_{2peak}) is expressed as a percentage of healthy age- and gender-matched sedentary subjects' values derived from normative data. On the left is shown Vo_{2peak} based on symptom-limited maximal exercise tests (grey bars); on the right is portrayed Vo_{2peak} predicted from a submaximal exercise test (blue bar). Peak cardiorespiratory fitness was not significantly different between the two studies that used symptom-limited exercise tests. Data are mean ± SD.

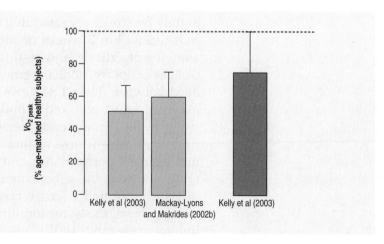

those obtained using cycle ergometry. This suggests that both task-specific (i.e. treadmill walking) and non-task-specific (e.g. seated cycling) modalities are appropriate for assessing levels of cardiorespiratory fitness in subacute patients.

Chronic stroke   Cardiorespiratory fitness continues to be reduced months and years afters the initial stroke (Bachynski-Cole and Cumming 1985, Macko et al 1997a, Potempa et al 1995, 1996). The low cardiorespiratory fitness of people affected by stroke has been widely attributed to residual hemiparesis, poor neuromuscular recruitment and an attenuated peak exercise heart rate (Bachynski-Cole and Cumming 1985, King et al 1989, Monga et al 1988, Potempa et al 1995, 1996). For example, during maximal effort, people with chronic stroke exhibit peak oxygen uptakes in the range of 13–21 ml/kg/min; Bachynski-Cole and Cumming 1985, Bjuro et al 1975, Fujitani et al 1999, Potempa et al 1995), usually less than 50% of the values obtained by a healthy age-matched population (Potempa et al 1995). It has been presumed that such low values of VO_{2peak} are due to reduced maximal heart rates (in the range of 100–130 beats/min; (Bachynski-Cole and Cumming 1985, King et al 1989, Monga et al 1988), although the exercise stroke volumes of these patients are also presumably worse due to a post-morbid physical deconditioning. In particular, low heart rate during peak effort represents both the consequence of hemiparesis and muscle deconditioning, but also the cause of reduced oxygen delivery to leg muscles during exercise. An attenuated peak exercise heart rate lowers cardiac output and reduces blood flow to working muscles, contributing to poor neuromuscular recruitment.

Interestingly, some authors (Bjuro et al 1975, Potempa et al 1995) have suggested that the proportion of patients achieving 85% of their age-predicted maximal heart rates was no different from a healthy cohort – an important characteristic of these studies was that patients were at least 6 months 'recovered' from their hemispheric stroke. Maximal heart rates for a similar age population of healthy individuals are in the range of 155–175 beats/min (for age 65 years; Franklin 2000), so there is merit to the view that reduced peak heart rates following acute stroke may lower exercise performance secondary to neuromuscular impairment.

During submaximal exercise after stroke, reduced cardiorespiratory fitness presents as a lower exercise tolerance at reduced cycle power outputs (36–50 W; Bachynski-Cole and Cumming 1985, Moldover et al 1984) or slower treadmill walking speeds (0.65 ± 0.27 m/s; Macko et al 1997b). At a given steady-state power output, heart rate, oxygen uptake and blood pressures are no different from healthy age-matched individuals (Bachynski-Cole and Cumming 1985, Monga et al 1988, Potempa et al 1996). However, the motor impairment with its associated negative sequelae in muscle morphology and histochemistry (reviewed in Potempa et al 1996) severely limits the quantity and quality of exercise that can be performed. Thus, the functional disability after stroke has consequences for submaximal and maximal exercise performance. Long-standing hemiparesis, a common residual neurological deficiency, reduces the number of recruitable motor units (Jakobsson et al 1992, Ragnarsson 1988) and may alter the recruitment pattern, with the usual endpoints being post-morbid sedentary behaviour and physical deconditioning. Reduced submaximal or peak exercise heart rates and lower stroke volumes both contribute to attenuated cardiac outputs, further impacting oxygen delivery to working leg muscles. The interaction of these neurological, neuromuscular and cardiovascular factors during exercise raises the question of whether 'central' or 'peripheral' factors limit aerobic exercise performance to a greater extent in chronic stroke.

WHY TRAIN CARDIORESPIRATORY FITNESS?

Improved aerobic fitness and 'cardiorespiratory reserve'

The value of exercise conditioning in the treatment of the symptoms of cardiovascular disease, particularly coronary heart disease, is well known (Halar 1999, Potempa et al 1996, Rimmer and Nicola 2002). Appropriate exercise training after stroke may improve aerobic fitness and ameliorate the symptoms associated with comorbid cardiovascular disease. However, the strongest reason for augmenting fitness with exercise training is the greater 'cardiorespiratory fitness reserve' conferred on the patient. By augmenting aerobic fitness, exercise conditioning improves tolerance to submaximal exertion, since patients are then able to perform physical tasks at a lower percentage of their $V_{O_{2peak}}$. Greater cardiorespiratory reserve also implies the ability to increase one's physical effort on demand, if the energy requirements of a given task unexpectedly increase.

Potempa and colleagues (1995) observed that, after a 10-week supervised aerobic training programme, mild–moderate hemiparetic patients augmented their $V_{O_{2peak}}$ by 13%. However, the authors noted that the increase of $V_{O_{2peak}}$ was not uniform amongst patients. Notably there was a 0–37% range of improvement in $V_{O_{2peak}}$, but all patients increased their exercise tolerance time and peak power output on the cycle ergometer.

Cardiorespiratory training both lowers the energy cost of submaximal exercise and increases the patient's $V_{O_{2peak}}$ – both of these contribute to higher cardiorespiratory fitness reserve. Macko et al (1997a, 2001) demonstrated that aerobic training reduced the energy costs of treadmill walking in people with chronic stroke. Their subjects ($n = 23$) underwent 6 months of low-intensity treadmill exercise at 40–60% of heart rate reserve. For those who were severely deconditioned, interval training was used initially, progressing to longer exercise periods and shorter recovery intervals as fitness improved. After 3 months, patients had improved their VO_{2peak} from 15.4 to 17.0 ml/kg/min (i.e. approximately 10%) and were able to undertake a standardized treadmill task at 20% less of their peak cardiorespiratory fitness.

In several studies, a common finding following aerobic training is a reduced steady-state heart rate (Brinkmann and Hoskins 1979, Wolman and Cornall 1994), systolic blood pressure (Potempa et al 1995), rate-pressure product (Fletcher et al 1994) and exercise recovery time (Wolman and Cornall 1994) at submaximal power outputs. Cardiorespiratory alterations at rest have been equivocal with the exception of a single study demonstrating a lower resting heart rate, an increased left ventricular ejection fraction and improved fractional shortening after exercise conditioning (Fletcher et al 1994). There have been no previous clinical or research studies which have documented possible changes of other cardiorespiratory or performance parameters at rest or during submaximal exercise (i.e. cardiac output, stroke volume, steady-state VO_2 or mechanical efficiency).

In a recent pilot study from our laboratory, nine people with chronic stroke (57 ± 5 years) were randomized to aerobic cycle training ($n = 5$) versus task-specific resistance training ($n = 4$) over 30 sessions of home-based exercise (Davis et al 2003). After training, the aerobic-trained subjects had increased their VO_{2peak} from 13.7 to 16.6 ml/kg/min, an improvement of 21% (Figure 7.2). In contrast, the strength-trained group did not change their aerobic fitness. The average VO_2 of the aerobic group during their 6-minute walk comprised 42% of the cardiorespiratory fitness reserve before training, but 36% of their reserve after training, a significant drop of 16% in their relative stress. In contrast, the strength-training group's cardiorespiratory reserve during the 6-minute walk was unchanged. These data highlight the tangible benefits of augmented aerobic fitness on reducing the relative stresses of Activities of Daily Living (ADL), as well as improving the cardiorespiratory fitness reserve during exertional tasks.

Improved walking ability

Within the rehabilitation process, physiotherapy intervention endeavours to maximize the ability to perform daily functional tasks such as walking and stairway ascent. Indeed, various studies have established that the majority of people affected by stroke

Figure 7.2   Change in cardiorespiratory fitness as a result of 10 weeks of training. Subjects ($n = 9$) underwent 10 weeks of either leg cycling exercise aimed at improving their aerobic fitness or box-stepping exercises intended to strengthen lower limb muscles. Only subjects who trained aerobically significantly improved their peak oxygen uptake (VO_{2peak}) ($P < 0.05$). Data are mean $\pm$ SD.

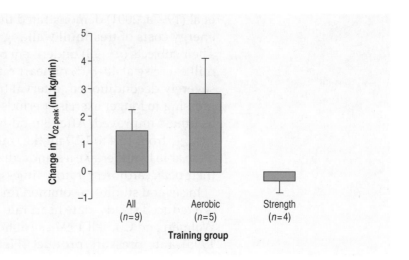

regain the ability to walk by the time they are discharged from physiotherapy (Dean and Mackey 1992, Hill et al 1997). However, walking is conducted at much higher energy expenditure than before their stroke (Olney et al 1986, Zamparo et al 1995).

The skill and efficiency with which an individual walks after stroke may be insufficient to facilitate ambulation within the community environment. Minimum criteria for successful community ambulation include an independent gait velocity of 0.8 m/s or greater, the ability to negotiate uneven terrain and kerbs, and gait endurance of 500 m or more (Hill et al 1997). These standards are well below the ability of healthy seniors (aged 60–80 years), who walk at velocities of $\geq$ 1.2 m/s (Waters et al 1988). In a recent review of 109 patients discharged from physiotherapy in an Australian hospital, only 7% achieved the minimum level (Hill et al 1997). The criterion that the majority of patients failed to achieve was gait endurance.

Evidence that walking endurance continues to be compromised after discharge from rehabilitation is evident from two studies. First, in a sample of community dwellers 1 year following stroke onset, poor walking endurance was the most striking functional deficit observed, and it was the only measure that was significantly associated with their quality of community reintegration (Mayo et al 1999). The energy cost and cardiorespiratory stresses required to perform tasks such as walking may limit the patient's ability successfully to undertake community activities. Second, in a 2-year follow-up study of 71 patients who 'were able to walk without personal help' on discharge, only 11 (8%) of the original cohort actually walked outside their homes (Wade et al 1985).

Cardiorespiratory fitness can address both the efficiency with which people affected by stroke can walk and the distance they can achieve. In the cohort of Macko et al (2001), treadmill walking economy (i.e. lower submaximal VO_2 during a standardized task) increased by 16% and the authors' estimate of 'peak ambulatory workload capacity' was higher by 39% after 6 months of aerobic training. Unfortunately, the authors failed to document beneficial changes in overground walking, as measures of self-selected gait and gait endurance were not assessed.

It is not just treadmill training that can improve walking endurance and ability. In our pilot study comprising a single-case design (Davis et al 2003), five people with chronic stroke underwent isokinetic cycle training for 30 minutes, three times per week over 8–10 weeks in their homes. Subjects commenced training at a heart rate (HR) equivalent to 50% of their VO_{2peak} during the initial 4 weeks; then proceeded to exercise at an intensity of 70–75% of VO_{2peak} (or their highest achievable workload) during the last 4–6 weeks. Interval training was employed during the first 2 weeks if subjects were unable to exercise continuously at the prescribed intensity, but by the end of the programme all subjects were training using continuous exercise. Subjects' walking endurance was assessed using the 6-minute walk test, over a baseline period, weekly during training, within 2 weeks of completion of training, and finally 3 months after the programme. As demonstrated in Figure 7.3, all subjects increased their walking distance over 6 minutes from a group mean of 245 ± 44 m to 276 ± 62 m, an

Figure 7.3 Time-series changes of 6-minute walk distance for five subjects who undertook cardiorespiratory training, three times per week over 10 weeks. During the baseline and training periods, the 6-minute walk test was performed weekly. Distance walked in 6 minutes did not change significantly during the baseline phase, but increased significantly during training and was retained after 3 months of follow-up.

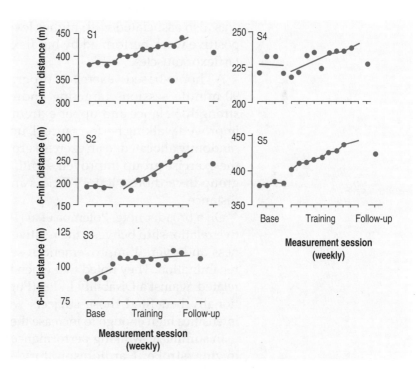

improvement of 13%. Self-selected and maximal walking velocities were increased by 18% and 17%, respectively, although these improvements did not achieve statistical significance. This pilot study was interesting because it suggested that there might be some 'cross-transfer of training effect' (i.e. 'cross-training') from aerobic cycling to walking endurance. A cohort group of patients in this study who were undertaking task-specific strength training (progressive height and repetition box stepping) in their homes did not show such marked improvements of gait endurance.

A few studies have examined the change in walking ability as a result of an exercise programme that includes an aerobic component. These studies have combined aerobic training with lower limb resistance training (Duncan et al 2003, Teixeira-Salmela et al 2001). Teixeira-Salmela and co-workers assessed the characteristics of walking in people with chronic stroke following a 10-week exercise programme. Each activity session comprised 5–10 minutes of warm-up consisting of stretching and callisthenics, aerobic exercise performed at an intensity equivalent to ~70% HR_{max}, progressive resistance training and a 5–10 minute cool-down period. The aerobic exercises included graded walking plus stepping or cycling, performed at an initial intensity of 50% HR_{max}, progressing up to 70% HR_{max}, and at an initial duration of 10 minutes proceeding to 20 minutes. After 10 weeks of training, people with chronic stroke walked faster by 37% (0.60 ± 0.39 to 0.76 ± 0.37 m/s) with associated improvements in their temporal–spatial and kinematic gait characteristics. The improvement in gait velocity was also associated with higher levels of leg muscle power and positive work performed by hip flexor/extensor and ankle plantarflexor muscles.

A home-based exercise programme that comprised 36 90-minute sessions targeting endurance as well as flexibility, strength, balance and upper extremity function also resulted in improved walking performance (Duncan et al 2003). Subjects were randomly allocated to an exercise group or control group. Those in the exercise group improved significantly more than the control group in cardiorespiratory fitness and their walking velocity and distance.

On a broader note, Potempa et al (1995) described a modest positive relationship between the relative gain in cardiorespiratory fitness and overall improvement in sensorimotor function during rehabilitation. They noted that when increases of VO_{2peak} were correlated against a Disability Index (Fugl-Meyer 1980), training functionally benefited those subjects who were able to exercise at intensities high enough to increase their cardiorespiratory fitness.

In summary, walking performance is usually compromised following stroke. Cardiorespiratory fitness training, performed either alone or as part of a multifaceted exercise programme, leads to improved walking ability with greater efficiency over longer distances and at a faster gait velocity.

Psychosocial improvement

The prevalence of depression is high among persons after stroke and, unlike other psychological problems, the depression is unlikely to be due to the location of the lesion (Carota et al 2002). Symptoms associated with diagnostic criteria for depression include insomnia, fatigue or loss of energy, feelings of worthlessness and a diminished ability to think or concentrate. Brinkmann and Hoskins (1979) provided evidence in a small sample of stroke subjects that some symptoms of depression may be influenced by aerobic exercise. Their particular interest was the effect of aerobic exercise on self-concept, as it influenced one's attitudes and behaviour. In this study, seven people with chronic stroke cycled at an intensity equivalent to 70% of the age-predicted maximal heart rate over 12 weeks. Six subjects attended regularly and completed the study. Following training, their predicted cardiorespiratory fitness was increased by two-thirds of initial values, and some measures of their self-concept returned to within 'normal' profiles. Especially marked were enhanced self-valuation and more positive self-attitudes held by the individuals following training.

A 12-week health promotion programme that consisted of fitness instruction and exercise, nutrition education and health behaviour changes also resulted in significant improvement in several psychological outcome measures associated with depression, including feelings of fatigue, 'blues', no interest in things and feeling that 'everything is an effort' (Rimmer et al 2000a). The exercise programme ranged from 45 to 70 minutes and included a 20–30-minute aerobic training component.

In our current randomized clinical trial of aerobic versus strength training, quality of life is assessed with the SF36 instrument (Hobart et al 2002) and the Stroke Impact Scale (Duncan et al 1999). In this prospective study of therapeutic exercise, all subjects attend training sessions three times per week over 10 weeks at our research centre. Individuals are randomly allocated to one of four arms of the study:

1. sham progressive resistance training (PRT) + sham aerobic training;
2. sham PRT + aerobic training;
3. PRT + sham aerobic training;
4. PRT + aerobic training.

At any one time, 4–6 subjects are at the centre, with cohorts of 10–14 attending daily. Regardless of which group the subjects were allocated to, quality of life scores have significantly improved. For example, the domains within the Stroke Impact Scale that significantly improved included strength, memory and thinking, mood and emotion, thinking, mobility and recovery from stroke, as well as the total score.

Quality of life was assessed using the Nottingham Health Profile following a 12-week exercise programme (Texeira-Salmela et al 1999). This scale assesses the individual's perceived level of distress in six domains, including physical ability, energy level, pain, emotional reactions, sleeplessness and social isolation. Similarly to other exercise trials, after 12 weeks of training the quality of life measures for the group (n = 13) showed a significant improvement of ~78% over pretraining baseline values.

These data would suggest that cardiorespiratory fitness training and the attendant socialization process that occurs when undertaking exercise with a cohort of similarly minded people affected by stroke has strong psychosocial impact. It would be interesting to assess whether subjects increase their physical activity patterns as a result of these training programmes – that is, does such exercise have habitual psychosocial 'carry over' effects to community life?

Carry over to primary impairments of weakness and loss of coordination

The primary aim of cardiorespiratory training, using lower limb muscles, is not to address either of the two primary impairments following stroke, that is, weakness and loss of dexterity. However, by the very nature of the tasks employed to address aerobic fitness, such exercise may have a 'transfer of training effect' onto the primary impairments. Hamstring and quadriceps muscle torques increased after a 3-month treadmill walking programme aimed at improving aerobic fitness (Smith et al 1998, 1999). Not only did subjects' fitness improve, but the eccentric and concentric torques produced by the quadriceps and hamstring muscles of the affected leg also significantly increased.

Loss of coordination for tasks such as walking may improve as a result of aerobic fitness training, particularly when a treadmill is used. Comparison of gait patterns from baseline measures with those after 10–12 weeks of training has revealed that subjects not only walk further, but there is a small trend towards a more symmetrical gait pattern (Silver et al 2000). To date, this crossover effect from treadmill training has not been fully investigated as there has been a reliance on measures of velocity and walking distance to reflect improvements. Physiotherapists and clinical biomechanists have been moving away from these measures in favour of temporal and spatial measures of gait. For

example, within our current randomized clinical trial of therapeutic exercise, subjects walk along a 9-m instrumented walkway during their assessments of self-selected gait velocity and
during their 6-minute walk test. During the 6-minute walk, data
are collected during the initial minute, halfway through the test
and during the final minute. From these data, we determine
whether subjects walk 'steadier' as a result of aerobic or strength
training.

CARDIORESPIRATORY EXERCISE PRESCRIPTION AND PROGRAMMING

A structured exercise
programme is
required

If one of the broad aims of rehabilitation soon after stroke is to
improve cardiorespiratory fitness, it needs to be specifically structured within the rehabilitation context. Evidence that current rehabilitation after stroke is not sufficiently potent to confer an aerobic
'stressor' has come from two studies.

Aerobic fitness and walking ability were assessed in 10 subjects
4 weeks post stroke and then 6–7 weeks later (Kelly et al 2000).
The subjects were in-patients at a rehabilitation centre, and were
receiving physiotherapy based loosely on the Motor Relearning
Program (Carr and Shepherd 1982) for approximately 1.5 hours a
day. In addition, they received other therapies, including occupational and speech therapy, as needed. Symptom-limited VO_{2peak}
did not change significantly between assessments during their
rehabilitation, being 1.17 ± 0.41 l/min and 1.23 ± 0.54 l/min at 4
and 11 weeks respectively. In contrast, the patients' walking velocity and 6-minute distance were significantly improved. Self-selected and maximal walking velocities, measured over a 10-m
distance, increased by 0.21 m/s and 0.28 m/s. Average 6-minute
walk distance also improved significantly by 77 ± 67 m, from an
initial distance of 292 ± 89 m to a final value of 369 ± 100 m.
Improvements in walking ability and endurance reflected the
focus of in-patient rehabilitation, that is, improvement in functional
outcomes.

Further evidence that current rehabilitation practice may be
insufficient to drive beneficial cardiorespiratory adaptations has
been suggested by a study in which heart rate was monitored
while patients received physiotherapy and occupational therapy
(MacKay-Lyons and Makrides 2002a). Individuals ($n = 20$) wore
heart rate monitors bi-weekly for 14 weeks during their therapy sessions. Neither physiotherapy nor occupational therapy
significantly stressed the cardiorespiratory system for extended
periods of time. For example, the average time per physiotherapy
session in which the heart rate was in the cardiorespiratory fitness

'training zone' was low (2.8 ± 0.9 min). Notably, as the patients were considered 'deconditioned' the training zone was set arbitrarily low, in the range of 40–85% HR_{max}. The physical activities that were coupled with elevating heart rate over 40% HR_{max} were associated with standing and walking.

Screening before commencement of training

In developing an aerobic exercise programme for patients soon after stroke, it is important to recognize that these patients are considered at high risk of a 'cardiac event'. The American College of Sports Medicine (Franklin 2000) has developed screening protocols for different populations, including those with pre-existing cardiomyopathy and known or suspected CAD. We advise adherence to these screening protocols for both assessment of cardiorespiratory fitness as well as for exercise training in subacute and chronic stroke. Before participation in an exercise test, all potential subjects should be medically assessed, and have undergone a resting 12-lead electrocardiogram (ECG). In our studies, in-patients are assessed by medical staff within the rehabilitation unit, with ECG interpretation performed by a clinician experienced in such analysis. In contrast, subjects who are living at home are referred to their general practitioner or to a diagnostic clinic for the prescreening ECG. During the maximal effort exercise tests, a medical practitioner is present and a 'crash cart' located nearby.

A maximal effort test is important for two main diagnostic outcomes. First, maximal exercise may reveal ECG abnormalities not observed on the resting 12-lead ECG. Our prudent view is that any exercise-induced ECG abnormalities (or other signs and symptoms of exertional intolerance) are better discovered during medically supervised pretraining assessment than during less monitored conditions of exercise in the physiotherapy clinic. Second, to establish the heart rate range within which a person may safely exercise, knowledge of symptom-limited or peak heart rate is valuable. For example, after stroke, if a 62-year-old man only achieves a maximal heart rate of 83 beats/min during a maximal effort test, the exercise prescription can only be at an intensity below that level. Training at 50% of age-predicted heart rate reserve would probably be lower than his peak heart rate [e.g. (220 – age) – resting heart rate × 0.5]; however, 70% age-predicted heart rate reserve might exceed an exercise heart rate for which he has been previously cleared. To progress this person during training from 50% of age-predicted heart rate reserve, a second maximal effort test would be necessary. In our 10-week randomized clinical trial of exercise therapy, subjects are reassessed during week 7.

Criteria for commencing a training programme

In general, inclusion criteria for cardiorespiratory exercise training should first establish that patients are deemed medically safe to undertake vigorous exercise (Franklin 2000) (see preceding section). In addition, we require our subjects who have had a stroke to achieve at least a score of 3 out of 6 on the walking category of the Motor Assessment Scale (Carr et al 1985) (i.e. walk 3 m unassisted, but may use a walking aid). With that as one criterion, the distance walked over 6 minutes at the time of their initial assessment has ranged between 45 and 507 m for patients attending our centre. Other researchers have specified that subjects were required to walk at least 3 minutes at a velocity of 0.22 m/s or greater (Macko et al 2001), able to sit on an exercise cycle (Brinkmann and Hoskins 1979), able to walk 15.24 m (50 feet) in an unspecified time (Rimmer et al 2000a, 2000b), able to walk 7.62 m (25 feet) (Duncan et al 2003) or were greater than Stage 3 of the Chedoke–McMaster Stage of recovery (Mackay-Lyons and Makrides 2002). If a person cannot achieve these criteria, the emphasis for this older and frail cohort should be on increasing muscle power and strength (Mazzeo et al 1998; see also Chapters 4 and 5).

Choice of exercise mode

Ideally, exercises selected for cardiorespiratory training must utilize the large muscles of the lower limbs and trunk (Franklin 2000). People affected mildly by stroke are probably able to use the traditional equipment found in commercial gyms for cardiorespiratory fitness training. In addition to traditional stationary cycles and treadmills, the mildly impaired might use stepping machines, vertical climbers or elliptical trainers. These devices do not require subjects to lift their feet off the footplates and so may, in fact, be safer than treadmill walking. For the individual with moderately impaired lower limbs, the challenge is to identify an exercise modality that can be undertaken, and yet not encourage maladaptive strategies.

In practice, treadmill walking (with or without partial body weight support), overground walking and stationary cycling all present particular advantages and disadvantages. Treadmill and overground walking may have high task specificity to community-based ambulation, but suffer from the requisite speed of gait necessary to elicit an adequate cardiorespiratory stress for fitness training (Duncan et al 1998). Stationary or recumbent cycling is safe for patients with balance disorders and removes the need to support body mass during aerobic training, but the cross-transfer of cycle training to gait is unknown – the single study cited previously (Kelly et al 2000) is the only example of a positive cross-training effect shown. Another factor that will influence the choice of exercise mode is the minimum setting available on the equipment; many treadmills and exercise cycles are not appropriate for a moderately impaired person because they do not cater for weak or very slow performances. Community ambulation may also not be appropriate, as Duncan et al (1998) noted that people affected mildly and moderately after stroke were unable to perform this activity at sufficient intensity and duration to challenge their cardiorespiratory system. Ultimately, the choice of exercise for aerobic training is dependent on the patient's status and equipment available.

For our training studies after stroke (Kelly et al 2000), we have used an isokinetic cycle ergometer with success. Subjects are required to demonstrate some strength and coordination of their leg muscles to use the isokinetic exercise cycle, but its primary advantage over traditional stationary cycle ergometers is its ability to permit very low power outputs as well as affected to unaffected side inequities.

Exercise prescription

Based on reports from the previous literature (Bachynski-Cole and Cumming 1985, Macko et al 2001, Potempa et al 1995, Rimmer et al 2000b, Teixeira-Salmela et al 1999) as well as the American College of Sports Medicine guidelines (Franklin 2000), it is possible to make some recommendations about exercise prescription after stroke. Table 7.1 summarizes the basic exercise prescription principles.

One caveat is to give careful consideration to the population's risk of misadventure due to unstable hypertension, cardiac disease comorbidity and the general advanced age or frailty of most people affected by stroke. In his review, Roth (1993) pointed out that up to three-quarters of people affected by stroke might have comorbid clinical or asymptomatic CAD, and others (Potempa et al 1996, Roth 1993) have suggested a high prevalence of myocardial perfusion defects in the population. As most people with subacute stroke may have elevated blood pressures at rest and during physical exertion, patients need to be carefully monitored during the first 3–4 weeks of their exercise programme (American College of Sports Medicine Committee on Certification and Education 1999, Rimmer et al 2000b). In particular, Rimmer et al (2002) have proposed blood pressure guidelines of a resting diastolic pressure under 100 mmHg to commence exercising, and exercise termination if blood pressures exceed 220/110 mmHg during cardiorespiratory training.

Of the major components of a clinical exercise prescription (Table 7.1), exercise intensity has received the most attention. In recent years, there has been a growing practice to prescribe

Table 7.1   Recommended dose of aerobic exercise after stroke.

Programme component	Subacute stroke		Chronic stroke	
	Threshold[a]	Recommended[b]	Threshold[a]	Recommended[b]
Frequency	2 times weekly	2–3 times weekly	2–3 times weekly	3–4 times weekly
Intensity	>40% Vo_{2peak}, 40% HRR[c]	>50% Vo_{2peak}, >50% HRR[c]	40–50% Vo_{2peak}, 40–50% HRR[c]	>60% Vo_{2peak}, >60% HRR[c], RPE[d] 12–14
Duration	Minimum 15 min	30+min	Minimum 20 min	30–45 min
Mode	Interval training	Interval training proceeding to continuous exercise	Interval training	Continuous exercise
Type	Isokinetic cycling, PBWS[e] - treadmill walking	Stationary cycling (semirecumbent or upright), isokinetic cycling, treadmill or overground walking, elliptical stepping	Treadmill walking (if needed PBWS[e]), isokinetic cycling, stationary cycling (semirecumbent or upright), overground walking, elliptical stepping	Treadmill walking, overground walking, isokinetic cycling, stationary cycling (semirecumbent or upright), elliptical stepping, other types for leg muscles based on patient preference
Monitoring	ECG, heart rate, blood pressures (3–5 min), signs and symptoms[f], RPE[d]	ECG (if appropriate), heart rate, blood pressures, signs and symptoms[f], RPE[d]	Heart rate, blood pressures (3–5 min), RPE[d]	Heart rate, blood pressures, RPE[d]
Comments				RPE[d] 12–14 ('Somewhat hard') may be used with experienced patients to estimate an appropriate exercise intensity (Borg 1998)

[a]Generally defined as the minimum 'dose' of an exercise programme component to elicit a gain of cardiorespiratory fitness in previously sedentary patients.
[b]Generally defined as the 'optimum dose' of an exercise programme component to elicit a gain of cardiorespiratory fitness in patients currently undertaking exercise.
[c]Heart rate reserve ($HR_{peak} - HR_{REST}$).
[d]Rating of perceived exertion (Borg 1998).
[e]Partial body weight supported.
[f]For example, clinical symptoms of exertional intolerance, dyspnoea, chest pain, pallor, nausea, headache or other symptoms associated with unstable hypertension.

exercise intensity on the basis of 'heart rate reserve' instead of a fixed percentage of HR_{max} or % VO_{2peak} (Franklin 2000). Heart rate reserve (HRR) is calculated as the difference between age-predicted (or measured) peak HR and the observed resting HR. The fractional component of HRR bears a close relationship to the fractional elevation of VO_2 reserve (i.e. $VO_{2peak} - VO_{2REST}$) in the range of 25–85% $V_{O_{2peak}}$. Thus, HRR presents a superior method for assigning intensity within an exercise prescription based on heart rate. For example, after stroke, a 60-year-old female with peak HR of 150 beats/min and resting HR of 80 beats/min would possess an HRR of 70 beats/min. If her exercise prescription was recommended to be at an intensity of 60% V_{O_2} reserve from her preceding exercise test, this would be equivalent to an HRR-derived training heart rate of ~122 beats/min (calculated from [peak HR − HR_{REST}] × 0.60 + HR_{REST}). HRR-established exercise prescription is free of 'floor effects', prevalent when using HR_{max} to determine aerobic training heart rate (i.e. a low fixed %HR_{max} assumes that the patient could exercise at an HR below his or her resting heart rate), or 'ceiling effects', when $V_{O_{2peak}}$ is very low in proportion to resting V_{O_2}.

A further complication for exercise prescription after stroke is the difficulty in prescribing an appropriate exercise intensity based on heart rate or heart rate reserve when patients are pharmacologically managed. Some medications (e.g. beta-blockers, some calcium-channel blockers, most antiadrenergic agents) reduce exercise heart rate or blunt cardioacceleration during exercise onset and in steady-state effort (Franklin 2000). People on these medications have been typically excluded from participating in research studies as outcome measures have usually included training-induced changes of heart rate; however, use of cardioactive medications does not preclude participation in an aerobic exercise programme. Some alternative approaches to prescribing exercise intensity have been proposed, for example, rating of perceived exertion (RPE) in the range 12–14 (Borg 1998), but RPE descriptions of 'somewhat hard' may be misunderstood or misreported by elderly people affected by stroke. Others have proposed using an age-adjusted heart rate, for example 85% × [220 − age] (MacKay-Lyons and Makrides 2001), although this approach is problematical, because it does not take into consideration heart rate 'floor effects'. An alternative for patients on beta-blockers or antiadrenergic agents is to set their exercise intensity using systolic blood pressure criteria. The heart rate reserve equation can be modified for such individuals, or with any person for whom blood pressure control is the most important determinant for exercise intensity, by using systolic blood pressure (SBP) responses derived from a maximal effort exercise test (Franklin 2000): Training SBP = [(SBP_{max} − SBP_{REST}) × 0.5 − 0.8] + SBP_{REST}. The best approach is probably a combination of routine monitoring of 'feelings', careful attendance to a prescribed cycle power output and conjoint use of RPE + heart rate to maintain the target exercise intensity. For this purpose, and for reasons of medical safety, we recommend each patient keep a training journal wherein the details of their exercise prescription are recorded on a daily basis.

Which patient responses are monitored and how much monitoring is appropriate represent a trade-off between prudent medical surveillance and pragmatic issues for the physiotherapist. At a minimum, HR must be monitored during all training sessions so that exercise intensity (i.e. walking speed, cycle power output) can be modified to keep the patient in the desired range. Blood pressures should be measured during the first week, and at random intervals in the next 2–4 weeks of exercise training, or when patients display signs or symptoms of exertional intolerance during an exercise session. Exercise termination criteria for blood pressures should be clearly established a priori, so that patients do not exceed 220/110 mmHg (Rimmer and Nicola 2002) or 240/110 (Franklin 2000) during cardiorespiratory training. The ECG may be monitored in some patients, particularly if the exercise stress test ECG was borderline negative (e.g. nearly 1.5 mV ST-segment depression, less than 6 VPBs/min, etc.; Franklin 2000), but clinicians trained in ECG diagnosis should be available for these patients.

Implementation of training regimens

In general, subjects have been encouraged to train for 20–40 minutes, three sessions per week, for 10 or more weeks. In the first few weeks of training, the target heart rate is relatively low (e.g. 40–50% of heart rate reserve), and as the person becomes habituated to exercise, exercise intensity may be progressed to about 70% of HRR. Feedback regarding heart rate is generally provided using a heart rate monitor. Heart rate monitors range from basic inexpensive models that provide the instantaneous heart rate to sophisticated and expensive models that store data collected over training sessions and can interface with computers.

Some individuals may be unable to sustain 30–45 minutes of continuous physical activity. For those persons, interval training programmes can be employed. In our 10-week randomized clinical trial of aerobic versus strength training, the majority of subjects undergoing cycling exercise typically required interval training for the first 2 weeks, with progressively fewer intervals over these initial weeks. By the third week of training, the majority of subjects were able to cycle continuously for 30 minutes. Figure 7.4 portrays the power output from a sample of sessions over the 10-week training programme and the number of rest periods required from two people moderately affected by stroke, taken from our current randomized clinical trial. Subject A walked 79 m in 6 minutes at her baseline assessment, whereas subject B walked 94 m. Two major improvements that are notable

Figure 7.4   Power output, averaged over the 30 minutes of training from individual training sessions. Data shown are from two moderately disabled stroke subjects. Box plots from single sessions of training display the median, interquartile ranges and whiskers for the 10th and 90th percentiles. The diamonds indicate the number of rests required to achieve 30 minutes of training for that session. Subject A required 14 rests at the first session, 9 at the second, and was able to cycle continuously by the 20th session. Subject B required three rests in the first session, and none by the 15th session. Subjects improved in both absolute power output and the consistency with which they cycled, suggested by the smaller interquartile ranges.

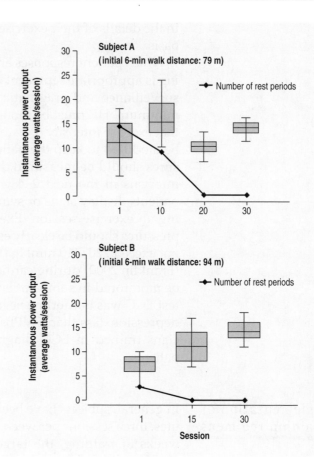

are: (1) the reduced number of recovery intervals required to complete a 30-minute training session and (2) the progressively higher power output at which the subjects cycled over time. In our training programme, we have kept the pedal cadence constant (40 r.p.m.) and increased resistance, in contrast to Duncan et al (2003) who used a standardized progression in which both speed and resistance increased.

Finally, there may be a useful trade-off between exercise intensity and duration that might benefit specific patients' aerobic fitness goals. Some individuals may prefer to exercise at the low end of their HRR-derived exercise intensity range to focus on longer durations of exercise. The 'total exercise dose' is the product of intensity and duration, so reinforcing this option may encourage continued patient participation – a primary goal of any cardiorespiratory fitness programme.

FUTURE DIRECTIONS FOR CARDIORESPIRATORY EXERCISE TRAINING

Certain kinds of assistive technology can significantly increase the potency of the cardiorespiratory exercise response and should be considered as a component of exercise prescription. These technologies include partial body weight support gait training, isokinetic cycling, use of biofeedback to 'pace' exercise intensity and use of functional electrical stimulation devices to aid walking speed.

Partial body weight support (PBWS) gait training

In the motor learning and sports literature, the importance of task specificity in training has been well accepted. Carr and Shepherd (1982) pioneered the application of task specificity during training in stroke rehabilitation. Based on task specificity, overground or treadmill walking is preferable to cycle ergometry to achieve outcomes of community ambulation. Furthermore, PBWS-treadmill training has demonstrated that overground walking speed and endurance can be restored (Hesse et al 1994) or significantly improved (Visintin et al 1998) after stroke. However, limiting factors in the use of treadmill walking are issues related to patient safety and the deterioration of gait quality while walking at velocities high enough to promote cardiorespiratory fitness. MacKay-Lyons and Makrides (2002b) addressed the issue of safety in testing persons soon after their stroke. They found that 15% BWS via an overhead suspension did not change the endpoints of testing in a neurologically normal cohort (MacKay-Lyons et al 2001), and so used this method with a group of subacute people affected by stroke (MacKay-Lyons and Makrides 2002b). With 15% BWS, the subjects' gait velocity ranged from 0.39 ± 0.12 m/s at the initial stage to 0.54 ± 0.30 m/s at the final stage of a symptom-limited exercise test. To date, although PBWS training has been used with some success for rehabilitation after stroke (Hesse et al 1994, Visintin et al 1998) and other neurological conditions (especially incomplete spinal cord injury and cerebral palsy – Barbeau et al 1999, Harkema 2001, Richards et al 1997), the desire for higher exercise intensities or longer durations available with PBWS-treadmill training versus the negative sequelae of poor gait mechanics remains unresolved. In our view, soon after stroke when the focus of rehabilitation is on improving the quality and quantity of gait, training that might reinforce maladaptive behaviours should be avoided; thus, for the moderately impaired individual soon after stroke, treadmill walking may not be the appropriate selection for aerobic training. In contrast, for people with chronic stroke with gait deficits that have been resistant to improvement, treadmill training might be a useful adjunct therapy to promote cardiorespiratory fitness.

Isokinetic cycling   The cycle ergometer that we use in our research is particularly good for people after stroke. It is an electronically braked isokinetic (i.e. constant-velocity) ergometer, which by its construction, can precisely measure power output (with ± 2 W resolution; Fornusek et al 2004) up to ~180 W over a range of cycling velocities between 5 r.p.m. and 60 r.p.m. (Figure 7.5a). The advantages of this bike are several, with specific features that are useful to a population who wish to undertake aerobic exercise after stroke. First, by virtue of its motorized design, it will passively move the affected leg forwards if the person does not apply sufficient pressure to the pedal. Second, with the addition of biofeedback software running on a laptop computer (described below), the cycle can measure affected:unaffected leg power outputs in real time. This feature permits the patient to train at a specific power output appropriate to their desired exercise intensity prescription, while consciously matching leg forces produced by affected and unaffected limbs (Figure 7.5b). Finally, the cycle, being isokinetic, can be used either to train at high pedal cadences (40–60 r.p.m.) appropriate for cardiorespiratory exercise, or to slow pedal cadences (5–20 r.p.m.) for emphasis on leg strength development.

(a)   (b)

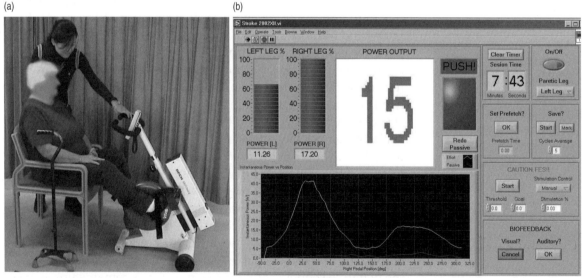

Figure 7.5   Cardiorespiratory isokinetic cycle training. (a) Overview of subject training using the isokinetic mode of the cycle ergometer. The affected leg is strapped to the calf support as well as the foot pedal. (b) The screen from the computer interface displays the total power output achieved by the individual, averaged over three cycles, in large easy-to-read numbers. In addition, the proportion of power produced by each leg is displayed, with the power produced from the unaffected leg represented as 100% and that from the affected leg represented as a percentage of the unaffected leg. The signal to 'push' is displayed sufficiently early to enable the individual to achieve peak force at the appropriate time in the cycle. On the right are the settings used to interface with the electrical stimulator to produce a stronger quadriceps contraction than the person is able to achieve voluntarily. Lastly, the instantaneous power output is graphically displayed.

Biofeedback-paced
cycling

We have identified three problems that can occur during cycling in people affected by stroke who have moderately impaired lower limbs. The first problem, and the easiest to address, is that the foot and leg may require assistance in maintaining the correct alignment. A pillow placed along the outside of the thigh will prevent the thigh from falling into external rotation, and calf supports with foot straps can keep the lower limb in place. Second, peak forces may be exerted on the pedals at inappropriate times during the pedal cycle. The individual may be slow in building up their leg force, such that muscle contractions (usually quadriceps) occur too late during the 'push' phase of cycling to effectively accelerate the pedal forwards for equal bilateral torque production. Thus, the unaffected limb receives relatively greater stress than the affected limb for a given power output. This problem probably reflects the decreased rate of torque development that can occur as a consequence of a stroke (Canning et al 1999). Tena et al (2002) overcame this problem by designing biofeedback software that displayed the instantaneous right and left leg power outputs, and elicited a visual + auditory biofeedback signal to 'cue' the individual when to push against the pedals (Figure 7.5b). The signal occurred 83 ms before the time when the subject was required to push, to allow for delayed reaction and movement times in this population. In the clinical environment, a metronome might be used to cue a patient when to push.

The third problem is the inability of some people affected by stroke to produce sufficient power output due to weakness of their quadriceps on the affected side. To address this problem, Tena et al (2002) also piloted a laboratory-grade skin surface functional electrical stimulation (FES) system that was triggered by exceeding a preset instantaneous torque threshold. The FES unit was controlled by the same 'virtual instrument' that provided feedback regarding the instantaneous power output and when to commence pushing with the affected leg. In a manner similar to use of commercial EMG-triggered neuromuscular stimulators, subjects were required to exceed a preset threshold prior to the FES unit activating to evoke larger peak torques than the individual was capable of producing voluntarily. Isokinetic synchronous force matching plus biofeedback pacing of the 'push' phase increased total power output in two of four chronic stroke subjects, and the addition of FES further augmented power output in these two individuals (Figure 7.6). In three of the four individuals, exercise heart rates were increased using biofeedback pacing by 4 beats/min, and using pacing plus FES by 8 beats/min, although the results for the fourth subject were equivocal. Clearly, interindividual differences exist within the stroke population with respect to biofeedback pacing of movement and FES tolerance, so further

Figure 7.6   Change in total power output under varying conditions of isokinetic cycling for four people with chronic stroke. Voluntary cycling (dark blue bars) is compared with addition of biofeedback pacing of force production (visual + auditory 'cues'; mid-blue bars) and with biofeedback plus function electrical stimulation (FES)-evoked muscle contractions (light blue bars). In subjects 3 and 4, power output increased with the addition of biofeedback and further increased with the addition of FES.

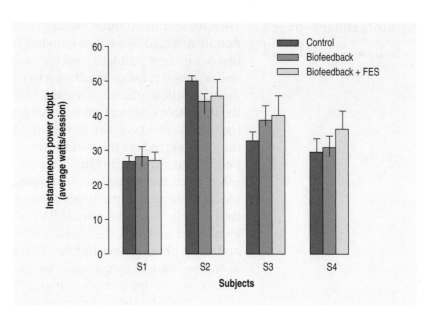

research is required before these techniques are widely deployed to augment cardiorespiratory fitness.

Odstock FES system to promote faster walking

A more traditional use of functional electrical stimulation (FES), with the primary purpose of reducing foot-drop gait, has been suggested as helpful for cardiorespiratory fitness training. Taylor et al (1999) undertook a randomized control trial of 111 stroke subjects who used the Odstock dropped foot stimulator over 4.5 months. The authors observed that self-selected gait velocity significantly increased by 27%. These data suggest that increasing the gait velocity by using the Odstock FES system may be a useful intervention during cardiorespiratory training, because Duncan et al (1998) identified slow gait velocity and poor walking endurance as limiting factors for community-based aerobic fitness conditioning.

CONCLUSION

One of Janet Carr and Roberta Shepherd's enduring legacies was to demand change in rehabilitation practice based on current scientific evidence. There is now a body of evidence that indicates cardiorespiratory fitness is impaired soon after stroke, and it does not improve with rehabilitation or over time. There is also evidence that this impairment is amenable to aerobic training, either in a cardiorespiratory fitness programme alone (Davis et al 2003, Macko et al 2001, Potempa et al 1995), or preferably in a conditioning programme that combines cardiorespiratory and strength-resistance training (Duncan et al 2003, Rimmer et al 2000b, Teixeira-Salmela et al 2001). Moderately disabled persons who have survived a stroke are capable of exercising for 30 minutes, and up to 90 minutes in fitness programmes that include both aerobic and resistance training components (Duncan et al 2003). Not only does cardiorespiratory fitness improve, but quality of life and other physical factors, such as mobility and strength, are also augmented. Thus, it would appear timely for cardiorespiratory training programmes to be fully integrated as a necessary component of post-morbid rehabilitation, with the expectation that patients would continue to receive the benefits of exercise after discharge.

ACKNOWLEDGEMENTS

We would like to thank our colleagues, Dr Brian Zeman, Dr Jacqui Raymond and Professor Maria Fiatarone Singh, as well as our students, Ms Joanna Kelly, Ms Mi-Joung Lee and Mr Raphael Tena, who have contributed to our research projects. In addition, our work has been supported by research grants from National Health and Medical Research Council and NSW Brain Foundation.

References

American College of Sports Medicine. Committee on Certification and Education. Health/Fitness Subcommittee 1999 ACSM Health and Fitness Track Certification Study Guide 1999: Exercise Leader, Health/fitness Instructor, Health/fitness Director. Williams and Wilkins, Baltimore.

Bachynski-Cole M, Cumming G R 1985 The cardiovascular fitness of disabled patients attending occupational therapy. Occupational Therapy Journal of Research 5:233–242.

Barbeau H, Ladouceur M, Norman K et al 1999 Walking after spinal cord injury: evaluation, treatment, and functional recovery. Archives of Physical Medicine and Rehabilitation 80:225–235.

Bjuro T, Fugyl-Meyer A R, Grimby G et al 1975 Ergonomic studies of standardized domestic work in patients with neuromuscular handicap. Scandinavian Journal of Rehabilitation Medicine 7:106–113.

Borg G 1998 Borg's Perceived Exertion and Pain Scales. Human Kinetics Publishers, Champaign, IL.

Bouchard C, Shephard R J, Stephens T et al (eds) 1990 Exercise, fitness and health. A consensus of current knowledge, 3rd edn. Human Kinetics, Champaign, IL.

Brinkmann J R, Hoskins T A 1979 Physical conditioning and altered self-concept in rehabilitated hemipelegic patients. Physical Therapy 59:859–865.

Burke D 1988 Spasticity as an adaptation to pyramidal tract injury. Advances in Neurology 47:401–423.

Canning C G, Ada L, O'Dwyer N 1999 Slowness to develop force contributes to weakness after stroke. Archives of Physical Medicine and Rehabilitation 80:66–70.

Carota A, Staub F, Bogousslavsky J 2002 Emotions, behaviours and mood changes in stroke. Current Opinion in Neurology 15:57–69.

Carr J H, Shephard R J 1982 A motor relearning programme for stroke. Heinemann Medical, London.

Carr J H, Shepherd R B 1998 Neurological rehabilitation: optimizing motor performance. Butterworth-Heinemann, Oxford.

Carr J H, Shepherd R B 2003 Stroke rehabilitation: guidelines for exercise and training to optimize motor skill. Butterworth-Heinemann, New York.

Davis G, Kelly J, Kilbreath S L et al 2003 Home-based exercise training improves walking endurance in chronic stroke patients: a pilot study. Medicine and Science in Sports and Exercise 35(Suppl. 5):S232.

Dean C, Mackey F 1992 Motor assessment scale scores as a measure of rehabilitation outcome following stroke. Australian Journal of Physiotherapy 38:31–35.

Duncan P, Richards L, Wallace D et al 1998 A randomized, controlled pilot study of a home-based exercise program for individuals with mild and moderate stroke. Stroke 29:2055–2060.

Duncan P W, Wallace D, Lai S M et al 1999 The stroke impact scale version 2.0. Evaluation of reliability, validity, and sensitivity to change. Stroke 30:2131–2140.

Duncan P, Studenski S, Richards L et al 2003 Randomized clinical trial of therapeutic exercise in subacute stroke. Stroke 34(9):2173–2180.

Esmonde T, McGinley J, Wittwer J et al 1997 Stroke rehabilitation: patient activity during non-therapy time. Australian Journal of Physiotherapy 43:43–51.

Fletcher B, Dunbar S, Felner J et al 1994 Exercise testing and training in physically disabled men with clinical evidence of coronary artery disease. American Journal of Cardiology 73:1558–1564.

Fornusek C, Davis G, Sinclair P et al 2004 A new Functional Electrical Stimulation cycle ergometer. Journal of Neuromodulation 7:56–74.

Franklin B (ed) 2000 American College of Sports Medicine guidelines for exercise testing and prescription, 6th edn. Williams and Wilkins, Philadelphia.

Fugl-Meyer AR 1980 Post-stroke hemiplegia assessment of physical properties. Scandinavian Journal of Rehabilitation Medicine 7(Suppl.):85–93.

Fujitani J, Ishikawa T, Akai M et al 1999 Influence of daily activity on changes in physical fitness for people with post-stroke hemiplegia. American Journal of Physical Medicine and Rehabilitation 78:540–544.

Gordon J 1987 Assumptions underlying physical therapy intervention: theoretical and historical perspectives. In: Carr J H, Shepherd R B (eds) Movement science: foundations for physical therapy in rehabilitation. Heinemann Physiotherapy, London, pp 1–30.

Halar E 1999 Management of stroke risk factors during the process of rehabilitation. Secondary stroke prevention. Physical Medicine and Rehabilitation Clinics of North America 10:839–856

Harkema S 2001 Neural plasticity after human spinal cord injury: application of locomotor training to the rehabilitation of walking. Neuroscientist 7:455–468.

Hertzer N R, Young J R, Beven E G et al 1985 Coronary angiography in 506 patients with extracranial cerebrovascular disease. Archives of Internal Medicine 145:849–852.

Hesse S, Bertelt C, Schaffrin A et al 1994 Restoration of gait in nonambulatory hemiparetic patients by treadmill training with partial body-weight support. Archives of Physical Medicine and Rehabilitation 75:1087–1093.

Hill K, Ellis P, Bernhardt J et al 1997 Balance and mobility outcomes for stroke patients: a comprehensive audit. Australian Journal of Physiotherapy 43:173–180.

Hobart J C, Williams L S, Moran K et al 2002 Quality of life measurement after stroke: uses and abuses of the SF-36. Stroke 33:1348–1356.

Jakobsson F, Grimby L, Edstrom L 1992 Motoneuron activity and muscle fibre type composition in hemiparesis. Scandinavian Journal of Rehabilitation Medicine 24:115–119.

Kelly J, Kilbreath S L, Davis G et al 2000 Cardiorespiratory fitness and ambulation in acute stroke patients. In: Fifth Scientific Congress, Sydney 2000 Paralympic Games, p 52.

Kelly J, Kilbreath S, Davis G et al 2003 Cardiorespiratory fitness and walking ability in subacute stroke patients. Archives of Physical Medicine and Rehabilitation 84(12):1780–1785.

King M L, Guarracini M, Lennihan L et al 1989 Adaptive exercise testing for patients with hemiparesis. Journal of Cardiopulmonary Rehabilitation 9:237–242.

Landin S, Hagenfeldt L, Saltin B et al 1977 Muscle metabolism during exercise in hemiparetic patients. Clinical Science and Molecular Medicine 53:257–269.

MacKay-Lyons M J, Makrides L 2002a Exercise capacity early after stroke. Archives of Physical Medicine and Rehabilitation 83:1697–1702.

MacKay-Lyons M J, Makrides L 2002b Cardiovascular stress during a contemporary stroke rehabilitation program: is the intensity adequate to induce a training effect? Archives of Physical Medicine and Rehabilitation 83:1378–1383.

MacKay-Lyons M, Makrides L, Speth S 2001 Effect of 15% body weight support on exercise capacity of adults without impairments. Physical Therapy 81:1790–1800.

Mackey F, Ada L, Heard R et al 1996 Stroke rehabilitation: are highly structured units more conducive to physical activity than less structured units? Archives of Physical Medicine and Rehabilitation 77:1066–1070.

Macko R F, DeSouza C A, Tretter L D et al 1997a Treadmill aerobic exercise training reduces the energy expenditure and cardiovascular demands of hemiparetic gait in chronic stroke patients. A preliminary report. Stroke 28:326–330.

Macko R F, Katzel L I, Yataco A et al 1997b Low-velocity graded treadmill stress testing in hemiparetic stroke patients. Stroke 28:988–992.

Macko R F, Smith G V, Dobrovolny C L et al 2001 Treadmill training improves fitness reserve in chronic stroke patients. Archives of Physical Medicine and Rehabilitation 82:879–884.

Mayo N E, Wood-Dauphinee S, Ahmed S et al 1999 Disablement following stroke. Disability and Rehabilitation 21:258–268.

Mazzeo R, Cavanaugh P, Evans W et al 1998 American College of Sports Medicine Position Stand: exercise and physical activity for older adults. Medicine and Science in Sports and Exercise 30:992–1008.

Moldover J R, Daum M C, Downey J A 1984 Cardiac stress testing of hemiparetic patients with a supine bicycle ergometer: preliminary study. Archives of Physical Medicine and Rehabilitation 65:470–473.

Monga T N, Deforge D A, Williams J et al 1988 Cardiovascular responses to acute exercise in patients with cerebrovascular accidents. Archives of Physical Medicine and Rehabilitation 69:937–940.

Olney S J, Monga T N, Costigan P A 1986 Mechanical energy of walking of stroke patients. Archives of Physical Medicine and Rehabilitation 67:92–98.

Potempa K, Lopez M, Braun L T et al 1995 Physiological outcomes of aerobic exercise training in hemiparetic stroke patients. Stroke 26:101–105.

Potempa K, Braun L T, Tinknell T et al 1996 Benefits of aerobic exercise after stroke. Sports Medicine 21:337–346.

Ragnarsson K T 1988 Physiological effects of functional electrical stimulation-induced exercises in spinal cord-injured individuals. Clinical Orthopaedics 126:53–63.

Richards C, Malouin F, Dumas F et al 1997 Early and intensive treadmill locomotor training for young children with cerebral palsy: a feasibility study. Pediatric Physical Therapy 9:158–165.

Rimmer J H, Nicola T 2002 Stroke. In: Myers J, Herbert W, Humphrey R (eds) ACSM's resources for clinical exercise physiology: musculoskeletal, neuromuscular, neoplastic, immunologic, and hematologic conditions. Lippincott, Williams and Wilkins, Baltimore, pp 2–15.

Rimmer J H, Braunschweig C, Silverman K et al 2000a Effects of a short term health promotion intervention for a predominantly African-American group of stroke survivors. American Journal of Preventative Medicine 18:332–338.

Rimmer J H, Riley B, Creviston B et al 2000b Exercise training in a predominantly African-American group of stroke survivors. Medicine and Science in Sports and Exercise 32:1900–1996.

Roth E J 1993 Heart disease in patients with stroke: incidence, impact, and implications for rehabilitation. Part 1: classification and prevalence. Archives of Physical Medicine and Rehabilitation 74:752–760.

Silver K H C, Macko R F, Forrester L W et al 2000 Effects of aerobic treadmill training on gait velocity, cadence, and gait symmetry in chronic hemiparetic stroke: a preliminary report. Neurorehabilitation and Neural Repair 14:65–71.

Smith G V, Macko R F, Silver K H et al 1998 Treadmill aerobic exercise improves quadriceps strength in patients with chronic hemiparesis following stroke: a preliminary report. Journal of Neurological Rehabilitation 12:111–117.

Smith G V, Silver K H, Goldberg A P et al 1999 'Task-oriented' exercise improves hamstring strength and spastic reflexes in chronic stroke patients. Stroke 30:2112–2118.

Taylor P, Burridge J, Dunkerley A et al 1999 Clinical use of the Odstock dropped foot stimulator: its effect on the speed and effort of walking. Archives of Physical Medicine and Rehabilitation 80:1577–1583.

Teixeira-Salmela L F, Olney S J, Nadeau S et al 1999 Muscle strengthening and physical conditioning to reduce impairment and disability in chronic stroke survivors. Archives of Physical Medicine and Rehabilitation 80:1211–1218.

Teixeira-Salmela L F, Nadeau S, McBride I et al 2001 Effects of muscle strengthening and physical conditioning training on temporal, kinematic and kinetic variables during gait in chronic stroke survivors. Journal of Rehabilitation Medicine 33:53–60.

Tena J, Davis G, Kilbreath S L 2002 Development of an FES biofeedback cycling system for exercise training of hemiplegic stroke patients. In: Cruchley G (ed) From cell to society conference 3. Leura, Australia, Poster 25-11.

Visintin M, Barbeau H, Korner-Bitensky N et al 1998 A new approach to retrain gait in stroke patients through body weight support and treadmill stimulation. Stroke 29:1122–1128.

Wade D, Lanton Hewer R, Skilbeck C et al 1985 Stroke: a critical approach to diagnosis, treatment and management. Chapman and Hall, London.

Waters R L, Lunsford B R, Perry J et al Energy–speed relationship of walking: standard tables. Journal of Orthopaedic Research 6:215–222.

Wolman R, Cornall C 1994 Aerobic training in brain-injured patients. Clinical Rehabilitation 8:253–257.

Zamparo P, Francescato M P, De Luca G et al 1995 The energy cost of level walking in patients with hemiplegia. Scandinavian Journal of Medicine and Science in Sports 5:348–352.

Chapter **8**

Training gait after stroke: a biomechanical perspective

Sandra J. Olney

Although I have spent many years studying walking I am still awed by the intricacy and perfection of this fundamental activity. I am particularly impressed by the balancing of a large upper body on one tiny freely movable point, the hip, with its tenuous toe-tip connection to the ground many centimetres behind while at the same time propelling it forwards. It is no wonder that gait retraining after stroke can be a difficult and demanding venture.

Therapists working with persons who have residual deficits as a result of stroke ask themselves many questions with respect to gait in general and even more in determining the best course of action they should take in re-educating the gait of their clients. In so doing they draw upon not only their own clinical experience but also relevant bodies of literature in motor learning, motor control, exercise physiology and biomechanics. Of these four, I believe biomechanics is the most difficult to apply effectively. There are several reasons for this. First, an overall understanding of the patterns of biomechanical variables of moments, energies and powers throughout the gait cycle is required, and these are not obvious or intuitive. Second, all too often we as researchers publish biomechanical findings with only the bare minimum of discussion devoted to the clinical implications of the findings, leaving the educated practitioner unable to make full use of the findings. Third, although usual deviations from these patterns have been published and give some guidance to general approaches, individual patients display many deviations from these patterns. Gait analyses for individual patients are rarely available for the practitioner to use in determining specific treatment, or for becoming familiar with improvement with treatment.

Several texts give excellent descriptions of gait deviations, their causes and methods of treatment, and readers of this text will be familiar with them (Carr and Shepherd 2003, Olney and Richards 1996, Richards and Olney 1996). Other publications show patterns of energies, joint moments and powers. What is missing is the biomechanical understanding to connect the two, the understanding that permits the therapist to judge how important a particular deficit or deviation is to gait competence, and hence what to emphasize in treatment. This chapter will attempt to address the first and second barriers to understanding. The aim is to provide an overall understanding of the patterns of the biomechanical variables of moments, energies and powers through the gait cycle of people affected by stroke by considering a range of clinical questions, both general and particular, that can be addressed from a biomechanical point of view. Many of the problems discussed are those identified by Carr and Shepherd (2003). Because the direction of progression of walking is our focus of interest, I will concentrate on the sagittal plane. It is the expectation of the author that the biomechanics will be understood as the reader uses it to understand the answers to the questions. This problem-solving approach is the reverse of the usual manner of presentation, but one with which clinicians are particularly comfortable.

GENERAL QUESTIONS ABOUT GAIT

What is good walking?

The therapist and patient must make explicit their aims in achieving walking competence or they run the risk of dispersing efforts counterproductively. Without discussion, aims may not be the same for therapist and patient. There is little disagreement about safety: patients and therapists alike agree that safety must take priority over most other considerations as a result of the high health and personal cost of falls (Stokes and Lindsay 1996, Wilkins 1999). Perhaps the greatest disagreement is between those who uphold the primary aim of gait retraining as 'a good pattern of walking' and those who vote for speed as though they were mutually exclusive. Biomechanically the answer is more subtle than a simple choice and this will be evident in the following discussions.

There are many good arguments to favour speed. Perhaps most obvious is the argument of logic. What is walking for? Most would agree it is to transport the body through one's environment at a pace that permits accomplishment of daily tasks. Although adults can often be persuaded that speed is not of primary importance, we have all had the experience of watching a child dash out of the clinic with all the training in good patterns taking second place to eagerness for the next activity.

A second argument emerges from the fact that walking speed has been found to relate to many measures of disablement, including impairment, function (Friedman 1990), disability (Potter et al 1995) and health outcomes (Cress et al, 1995). Of course the presence of a correlation does not infer a causal relationship, which must be supported by randomized control trials with an intervention directed to increasing walking speed. At least one recent study (Teixeira-Salmela et al 1999) in which speed of walking was targeted in treatment has shown similar gains in health outcomes, and further support awaits completion of relevant research.

A third argument is a biomechanical one showing that normal walking speeds are necessary for walking efficiency and are therefore desirable. The following few paragraphs will give the background needed to make the explanation clear. There are many different motion analysis systems that can give position and timing information about movement of the body in space. Furthermore, anthropometric information such as weights of body parts, locations of centres of mass and moments of inertia can be calculated by proportions of the body of interest using known mathematical constants (Winter 1990). This information is needed to perform the biomechanical analyses that support this argument. Further information may be found in Winter (1990) and Sheirman and Olney (1997).

The total energy of the body at any instant in time is the sum of the energy of each of its parts, which we call 'segments', for example, lower leg, thigh, head, arms and trunk. The energy of each of the segments at any instant in time is the sum of its potential energy (mass × gravitational constant (9.8) × height) and its kinetic energy. Its kinetic energy is the sum of its linear kinetic energy ($\frac{1}{2}$ × mass × velocity^2) and its rotatory kinetic energy ($\frac{1}{2}$ × mass × moment of inertia × angular velocity^2) (Figure 8.1). The masses are obtained by taking a proportion of the person's body weight; the locations of the centres of mass and the moments of inertia are obtained by using constants expressing a proportion of the limb length. Velocities are calculated by dividing the distance between two sequential locations of body markers by the time, and accelerations by dividing the velocities by that time. The potential and kinetic components for each segment are calculated for each instant in time. If either potential or kinetic energy goes up and the other down in two successive instants there has been an exchange between kinetic and potential types and what remains is the net change in energy level of the segment. The total energy of the body is calculated as the sum of the net energies of all the segments for each instant in time, assuming that between-segment transfers occur between segments. The change between the two intervals represents the total energy added to the body over that time (if higher) or absorbed (if lower).

Figure 8.2 shows the total energy of the upper body (at the top), which is the sum of the potential energy portion which varies with height changes (middle) and the kinetic energy portion, which varies with velocity squared (lower). Like a ball rolling down a hill (mid-stance to initial contact) and then going up the next hill (initial contact to mid-stance of the other foot), there is an exchange between kinetic and potential energy. The result is shown in the

Figure 8.1 Simple four-segment link segment model of half-body with links at ankle, knee, hip joint centres and head, arms and trunk bundled into one. PE = potential energy, M = mass, g = gravitational constant, h = height, KE = kinetic energy, v = velocity, I = moment of inertia, ω = angular acceleration.

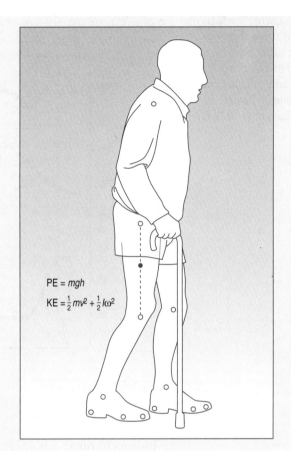

$$PE = mgh$$
$$KE = \tfrac{1}{2}mv^2 + \tfrac{1}{2}I\omega^2$$

total curve – the changes are much smaller than they would be if no exchange had taken place. In other words the exchange promotes efficiency. However, if the speed of walking is low, very little exchange can take place and the person will have much higher total energy costs per metre walked. You can see that in some cases a person walking slowly may be able to walk faster with no extra total energy costs just because they are doing so more efficiently.

Figure 8.3 shows, however, that the total 'ups and downs' of energy generations and absorptions of the upper body are much less than those of the lower limbs, which are the most costly part of gait. Figure 8.3 shows the total energy of the whole body (at the top), which is the sum of the total of the upper body (head, arms and trunk together – middle) and the energy levels of the two lower limbs (bottom).

There are instances in which maintaining a 'good pattern of walking' can be argued. First, walking patterns that put high forces on vulnerable structures are clearly to be avoided; an example of this is the hyperextended knee during stance phase. Furthermore, there are a number of 'good patterns' that are related

Figure 8.2 Energy levels (J) over one gait stride showing total for the upper body (at the top) and its components: potential energy (middle) and the kinetic energy (lower). (From Quanbury et al 1975.)

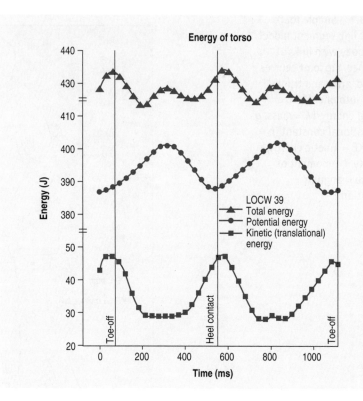

to biomechanical advantages. Although more of these patterns may emerge with further research, the following are supported by current literature:

- avoiding of hip hiking on either side;
- avoiding high limb swing for toe clearance;
- avoiding jerky movements;
- achieving good hip extension in late stance on the affected side;
- achieving dorsiflexion of the ankle during stance phase and good ankle joint excursion during push-off;
- bending the knee at the end of stance (avoiding hyperextension);
- bending the knee and hip during swing phase.

Some of these are discussed below. However, maintaining a pattern for pattern's sake is inherently indefensible.

Are Saunders' 'determinants' in gait still meaningful?

Many gait re-education practices have been based on Saunders' classic paper, 'The major determinants in normal and pathological gait' (Saunders et al 1953). A determinant, by definition, must be causal. In the context of knowledge gained during the last half

Figure 8.3   Energy levels (J) over one gait stride of each of the two lower limbs (bottom), the total of the upper body (middle) and their sum (top). (From Quanbury et al 1975.)

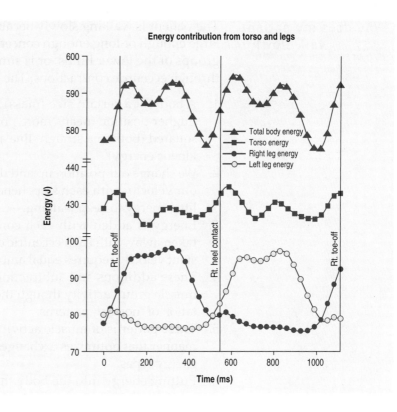

Energy contribution from torso and legs

century, Saunders' determinants should be renamed descriptors. All of the factors identified by Saunders are kinematically based, that is, they are derived from position data. As such they cannot be determinants. They are, rather, descriptors, and should never be mistaken for causes. Saunders' central assumption, that 'the displacement pattern of the centre of gravity may be regarded as constituting the summation or end result of all forces and motions acting upon and concerned with the translation of the body' and his consideration of the limbs as 'weightless levers of the body' contains grave errors. As shown in Figure 8.3, movement of the limbs requires considerably more energy than is reflected in movement of the upper body. The upper body accomplishes considerable savings by exchanging potential and kinetic energy with every step. Assumptions based on Saunders' descriptors, for example, that bending the knee in stance phase decreases the energy costs of walking, are simplistic or misleading at best and incorrect at worst (see below). I am sure Saunders himself would agree that the insight given by current analyses surpasses what was available to him at the time of writing of his classic, but now thoroughly misleading, article. No, they are not meaningful!

Why does my patient walk slowly?

The patient is walking slowly because she or he is not performing large enough or long enough concentric contractions of the muscle groups of the lower limbs, or is simultaneously removing energy through eccentric contractions. The rationale is as follows:

1. A body of a certain size (mass) has energy due to its position (higher position means more potential energy) and its velocity squared (both in a straight line and turning; faster means more kinetic energy).
2. We change our position up and down and increase and decrease our velocity with each step, hence we have to keep putting in a little energy to keep walking.
3. Energy is added with each concentric contraction; energy is taken away with each eccentric contraction. Maintaining a constant velocity requires equal amounts of both.
4. These additions and subtractions occur in typical patterns of muscle group activity though there are many options for adaptation of 'normal' patterns.
5. These patterns of muscle activity occur in normal walking in a manner that optimizes exchanges between potential and kinetic energy types.
6. Putting energy into the body through concentric contractions must result in increase of velocity or increase in height or both unless the energy is removed by eccentric muscle activity.

A direct method for increasing speed, then, is to increase the amplitude and/or the duration of concentric muscle contractions of the lower limbs of either side of the body. This is an unfocused approach, however, and further information will permit a therapist to use a more targeted approach. However, if one simply directs a patient to walk faster, the patient probably intuitively increases the concentric activity of available muscle groups. A second way of increasing speed is to reduce simultaneous eccentric activity.

Which muscle groups perform the work of walking?

To answer this question we need to understand how kinetic information from gait is obtained. We need the spatial information discussed above, as well as the size of the force applied to the foot, its direction and exactly where on the foot it is applied. These are obtained from force plates embedded in the floor. To derive moments (the 'turningness' of muscle groups), we obtain solutions for what forces and moments had to be applied to the foot for it to move in the way it was, hence, that particular mass had that particular acceleration and direction of acceleration. If we isolate the foot as shown in Figure 8.4, basic Newtonian mechanics tells us that the sum of all forces in the direction designated X or Y must equal the

Figure 8.4   Model of the foot for kinetic analysis. Note we have all we need to know to solve for two net forces and one net moment at the ankle if we know masses and positions in space and use anthropometric constants. a, ankle; f, foot; I_f, moment of inertia about the centre of mass of the foot (kg/m^2); m_f, mass of the foot (kg); a_{fX}, horizontal acceleration of the centre of mass of the foot (m/s); a_{fY}, vertical acceleration of the centre of mass of the foot (m/s); ω, angular acceleration of the foot (rad/s). $\Sigma F_X = m_f a_{fX}$, the sum of the forces on the foot in the horizontal direction (= the product of mass and acceleration in the horizontal direction); $\Sigma F_Y = m_f a_{fY}$, the sum of the forces on the foot in the vertical direction (= mass times acceleration in the vertical direction); $\omega \Sigma M = I_f \omega_f$, the sum of the moments on the foot acting about the centre of mass (= moment of inertia times angular acceleration of the foot).

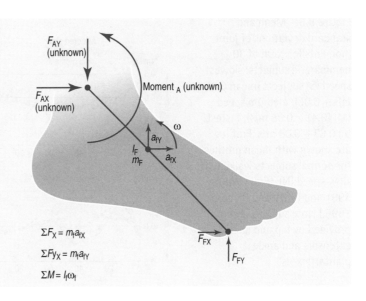

product of the mass and the acceleration in that direction. Likewise the tendency of the body to turn about its centre of mass must equal the product of the moment of inertia (the 'turning' equivalent of mass) and the angular acceleration (rotatory acceleration). Each of these can be derived from measured position information, calculations from it or from using anthropometric constants. The force being impressed from above on the talus and the moments caused by the muscles are derived from these three equations. Note that only one value can be obtained for the muscle moment so if both ankle dorsiflexors and plantarflexors are active this calculation will only 'see' the net effect. Having made the calculation for the ankle, one simply moves up a segment and in exactly the same way deals with the lower leg, etc., one segment at a time. Normal net moments are shown in Figure 8.5, with net moments from people affected by stroke of varying levels of ability walking at three different speeds. Note that the presence of a positive or negative moment about a designated point, the joint, does not necessarily involve any joint angular change.

If a muscle group is exerting a moment across a joint in such a way as to perform a concentric contraction, the energy per unit time (the power) is the product of that moment and the net angular velocity between the two segments. Therefore, if the ankle plantarflexors are plantarflexing the ankle there is positive power generation. Normal powers are shown in Figure 8.6, and Figure 8.7 depicts powers from people affected by stroke of varying levels of ability walking at three different speeds compared with normal. Because power multiplied by time is work, the area under the curve

Figure 8.5 Mean and standard deviations of joint moments for total of 30 hemiparetic subjects: slowest speed (S) subjects (mean 0.25 m/s ± 0.05); medium speed (M) (0.41 ± 0.08 m/s); fastest (F) 0.63 ± 0.08 m/s. Profiles are shown with mean profiles for normal subjects walking at slow speed (N). (From Winter 1991 and Olney and Richards 1996.) Note support is sum, provided by hip and knee extensors and ankle plantarflexors.

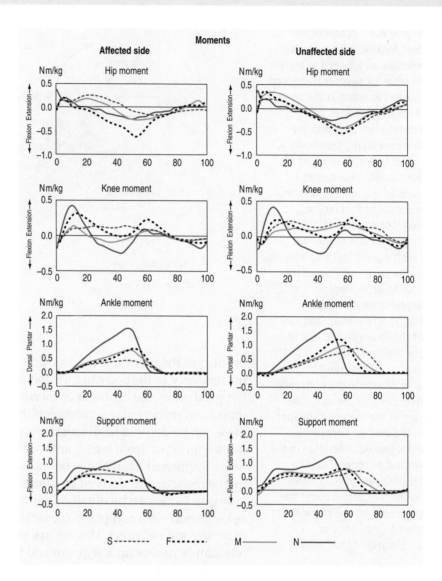

is the work performed, with work gained by the body through concentric contractions shown positively and that which is lost through eccentric or lengthening contractions shown below the line.

Figure 8.7 shows normal power patterns plotted over the gait cycle for the hip, knee and ankle, beginning and ending with initial contact of the foot to the floor for normal subjects. Note at which joint the biggest areas under the curves occur. This is work (power over time). The area occurring above the line is adding to the energy of the body and means that a concentric contraction is being performed by that muscle group. With the scale on the vertical axis kept the same for all joints, it is apparent that there are two ways of getting a bigger area of work – either increase the amplitude or increase the time over which the muscle contraction is

Figure 8.6   Mean and standard deviation of normal power patterns (W/kg) plotted over the gait cycle for the hip, knee and ankle, beginning and ending with initial contact of the foot to the floor. (From Winter 1991.)

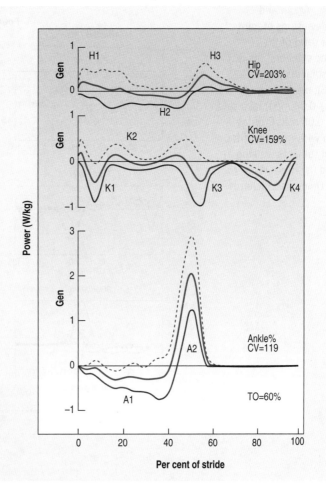

active. This is clinically important. To increase the amplitude we exert a higher level of contraction (force), resulting in a larger moment, or 'turningness', around the joint. Now to return to the original question – at which joint do the biggest areas under the curves occur? Looking first for positive areas, it can be seen that the largest is at the ankle around mid-cycle (A2), and two other important ones occur at the hip, one early in stance (H1) and one a little after mid-cycle (H3). This figure does not tell us whether, for example, the A2 burst is the result of ankle dorsiflexors dorsiflexing or the plantarflexors plantarflexing, and for this we can refer either to the moment or to the joint angle curves. In this case the plantarflexors are turned on and the ankle is plantarflexing; push-off is occurring. Similarly, around the same time at the hip, the hip flexors are on and hip flexion is occurring, and we sometimes refer to this as pull-off. Early in stance the hip extensors are dominant and the hip is extending ('push-from-behind'). Note K2, the result of knee extensors extending, is relatively unimportant. However, a

Figure 8.7 Mean and standard deviations of joint powers for total of 30 hemiparetic subjects: slowest speed (S) subjects (mean 0.25 m/s ± 0.05); medium speed (M) (0.41 ± 0.08 m/s); fastest (F) 0.63 ± 0.08 m/s. Profiles are shown with mean profiles for normal subjects walking at slow speed (N) (from Winter 1991 and Olney and Richards 1996).

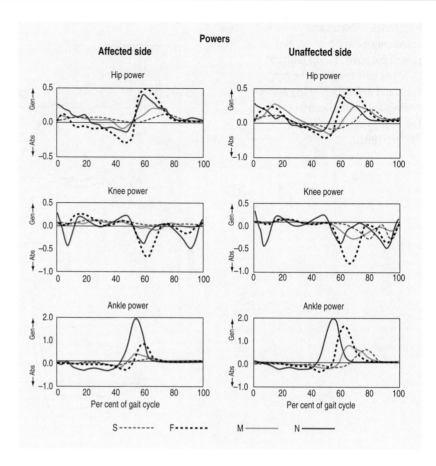

considerable amount of eccentric work or absorption is performed by the knee. Notable is K3, caused by a very small extensor moment at the end of stance while the knee is flexing rapidly. This is mentioned because K3 is often increased in pathologies and, occurring at nearly the same time as A2, is responsible for inefficiency if it is larger than normal. Thus, the answer to the question, 'Which muscle groups perform most of the work of walking?' is the ankle plantarflexors at push-off, the hip flexors at pull-off and the hip extensors in early stance.

Do the muscle groups performing the work of walking change with speed or with age?

In general, increased speed simply 'turns up the gain' of the muscle contractions. Correlations between curves at different speeds, which are measures of their similarity in shape, have been reported to range from 0.87 to 0.99 (Winter 1991, p. 48). There are also differences in timing with which we are familiar – shortening of the stance phase and double-support phase.

Data from older adults have shown that general shape and timing of power profiles is similar to that of younger people. However, two significant differences have been reported. The ankle plantarflexor burst A2 was lower, and the knee absorption power caused by the hamstrings at the end of swing (K4) was lower (Winter 1991, p. 93). The effect of the first is obvious – less work is done by the ankle plantarflexors.

Reduction in K4 results in less slowing of the swinging leg, with the result that the elderly person's foot makes initial contact with higher velocity, a situation that compromises their balance in a manner similar to that encountered when stepping off a moving walkway.

GENERAL QUESTIONS ABOUT GAIT IN PEOPLE AFFECTED BY STROKE

Are the muscle groups performing the work of walking in people affected by stroke different from those of normal older adults?

We examined the kinematics and kinetics of gait of 30 people affected by stroke and grouped the results into three levels of competence (mean gait speed 0.25 ± 0.05 m/s; 0.41 ± 0.08 m/s; 0.63 ± 0.08 m/s) (Olney et al 1991). One must bear in mind that individual data are washed out in these analyses, and yet the subtleties of adaptations and compensations are most apparent in individual subjects. We found the average power patterns to be of the same shape as those of able-bodied subjects but amplitudes were lower (Figure 8.7). In fact, amplitudes for the slowest group were barely apparent. The positive A2 burst by the ankle plantarflexors during push-off was a major contributor to the positive work accomplished on both sides with one exception: it was barely evident on the affected side in the slowest speed group. The muscles of the knee, like their able-bodied counterparts, acted primarily eccentrically with K3 in the fastest speed group on the unaffected side shown to be even larger than normal. A small burst of positive work by the knee extensors (K2) was evident on the affected side only in the fastest speed group. At the hip the pull-off phase (H3) was evident in all plots although the level was very low on the affected side of the slowest group. In contrast, the mean of the H1 phase, caused by hip extension in early stance, was evident only on the affected side. Events occurred earlier on the affected side, reflecting the shorter than normal stance phase but occurred later on the unaffected side. There seemed to be limits to the amount of work that could be substituted from the unaffected side, and the affected side, on average, contributed about 40% of the total. In summary, while the same muscles are responsible for performing the work of walking and the general patterns tend to be the same, a number of differences can be seen.

Which muscle groups show the greatest deficits after stroke?

We have not yet completed a study in which we express muscle strength of major muscle groups of the affected side as a proportion of the strength of the unaffected side, using a hand-held dynamometer. We have found that the greatest deficits occur in the ankle plantarflexors (approximately 60% of unaffected side), followed by knee flexors and ankle dorsiflexors (64% and 66% respectively), hip abductors and knee extensors (72% and 73%) and hip flexors (78%) and hip extensors (83%). Although these subjects represented a range of abilities and variance was high, the mean level was also fairly high. A previous study showed the same relative distribution of strength, with ankle plantarflexors 'worst' and hip extensors 'best' on average. We should also bear in mind that normal level walking requires a relatively small proportion of the maximum capability of all major muscle groups except for the ankle plantarflexors.

Do other muscle groups compensate for deficient muscle groups in gait?

The wonderful redundancy of muscles acting across one or two joints means that adaptations and compensations may occur in the affected limb (intra-limb compensation) or in the unaffected limb (inter-limb compensation) (Winter et al 1990). With deficits greater in the affected ankle plantarflexors, individual subjects frequently increase H3 on the same limb and, less frequently, H1. Inter-limb compensations are almost always evident, with increases in A2, H1 and H3 frequently reaching above normal values.

When gait speed improves with training, do the work/power changes occur in particular muscle groups or in particular patterns?

Recent work (Parvataneni 2002) has analysed kinetic gait derived before and after a strengthening and conditioning programme administered to 28 subjects with residual effects of stroke. The group was generally high-performing with average speed of walking 0.70 m/s before training and 0.83 m/s following training. The slowest speed pretraining was 0.17 m/s and the fastest gait speed recorded was 1.54 m/s. Although this is clearly a high-performing group and deviations are large, the information may be helpful in suggesting where gains are likely to occur. Table 8.1 shows that, on average, A2 and H1 on both sides tended to increase with change in speed by 0.04 or 0.05 J/kg, as did H1 (by 0.03 or 0.04 J/kg), but H3 increased on average only on the unaffected side (by 0.04 J/kg). It is also noteworthy that prior to treatment A2, H1 and H3 of the unaffected side showed average values higher than Winter's normal data, consistent with the expectation of compensation for affected-side deficits in this high-performing group. To give an impression of individual subject data, of the 28 subjects who showed increases in their speed of walking, 18 showed trends to increases in positive work on the affected side in

Table 8.1   Mean and standard deviations of work (normalized to body mass, J/kg) for major ankle, hip and knee power bursts during walking, for affected and unaffected sides, before and after treatment, compared with Winter's subjects walking at mean speed of 1.2 m/s. (From Parvataneni, 2002, with permission.)

Activity phase	Winter 1990	Affected		Unaffected	
		Before	After	Before	After
A2	0.19 ± 0.05	0.12 ± 0.08	0.17 ± 0.09	0.24 ± 0.18	0.29 ± 0.15
H1	0.07 ± 0.04	0.07 ± 0.08	0.11 ± 0.10	0.11 ± 0.09	0.14 ± 0.11
H3	0.10 ± 0.03	0.12 ± 0.14	0.11 ± 0.04	0.12 ± 0.05	0.16 ± 0.07
K2	0.04 ± 0.24	0.02 ± 0.03	0.03 ± 0.03	0.03 ± 0.03	0.03 ± 0.03
K3	0.09 ± 0.05	0.08 ± 0.07	0.11 ± 0.09	0.14 ± 0.08	0.22 ± 0.13

A2, ankle power burst at push-off; H1, hip power burst at early stance; H3, hip power burst at early swing; K2, knee power burst at mid-stance; K3, knee power burst at early swing.

A2, 16 in H1, 15 in H3 and 12 in K2. On the unaffected side, 21 subjects showed increases in A2, 20 in H3, 18 in H1 and 9 in K2. Increases in negative work at K3 were observed in 12 subjects on the affected side and in 21 subjects on the unaffected side.

The proportion of positive work performed by the ankle expressed as a proportion of the work of the whole affected limb tended to be higher after treatment for the affected side (40% cf. 37%) but not the unaffected (44% cf. 45%). The reverse was true of the hip, with the unaffected side showing a trend to assuming a greater proportion of the total work (46% after, 43% before). The total amount of positive work performed by the major contributors on the affected side increased by 33% with training, and on the unaffected side by 40%, but the overall proportion of work done by the unaffected limb remained very close to 40% of the total for the two limbs. The price paid in terms of changes in negative work was largely during the K3 phase, with absorption from the unaffected side eating up a large proportion of the profit from gains in A2 and H3 of the affected side (−0.14 to −0.22 J/kg).

GENERAL QUESTIONS ABOUT GAIT TRAINING FOR PEOPLE AFFECTED BY STROKE

Which muscle groups should we target for gait training?

Fundamentally there are six possible target muscle groups, three on each side:

- ankle plantarflexors at push-off;
- hip flexors at pull-off;
- hip extensors in early stance.

It seems most consistent with accepted practice to target muscle work on the affected side early in treatment. While we traditionally have spent a great deal of time concentrating on the knee, and it certainly deserves attention for reasons to be discussed below, it will never help the patient increase gait speed. For this we want to stress as high a level of contraction as we can achieve (high moment at fast speed). Remember that energy varies as velocity squared, so speed is worth encouraging. To achieve speed over a range one needs to move through a good joint range.

Let us first consider increasing A2. One reason that we encourage a big step forward by the unaffected limb is that this positions the ankle of the affected side in more dorsiflexion from which to push off. The other reason is that the direction of the push is more forward than upward, which obviously is an advantage when one is looking to increase forward velocity! We like them to PUSH, not just lift the leg using H3.

Considering H3 has great capacity to add to the energy of the body it is surprising that we have not yet seen studies in which it has been exploited. Again both force and the velocity are important. Recall that this movement begins when hip extension ceases at the end of stance phase. Thus, in order to achieve high velocity it is particularly important to have a good range of hip extension from which to accelerate. To achieve the speed of pull-off, some of my colleagues (R W Bohannon, personal communication) ask their patients to yank their foot off the ground. You may wonder how yanking the foot off the ground can do useful work in moving the upper body forwards, and this is an excellent and perceptive biomechanical question. The answer lies in the transfer of energy from one part of the body to another, in this case from the thigh to the upper body (Winter 1990). In brief, following its acquisition of energy, the swinging limb slows down and during this time a major portion of its energy is transferred to the trunk, which must end up as an increase in velocity (kinetic energy) or a raising of the body (potential energy), or both.

H1 is sometimes called the 'push from behind'. Note that in able-bodied walking it is quite small, but has a long duration. Remember also that use of these big hamstring muscles augmented by gluteal muscles enables an above-knee amputee to walk effectively with a prosthesis. Furthermore, in people affected by stroke the hip extensors frequently have good residual strength. This muscle group also appears to be very responsive to training. Figure 8.8 shows power patterns of one subject before and after a strengthening and conditioning programme. Again one should stress the force of the muscle contraction (beginning with the ending of swing phase through initial contact and into stance phase), the speed of the movement and the continuation of the 'push from behind' to increase its duration, each of which will increase the work done on the body.

Should I use direct means of strengthening muscle groups

Although muscle weakness is recognized as a limiting factor in the rehabilitation of people affected by stroke, strength training and strength measurement have been controversial issues. However, measures of muscle strength have been established as predictors of gait performance, and the torques generated by the hip extensors, hip flexors, knee flexors, knee extensors, ankle plantarflexors and ankle dorsiflexors have been shown to correlate positively with gait performance (Bohannon 1986, Bohannon and Walsh 1992, Nakamura et al 1988). Some studies have shown increases in health outcomes as well as measures of motor performance when direct strengthening has been included in the exercise programme (Teixeira-Salmela et al 1999, 2001). Assessment of spasticity following strength training has not identified any adverse effects (Sharp and Brouwer, 1997, Teixeira-Salmela et al 1999).

Figure 8.8   Power patterns of one subject before and after a strengthening and conditioning programme. Note increases in H1 on the affected limb (intra–limb compensation for deficits) and unaffected limb (inter–limb compensation).

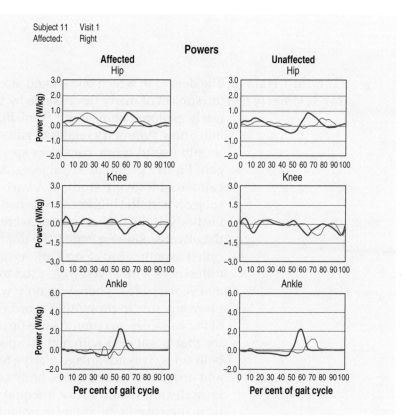

Continued

Figure 8.8 **Continued**

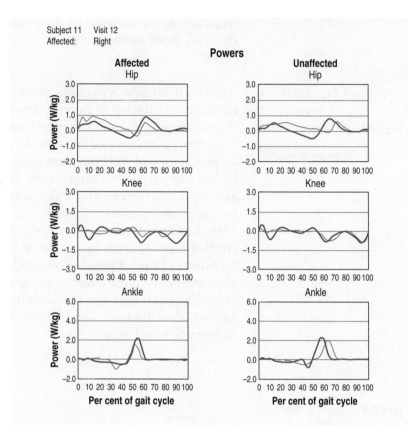

Should I train
for symmetry?

The degree to which one should stress symmetry in gait has been
the subject of many discussions by therapists, but the question is
rarely explored empirically. Some light was shed on this by examining how symmetry relates to gait speed (Griffin et al 1995). This
is only useful if one considers speed to be a valued attribute of
gait. From a group of 31 subjects, the symmetry properties of 34
gait variables were studied. A variable was called 'symmetric' if
subjects with the highest speeds had equal values on both sides of
the body. If the highest speeds were achieved when the values of
the affected side exceeded the unaffected side, the variable was
called 'asymmetric'. Correlations of the differences and absolute
differences with speed were used to detect symmetric and asymmetric variables. There was only weak evidence that symmetry
plays any role in promoting speed in this subject group; only one
of the variables, maximum knee flexion in stance, showed symmetry, that is, subjects with highest speeds showed similar values on
both sides. This advantage may be related to maintaining equal up
and down excursions of the body because a large discrepancy in
knee flexion would cause unequal excursions, which would, in
turn, increase fluctuations in potential energy. Asymmetric vari-

ables seemed to be somewhat more important: asymmetry of hip negative work, of hip maximum flexor moments, of hip maximum extension and of the sums of negative work were all associated with higher speeds. In each case speed was associated with larger values from the affected than the unaffected side. It seems consistent with therapists' aim of restoring normal function to attempt to obtain symmetry early in rehabilitation, but unless one suspects that adverse forces result from the particular asymmetry that is seen, asymmetric patterns may sometimes produce more functional gait than symmetrical ones.

Is walking speed or a normal gait pattern more important?

One must first determine on what factors the pattern can be said to be poorer, then tackle the question explicitly with the patient, who should decide upon priorities. At the same time, one must determine whether the 'poorer' pattern can be reduced or eliminated by making adjustments for the faster walking. For example, a somewhat stiff plantarflexor group may be perfectly adequate for slow-speed walking, but when faster speeds are attempted the ankle may not dorsiflex sufficiently, thrusting the knee into hyperextension. Increasing the heel height by a small amount may avoid the problem.

QUESTIONS ABOUT TRAINING DURING STANCE PHASE

Does limited ankle dorsiflexion matter?

Limited ankle dorsiflexion is an important energy consideration. A great deal of the efficiencies in walking occur through trade-offs between kinetic and potential energy of the trunk, with the changes in potential energy (reflecting rises and falls in height of the upper body) close in magnitude to the fluctuations in kinetic energy caused by velocity changes. Figure 8.9 shows the result of lifting up the leg and pelvis in order to clear the ground, an adaptation that is particularly costly. Although empirical data are not available, lifting only the limb itself higher would have less serious consequences, so training to minimize pelvic lift is important.

Should I stress knee bending in early stance?

One might think that the argument used in the previous question applies here, and there would be an inverse relationship between knee flexion and the energy cost, at least up to a point. This is what Saunders' logic would suggest (Saunders et al 1953). However, it is far more likely that the teleological reason for knee flexion in early stance is not minimization of energy costs but absorption of energy following swing phase. In early stance we have a 'reverse pendulum,' that is, the body is pivoting about the foot, with energy exchanging nicely between potential and kinetic types. Although

Figure 8.9 Costly energy pattern (J) resulting from inadequate lifting of the leg and pelvis in order to clear the ground with straight knee. Note that there is no opportunity to exchange potential and kinetic energy. (From Olney et al 1986.)

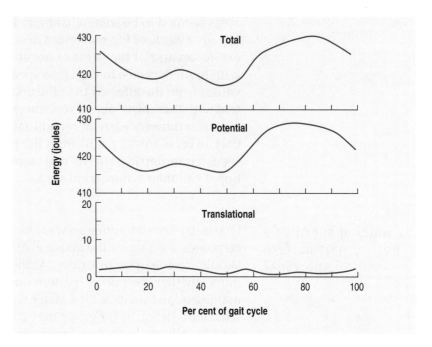

again there are no extensive empirical data, a small study by Winter (1983) assessed the mechanical work cost in seven normal subjects walking at a variety of speeds. The work costs were correlated with maximum knee flexion during stance. Results showed that energy costs were significantly positively related to maximum knee flexion, which means that at least under these circumstances the prediction of Saunders (1953) that stiff-legged weight bearing is more energy consuming than normal flexed-knee stance does not hold. Although the study was influenced by speed variations that might vary inversely with energy costs over at least part of the speed range, the findings nevertheless suggest that the knee flexion in early stance does not have a large influence on energy costs if other biomechanical variables remain the same.

There is a reason for stressing knee bending in early stance, however, unrelated to energy costs, and that is to avoid development of a tendency towards a hyperextended knee. The knee need not actually be hyperextended; the same tendency is present if the force of the floor proceeds too rapidly to the toe, or if the patient does not transfer the weight early enough in stance. In both of these cases, the reaction force from the floor develops a large moment tending to extend the knee, which must be broken in order for the patient to enter into the most important energy-generating phase of gait – push-off and pull-off, occurring at the end of stance and early swing phase.

Should I stress knee flexion towards the end of stance?

The answer is a resounding 'yes'. In fact I would go so far as to say that obtaining this opportunity for generation of energy, providing the patient has some muscle function in ankle plantarflexors and hip flexors, is the single most important gait training consideration following safety. I have mentioned that there is apparently a limit to the amount of work that can be substituted by the unaffected side (ratio for the two sides may be about 40:60). Maintaining a stiff leg in late stance, which is followed by little or no flexion in swing phase, makes it impossible to generate energy from either A2 or H3.

Does a flexed position throughout stance, and the ankle remaining in excessive dorsiflexion matter?

It is important only indirectly. 'Supportingness' of the thigh–lower leg–foot linkages during stance phase is provided by the hip extensors, knee extensors and ankle plantarflexors (Winter 1991, p. 40), which are responsible for the moments shown in Figure 8.5. In normal walking (Winter 1991, pp. 57–69) very early in stance this support is provided by the hamstrings, which are nearly at their peak of activity at initial contact, and the quadriceps, which are increasing their activity and both of which will approach near-zero values by 30% of the cycle. The calf muscle group has very low levels of activity early in stance and crescendos between 30% and 60% of the cycle providing support at that time. In pathologies the muscle groups substitute for each other. Consider the above-knee amputee who has no knee extensors and provides adequate support through hip extensors and a fairly stiff (moment contribution) foot–ankle complex. For the patient unable to generate a knee extensor moment it is important to attempt 'knee control' with the hip extensors. If the knee is flexed or flexes in early stance, the cause is not deficient ankle plantarflexors as they contribute later. The ankle that remains in excessive dorsiflexion through stance is usually caused by low or absent plantarflexion activity, but again, knee extensor and hip extensor activity can substitute to some degree. Fixing or partial fixing of the ankle by an orthosis will provide support, although it will also limit the amount of work from A2. If work is not being generated by A2, an orthosis may be a positive option.

After considering support, which is a non-dynamic issue, the therapist should examine the three power-generating phases, which are dynamic issues. Some recent evidence shows that therapists can discern the effectiveness of these phases (McGinley et al 2003). Is the patient achieving a good 'push from behind' in early stance, a firm push-off and rapid pull-off? Of these the least likely is the second, as the plantarflexors in early stance are one of the two 'supports' of the thigh–lower leg–foot linkages at that time. The other one is the hip extensors. If the therapist can see brisk generations occurring, the walking with flexion is of little concern. In a principal components analysis of gait data from people affected by stroke (Olney et al 1998), the third factor measured a tendency to adopt a postural flexion or extension bias. A subject showing flexion bias showed high flexion during stance, also ankle dorsiflexion, and the trunk inclined forwards. Note that the principal component analysis extracts factors independent of each other; in other words neither speed nor degree of symmetry, which were the first two components extracted, was related to whether the person walked with flexion or extension. In summary, walking with a somewhat flexed posture does not relate to walking competence as reflected in gait speed.

Why is there confusion about the importance of push-off?

No confusion remains. Earlier workers who did not have the benefit of sophisticated kinetic biomechanical analysis observed that persons with cerebral palsy and with amputations could walk perfectly well with a fixed ankle. Of course, we know now that a person without generation from the ankle plantarflexors can still walk as long as she or he generates work from somewhere else. A person who maintained normal values for hip generation would walk at a slower speed. If a person increased the available opportunities for compensation, he or she might even walk at normal speeds. 'Lift-off' reflects the H3 generation phase (though I favour the more dynamic 'pull-off') and is a more accurate description of the event if the ankle plantarflexors are not generating any energy.

Why is there decreased plantarflexion at the ankle joint during push-off?

Usually, reduced A2 results from weak ankle plantarflexors, as discussed above. To generate energy the muscle must perform a concentric contraction against the foot–floor force being applied to the forefoot: there must be sufficient force capability of the muscle to move the ankle through the range. Although adding an orthosis or otherwise fixing the ankle can produce a moment that will prevent the ankle from dorsiflexing, it can accomplish no A2 generation.

Does limited hip extension and limited ankle dorsiflexion on the affected side in late stance matter?

This also appears as a short step length on the unaffected foot and has serious biomechanical consequences, which can be summarized as reduced opportunity to generate positive work by both A2 and H3. Look first at the ankle and hip power profiles in Figures 8.6 and 8.7. At the end of stance phase, if the person has a short step length the ankle would be much less dorsiflexed, giving it less opportunity to acquire an effective velocity for push-off. A2 would be small. Similarly, the limited hip extension means that the hip flexors have less opportunity to acquire an effective velocity for pull-off (H3). In addition, there are costs associated with each step to raise and lower the body from one foot to the other, which must be 'paid for' regardless of how big the step is. Although there are no empirical data showing this, it is theoretically reasonable to assume that all else being equal, taking more steps to cover the same distance will have higher energy costs.

There is empirical evidence for the importance of several biomechanical events consistent with obtaining a well-extended hip in late stance. One study (Olney et al 1994) reported that of many kinematic variables, maximum hip extension on the affected side had the highest correlation ($r = 0.61$) with gait speed in 32 people affected by stroke. In a stepwise regression of gait variables on speed, the maximum hip flexor moment was the first variable selected and accounted for 74% of the variance. Other authors have noted the importance of the biomechanical events occurring with effective hip extension on the affected side (Nadeau et al 2001).

What are the guiding biomechanical principles for choosing an ankle–foot orthosis?

Orthoses are used for three reasons:

1. to facilitate foot clearance during swing phase when the ankle dorsiflexors are inadequate or if the plantarflexor complex is overactive or stiff;
2. to prevent excessive ankle dorsiflexion in late stance if ankle plantarflexors are inadequate; or
3. to hold the foot in a balanced position if it tends to invert or evert on contact.

An orthosis to fulfil outcome 1, above, is very simple; however, to do so without fixing the ankle in order that the ankle plantarflexors can make a contribution to positive work is more difficult. A very flexible ankle–foot orthosis or a hinged orthosis that permits as much ankle range as possible is best, providing the ankle plantarflexors are able to generate some force. Outcome 2 can be accomplished with a hinged orthosis with a dorsiflexor stop that permits as full movement into plantarflexion as possible. Outcome 3 likewise requires mediolateral stability without unduly limiting plantarflexion and dorsiflexion. If plantarflexors are very weak there is little to be lost by using an orthosis. In all cases it is recommended that the patient's natural speed of walking be assessed with each possible aid, as the chosen walking speed will give a good indication of the relative merits of each orthosis. Recently, energy-returning orthoses that store energy as the foot dorsiflexes in early stance and release it at push-off have appeared on the market. No studies to date have demonstrated their ability to return energy but when they do, this will be the orthosis of choice.

QUESTIONS ABOUT GAIT TRAINING DURING SWING PHASE

Does slow flexion of the hip of the affected side during swing matter?

Failure to initiate a brisk hip flexion in swing reduces the generation of energy of H3. As this is a good potential source of energy it should be encouraged whenever possible. H3 also occurs at a time of good stability on the unaffected limb, which should add to its ability to be effective.

Is knee bending during swing phase important?

Keeping the knee straight through swing frequently arises from a fear of being unable to catch the weight of the body with the affected limb rather than from the patient being unable to generate sufficient muscle contraction, an illustration of 'adaptive motor behaviour' of Carr and Shepherd (1998, p. 249). A walking stick or hiking pole may offer security. The mechanism of knee bending is often misunderstood. Knee bending is not caused by hamstrings – they are silent at this time. Knee bending is caused by active ankle plantarflexion augmented by hip flexion. Thus, a firm push-off is the most important means of obtaining knee flexion. A longer step on the unaffected side will also place the affected hip in an extended position, which favours good push-off. The energetic costs of carrying a straight leg through swing phase have been discussed above. In summary, the therapist should continue to attempt to obtain knee flexion during swing by encouraging push-off in stance.

QUESTIONS ABOUT GAIT TRAINING DURING DOUBLE–SUPPORT PHASE

What are the consequences of a very long double-support phase?

An extended period of double support is costly in terms of energy. During 50% to 60% of the gait cycle on the stance phase limb in normal gait, considerable energy is being generated from A2 and H3. Note only a very small amount of simultaneous absorption occurs from the first part of K1 (quadriceps eccentric activity) on the forward limb during the first 10% of its gait cycle. However, if stance phases of the two limbs overlap to a greater degree, more push-off from the stance limb and increasing amounts of K1 and A1 from the other stance limb would occur simultaneously, thus negating each other and creating inefficiencies.

An extended period of double support is frequently associated with a sense of poor balance by the subject. This instability may be responsible for the large K3 that we frequently see on the affected side in people with stroke (Figure 8.7). This results from a small knee extensor moment probably stabilizing the limb, while knee flexion occurs. This energy-absorbing inefficient manoeuvre is another reason for stressing a strong push-off and rapid 'yank' at the end of stance phase.

CONCLUSION

Consideration of the biomechanical issues that are relevant to gait training after stroke can assist in treatment decisions. This chapter has attempted to clarify the most commonly encountered issues. When assessing individual patients it is not possible, of course, to determine what moments and powers are present for that individual. However, there is limited evidence that the powers at push-off can be seen visually (McGinley et al 2003) and we have no reason to believe that the other phases would be different. Not recognizing their importance, we have not known how to look. There would doubtless be gains from individual analyses that would permit more precise targeting of treatment, but I believe these are less important than having an overall understanding of the principles upon which treatment can be based.

References

Bohannon R W 1986 Strength of lower limb related to gait velocity and cadence in stroke patients. Physiotherapy Canada 38(4):204–206.

Bohannon R W, Walsh S 1992 Nature, reliability, and predictive value of muscle performance measures in patients with hemiparesis following stroke. Archives of Physical Medicine and Rehabilitation 73(8):721–725.

Carr J, Shepherd R 1998 Neurological rehabilitation: optimizing motor performance. Butterworth-Heinemann, Oxford.

Carr J, Shepherd R 2003 Stroke rehabilitation: guidelines for exercise and training to optimize motor skill. Butterworth-Heinemann, Oxford, pp 76–128.

Cress M E, Schechtman K B, Mulrow C D et al 1995 Relationship between physical performance and self-perceived physical function. Journal of the American Geriatrics Society 43(2):93–101

Friedman P 1990 Gait recovery after hemiplegic stroke. International Disability Studies 12(3): 119–122.

Griffin M P, Olney S J, McBride I D 1995 The role of symmetry in gait performance of persons with hemiparesis resulting from stroke. Gait and Posture 3:132–142.

McGinley J L, Goldie P A, Greenwood K M et al 2003 Accuracy and reliability of observational gait analysis data: judgments of push-off in gait after stroke. Physical Therapy 83(2):146–160.

Nadeau S, Gravel D, Olney S J 2001 Determinants, limiting factors, and compensatory strategies in gait. Critical Reviews in Physical and Rehabilitation Medicine 13(1):1–25.

Nakamura R, Watanabe S, Handa T et al 1988 The relationship between walking speed and muscle strength for knee extension in hemiparetic stroke patients: a follow-up study. Tohoku Journal of Experimental Medicine 154(2):111–113.

Olney S J, Richards C 1996 Hemiparetic gait following stroke. Part I: characteristics. Gait and Posture 4(2):136–148.

Olney S J, Monga T N, Costigan P A 1986 Mechanical energy of walking of stroke patients. Archives of Physical Medicine and Rehabilitation 67:92–98.

Olney S J, Griffin M P, Monga T N et al 1991 Work and power in gait of stroke patients. Archives of Physical Medicine and Rehabilitation 72:309–314.

Olney S J, Griffin M P, McBride I D 1994 Temporal, kinematic and kinetic variables related to gait speed in subjects with hemiplegia: a regression approach. Physical Therapy (AM) 74:872–885.

Olney S J, Griffin M P, McBride I D 1998 Multivariate examination of data from gait analysis of persons with stroke. Physical Therapy (AM) 78(6):814–828.

Parvataneni K 2002 Kinetic factor responsible for gait speed increases in stroke after a training program. MSc thesis, Queen's University, Kingston, Ontario.

Potter J M, Evans A L, Duncan G 1995 Gait speed and activities of daily living function in geriatric patients. Archives of Physical Medicine and Rehabilitation 76(11):997–999

Quanbury A O, Winter D A, Reimer G D 1975 Instantaneous power and power flow in body segments during walking. Journal of Human Movement Studies 1:59–67.

Richards C, Olney S J 1996 Hemiparetic gait following stroke. Part II: recovery. Gait and Posture 4(2):149–162.

Saunders J B de C M, Inman V T, Eberhart H D 1953 The major determinants in normal and pathological gait. Journal of Bone and Joint Surgery 35A(3):543–558 .

Sharp S, Brouwer B J 1997 Isokinetic strength training of the hemiparetic knee: effects of function and spasticity. Archives of Physical Medicine and Rehabilitation 78:1231–1236.

Sheirman G, Olney S J 1997 Clinical analysis using the Peak Motus motion measurement system. Orthopaedic Physical Therapy Clinics of North America 6:17–43.

Stokes J, Lindsay J 1996 Major causes of death and hospitalization in Canadian seniors. Chronic Diseases in Canada 17:63–73.

Teixeira-Salmela L F, Olney S J, Nadeau S et al 1999 Muscle strengthening and physical conditioning to reduce impairment and disability in chronic stroke survivors. Archives of Physical Medicine and Rehabilitation 80(10):1211–1218.

Teixeira-Salmela L F, Nadeau S, McBride I et al 2001 Effects of muscle strengthening and physical conditioning training of temporal, kinematic and kinetic variables during gait in chronic stroke survivors. Journal of Rehabilitation Medicine 33:53–60.

Wilkins K 1999 Health care consequences of falls in seniors. Health Reports 10:47–55.

Winter D A 1983 Knee flexion during stance as a determinant of inefficient walking. Physical Therapy 63(3):331–333.

Winter D A 1990 Biomechanics and motor control of human movement. Wiley Interscience, Toronto.

Winter D A 1991 The biomechanics and motor control of human gait: normal, elderly and pathological. Waterloo Biomechanics, Waterloo.

Winter D A, Olney S J, Conrad J et al 1990 Adaptability of motor patterns in pathological gait. In: Winters DA, Woo SLY (eds) Multiple muscle systems: biomechanics and movement organization. Springer-Verlag.

Chapter 9

Assessment and training of locomotion after stroke: evolving concepts

Francine Malouin and Carol L. Richards

Both the assessment and therapy of locomotor disorders have evolved remarkably over the last 20 years. This evolution has heralded the coming of age of physiotherapy as a clinical science. The work of Carr and Shepherd (1982, 1987, 1998) and their colleagues had a major impact on the thinking of physical therapy academic researchers, who directed their efforts at better understanding the biomechanics and motor control mechanisms of locomotor-related tasks, the development of task-oriented training approaches and the evaluation of their efficacy. This paradigm shift to task-oriented training and the basic tenet of the need for 'appropriate' practice has led to multidisciplinary studies that have recruited the expertise of epidemiologists, neuropsychologists, engineers and computer programming experts to explore new and innovative ways to augment the type and intensity of locomotor practice. The importance of cognitive processes related to decision-making, anticipatory locomotor adjustments and goal-oriented behaviour has also been recognized. Taken together, these influences and interactions have led to a veritable explosion of knowledge in the field of neurological rehabilitation and more specifically the therapy of locomotor disorders.

This chapter will review studies that have contributed to the dramatic evolution of the task-oriented approach to gait training for people after stroke, and our contribution to this evolution over the last 15 years. The specific aims of the chapter are to:

1. review the evidence for a task-oriented approach and the role of sophisticated equipment in the success of this approach;
2. demonstrate the need for task-specific strength and endurance training;
3. review recent studies incorporating physical conditioning-related training;
4. explore ways of promoting augmented practice by:
   a. examining the potential of mental practice as an adjunct to physical practice, and
   b. investigating the promise of using virtual reality training methods to improve the quality of walking practice;
5. review recent work on two locomotor-related tasks;
6. emphasize the need to evaluate walking competency.

TASK-ORIENTED LOCOMOTOR TRAINING

Treadmill training

In 1987, when we began a randomized controlled pilot trial to compare a task-oriented with a conventional neurodevelopment treatment (NDT) (for reviews of traditional approaches see Gordon 1987, Horak 1991) physical therapy approach for the training of gait in people with acute stroke (Malouin et al 1992, Richards et al 1993), the use of a treadmill in this population was unusual. Five years later it still was not accepted practice and promoted much discussion as demonstrated by the long commentary accompanying the description of the task-oriented approach (Malouin et al 1992). Today, the treadmill is accepted as a basic component of gait training after stroke. In fact, use of the treadmill with or without body weight support, promoted by a number of studies (Finch and Barbeau, 1985; Hesse et al 1994a, 1995, 2001, Smith et al 1999, Visintin et al 1998), has led to the general acceptance of treadmill gait training.

Treadmill walking is seen as an efficient means of promoting task-specific training. Moreover, load on the musculoskeletal system can be varied by body weight support (BWS) and walking speed can be controlled. Treadmill walking has been said to be a motivational and safe way of promoting walking practice, and it has been assumed to be goal-directed. An underlying problem raised by people specialized in motor learning, such as Gentile (1987), has been the closed-loop nature of the repetitive task, which limits the engagement of the cognitive components of walking in a changing environment. The treadmill approach has been taken to the extreme with the introduction of robotized gait-trainers (Hesse et al 2001, Werner et al 2002b) that reduce the demands made on therapists by assisted treadmill walking. The concept that robotized assisted practice leads to the enhancement of locomotor skill remains to be demonstrated in a controlled study. Such a concept nevertheless contravenes the conceptual underpinning of the widely accepted motor learning approach (Carr and Shepherd 1987, 1998, Winstein, 1991) that recommends goal-directed, environmentally contextual and ever-changing locomotor training. The treadmill per se has also, to some extent, become equated with task-specific locomotor training. This is a serious misconception and negates the cognitive and motivational contribution of the patient and the guidance role of the therapist.

Is use of a treadmill and other sophisticated equipment necessary to offer task-oriented training? When the treadmill is part of an overall approach to task-oriented training, some results have suggested that such an approach is superior at enhancing walking capacity in people with acute stroke compared with conventional therapy (NDT) (Malouin et al 1992, Richards et al 1993) or in people with chronic stroke compared with sham therapy (upper extremity training) (Dean et al 2000, Salbach et al 2004). Although one may tend to attribute such positive results, at least in part, to the use of a treadmill and other sophisticated devices such as a Kinetron or limb load monitors, three recent randomized controlled trials have shown that the key factor is varied practice of locomotor-related tasks that are guided and monitored by a physical therapist. In the first study, Olney et al (1995, 1997) reported large improvements in the gait of both groups (with and without biofeedback) of people with chronic stroke but were unable to show the superiority of a sophisticated computer-controlled biofeedback system that targeted the 'push-off' activation of the ankle plantarflexors (electromyography, or EMG, feedback) at the end of the stance phase and the 'pull-off' movement (angle feedback) of the hip flexors at the initiation of the swing phase. In the second study, Nilsson et al (2001) compared two training regimens for people with acute stroke. They found that treadmill walking with body weight support training was comparable to overground walking training according to the motor relearning approach. The third study, designed as a sequel to the Richards et al (1993) study and involving people less than

92 days after stroke treated in a rehabilitation centre for 8 weeks, Richards et al (2004) found that both the task-oriented and conventional therapy groups more than doubled their walking speed after therapy and showed improvements in a number of secondary measures. They were unable, however, to show the superiority of the task-oriented approach that included treadmill training without weight support, training on a Kinetron isokinetic device and use of a limb load monitor during walking. On the basis of these studies, one must conclude that although sophisticated equipment such as treadmills or biofeedback systems are beneficial, and may in fact help make therapy more varied and interesting as well as reduce the physical demands on therapists, they are not essential for achieving success with the task-oriented approach to therapy.

The impact of these three studies on future therapy planning should not be underestimated. First, they give credence to the basic approach promoted by Carr and Shepherd (1982, 1998), which encourages task-specific practice of various locomotor-related tasks, including the task-specific strengthening of muscles (shortening, static or lengthening contractions of specific muscle groups) with the assistance of basic equipment available in most rehabilitation settings or in homes. Secondly, these results suggest that expensive and sophisticated equipment is not necessary to enable the application of the task-oriented motor learning approach – an important consideration in private practice and in cash-strapped physiotherapy departments worldwide. Other evidence promoting walking practice without the use of a treadmill comes from a recent meta-analysis by Wood-Dauphinee and Kwakkel (2003), who found that, after examining the four randomized controlled trials that compared treadmill training without BWS to conventional gait training, there was no evidence that treadmill training without BWS had additional effects on walking compared with conventional overground gait training programmes.

The question then arises as to whether treadmill training with BWS should be encouraged in people with acute stroke. In a large randomized controlled trial comparing the value of including treadmill walking with and without BWS, Visintin et al (1998) found both walking speed and the distance walked in 6 minutes to be superior in the BWS group after 6 weeks of therapy and 3 months later. These results, however, do not provide guidelines as to the need for treadmill practice early after stroke. For example, is the indication for treadmill practice the same for a non-independent walker as for an independent walker? It is evident that the postural and equilibrium requirements are quite different under BWS conditions, and one must ask whether such practice could impede locomotor recovery in independent walkers. It does appear, however, that it is to be recommended for non-ambulating people with chronic stroke (Hesse et al 1994a, 1995). Nevertheless, when using BWS it is important to consider the effect of this support on the muscle activations of the trunk and lower extremities. Hesse et al (1999) recommended a maximum of 30% BWS to enable activation of the extensor muscle groups of normal amplitude. They also demonstrated, as previously shown in people with spinal cord injuries (Fung and Barbeau 1989, Fung et al 1990), that BWS may reduce the expression of hyperactive stretch reflexes (spasticity) in the ankle plantarflexors of people with stroke. In their recent review, Wood-Dauphinee and Kwakkel (2003) reported that although the evidence for the overall effectiveness of treadmill training with BWS was weak, such training generated additional effects on gait endurance, but not on gait speed, balance or walking ability. They suggested that these findings were linked to the decreased oxygen demand because of the body weight support (Danielsson and Sunnerhagen 2000, Macko et al 2001, Nilsson et al 2001).

Strength training

Although paresis is a basic and well-documented component of the locomotor disorder in people with stroke (Knutsson and Richards 1979, Lamontagne et al 2002, Richards and Knutsson 1974), traditional physiotherapy approaches (Gordon 1987, Horak 1991) have not encouraged muscle strengthening because of the fear of increasing spasticity. Experience with the effects of dorsal rhizotomies aimed at reducing spasticity in children with cerebral palsy (for reviews see Richards and Malouin 1992, 1998) has improved our understanding of the relationship between spasticity and paresis. In many children, successful reduction of spastic reflexes unmasked the underlying paresis, and in many cases, because the 'spastic crutch' was removed, reduced the child's ability to walk. Such clinical results clearly demonstrated that spasticity reduction did not necessarily allow for more normal muscle activations and movement patterns to emerge. It is now generally recognized that paresis, or muscle weakness, is a major factor in the movement disorder of people with stroke, and task-specific muscle strengthening using the body weight as resistance is to be recommended (Carr and Shepherd 1998).

Kinetic analyses of muscle actions during the gait cycle have elucidated the key roles that the ankle plantarflexors and hip flexors, and to a lesser extent the hip extensors, play in gait propulsion and the generation of walking speed (Winter 1991). To simplify, one can say that nearly two-thirds of the power generation comes from the A2 push-off plantarflexor activation burst at the end of stance and about one-third from the hip flexor pull-off burst (H3) at the beginning of the swing phase (see Chapter 8). The work of Olney et al (1991) has shown that in people with chronic stroke, gait speed is highly correlated to the magnitude of the A2 plantarflexor power burst and that increased use of the hip flexors may compensate for poor plantarflexor power. Richards et al (1998) reported the effects of 2 months of rehabilitation on static hip flexor and ankle plantarflexor strength, ankle and hip power bursts during walking and walking speed in a cohort of 19 people with acute stroke. They confirmed the 'hip strategy compensation' (Olney et al 1991) even at baseline, and the tendency of this strategy to become even more marked after therapy when the static strength of the hip flexors was significantly increased. The moderate improvement in the A2 power burst, on the other hand, was associated with a lack of static strength increase in the ankle plantarflexors, suggesting that choice of a 'hip pull-off' or an ankle 'push-off' strategy may be dictated by the strength available from individual muscles (Richards et al 1998). As expected (Bohannon 1986, Kim and Eng 2003), Richards et al (1998) found the static and dynamic (H3 and A2 power burst peaks) strength of the hip flexors and ankle plantarflexors to be significantly correlated to walking speed ($r = 0.48$–0.85), with the A2 burst explaining about 72% of the speed.

The roles of the hip extensors in early stance, the ankle plantarflexors in late stance and the hip flexors in early swing in gait propulsion justify targeting these muscles in order to improve gait after stroke (Olney et al 1991, Olney and Richards 1996, Richards et al 1998; see also Chapter 8). According to the task-oriented approach to gait training, the most efficient means of promoting improved contributions of these muscles is by practising locomotor tasks or subcomponents of these tasks by using the body weight as resistance (Carr and Shepherd, 1998). However, are other strengthening methods to be recommended? For example, is muscle strength gained after training statically or with isokinetic devices transferred to improvements in locomotor tasks?

Significant increases in muscle strength after concentric training of the knee extensors and flexors have been reported in people with chronic (Engardt et al 1995, Sharp and Brouwer 1997) and acute (Kim et al 2001) stroke. Interestingly, only Sharp and Brouwer (1997) were able to relate the increased strength to a small but significant increase in walking speed. Kim et al (2001), in a double-blind study that compared a group of people with chronic stroke receiving concentric isokinetic training for the hip, knee and ankle muscles of the paretic leg with a control group receiving passive movements using the same isokinetic KinCom dynamometer, found that both groups had increased their strength and walking speed post intervention. The lack of a significant strength increase with isokinetic training over passive movements is surprising and may be due to the small sample size and the large variability, as suggested by the authors, which again emphasizes the need for control groups when testing in this population. Nevertheless, these authors were unable to specifically link the effects of the strengthening intervention to improvements in walking speed.

A possible explanation for the lack of marked effects of increased strength on walking speed, at least for the Engardt et al (1995) and Sharp and Brouwer, (1997) studies, is the relatively small contribution of the quadriceps to propulsive force during walking (Olney et al 1991, Richards et al 1999, Winter 1991). Rather, it acts to absorb power (eccentric contractions) during early stance phase at weight acceptance and in early swing phase to limit knee flexion as the plantarflexor 'push-off' burst creates a knee flexion thrust. Another possibility is that muscle strengthening may need to be accompanied by training that requires the use of these strengthened muscles during the performance of tasks in order to promote carry over of the effects of strengthening to function (Kim et al 2001).

Engardt et al (1995) compared strength gains between concentric and eccentric training. They reported superior gains with the eccentric training and were able to relate the improved eccentric strength of the knee muscles to improvements in the weight distribution during the sit-to-stand task. Furthermore, during eccentric contractions of the quadriceps, the spastic hamstring muscles are not stretched, as demonstrated by monitoring muscle activity (Engardt et al 1995), and this may allow the subject to generate a higher torque than during concentric contractions. However, even if concentric isokinetic movements do stretch potentially spastic muscles, there has been no report of deleterious effects on function (Engardt et al 1995) or muscle tone (Sharp and Brouwer, 1997) after concentric training of the knee extensors or reciprocal concentric training of the knee extensors and flexors.

Endurance training

Endurance training, like strength training for people after stroke, has long been neglected because of the dogma related to spasticity. The work of Potempa et al (1995) with bicycle training and that of Macko et al (1997, 2001) with treadmill training, which demonstrated the positive results of endurance training on the aerobic capacity of people with chronic stroke, helped promote the idea of the need for fitness in this population. Other studies (Brown and Kautz 1998, Smith et al 1999) have dispelled the fear about increasing spasticity in people with stroke using either bicycle training or treadmill walking. Furthermore, Smith et al (1999) were able to demonstrate in a cohort study that treadmill walking also led to improved strength of the thigh muscles.

The deficit in endurance, even in people with stroke capable of walking at a speed of 122–142 cm/s, should not be underestimated, as shown by Richards et al (1999) in a multiple single-case study. People with chronic stroke ($n = 3$) were evaluated before and after 9 hours of task-oriented individualized training focusing on their ability to push-off with the ankle plantarflexors at the end of the stance phase of walking. They increased their 6-minute walk distance by a mean of 110 m, corresponding to increases ranging from 27.6 to 28.5%, with all three covering a distance of more than 495 m (at an average speed of 140 cm/s), a distance close to normal values (Enright and Sherrill 1998). These results not only document the deficit in endurance in these high-performing subjects, but also the potential for recovery with a targeted locomotor-oriented therapeutic approach requiring only 9 hours on an outpatient basis. Dean et al (2001) further quantified the deficit in endurance in a group of 14 people with chronic stroke using a reference formula to compare stroke with healthy individuals (Enright and Sherrill 1998). They found that people with stroke walked only about 50% of the distance predicted for healthy individuals with similar physical characteristics. Moreover, given the inability of people with stroke to maintain a constant walking speed for 6 minutes, calculation of the distance walked in 6 minutes from the walking speed measured over 10 m overestimated the distance walked (Dean et al 2001). These results emphasize the need first, to train endurance in people with chronic stroke, and secondly, that endurance must be directly measured, not calculated from walking speed over 10 m. Eng et al (2002) have further cautioned that a measure of myocardial exertion, such as heart rate, should be used in addition to the distance walked (6- or 12-minute walk tests), given the contribution of stroke-specific impairments to the distance walked.

To date, little is known about the deficit in endurance or its capacity to improve in people with acute stroke. It appears, however, that the cardiovascular stress induced by a contemporary rehabilitation programme for acute stroke is not sufficient to induce a training effect as measured by heart rate monitoring during therapy (MacKay-Lyons and Makrides 2002). Given the usual intensity of rehabilitation in early stroke, compounded by the physical condition of many people prior to their stroke, it is likely that an endurance component should be added to the therapy approach if the person's cardiovascular status permits it. The decision, however, to include such a programme should only be taken by a consultant cardiologist or the treating physician. See Chapter 7 for guidelines on endurance training in acute stroke.

Combining strength and endurance training to promote physical conditioning

The general acceptance of the task-oriented approach to locomotor training after stroke and the increasing information on endurance deficits in people with stroke (Dean et al 2001, Macko et al 1997, 2001) have promoted the development of locomotor training programmes that promote physical conditioning in people with chronic stroke. In a pilot randomized controlled study, Dean et al (2000) compared the effects of a circuit training programme focusing on locomotor-related tasks in a group of people with chronic stroke to those obtained in a control group who practised tasks for the upper extremity. They reported significant increases in both gait speed and the distance walked in 6 minutes as well as other outcomes only in the group that trained on locomotor tasks. These results thus support the specificity of training concept (Richards et al 1993) and clearly demonstrate that 4 weeks of training three times a week for 1 hour can lead to important changes in the walking capacity of people with chronic stroke. Salbach et al (2004), in a multicentred randomized controlled trial involving 91 subjects, inspired by the results of Dean et al (2000), have also found that 6 weeks of mobility-related task training significantly improves the distance walked in 6 minutes.

Teixeira-Salmela et al (1999, 2001) have reported that a 10-week programme of muscle strengthening and physical conditioning leads to improved locomotor capacity in chronic stroke survivors. Although somewhat different from the Dean et al (2000) and Salbach et al (2004) studies, the rationale for this study was similar and the findings are in agreement. These three studies demonstrate the feasibility of out-patient-based training programmes aimed at improving walking competency and the potential for improvement in people with chronic stroke. Given the rapid return to home of people with mild and moderate stroke in the USA, Duncan et al (1998), prior to embarking on the large Kansas City Stroke Study, undertook a pilot study designed to compare usual care with a therapist-supervised home programme that included balance, strength and endurance training and varied walking practice. As expected, the latter regimen produced gains in balance, gait speed and endurance outcomes that were superior to the control group. It is interesting to note that the investigators found walking practice alone not intense enough to promote changes in endurance, and added an ergonomic bicycle to the programme for the later subjects.

Altogether, the results of these studies demonstrate once again that people with stroke discharged to their homes either have not attained their full walking potential or have not maintained gains reached during the active rehabilitation phase. The question is then whether such programmes should be made available to people with chronic stroke to help them maintain gains or to reach new levels of walking competency, defined as a level of walking ability that allows an individual successfully to navigate in their community. Criteria of successful navigation include the ability to:

- walk at speeds to safely cross streets (77–138 cm/s; Robinett and Vondran, 1988);

- walk long enough distances to accomplish tasks of daily living (about 300 m);

- negotiate raised curbs (Lerner-Frankiel et al 1986);

- demonstrate anticipatory strategies to avoid or accommodate for obstacles (McFadyen and Winter 1991, Said et al 1999, 2001).

If we remember that most people affected by stroke walk slower than 50 cm/s when discharged from in-patient rehabilitation (Goldie et al 1996, Richards et al 1999), and that Perry et al (1995) have found community-independent people after stroke to walk at about 80 (±18) cm/s, we must find ways to help people with stroke improve their walking competency.

The emphasis on muscle strengthening should not imply that spasticity during walking is not a crucial problem in some people with stroke (Knutsson and Richards 1979, Lamontagne et al 2001), but rather that, in most, paresis will dominate. Excessive coactivation of antagonistic muscles may also dominate the motor control disorder in a minority of the cases (Knutsson and Richards 1979) and excessive coactivation of antagonist muscles at the ankle may also occur on the non-paretic limb as a compensatory mechanism to promote stability (Lamontagne et al 2000a). Interestingly, the excessive stiffness of the paretic plantarflexors that has been shown to be present in the first months after stroke (Malouin et al 1997) may augment the resistance to dorsiflexion in mid- and late-stance phases of the gait cycle, to compensate for weak plantarflexors (Lamontagne et al 2000b). On the other hand, excessive plantarflexor stiffness may impede dorsiflexion in early swing phase (Lamontagne et al 2002).

AUGMENTING PRACTICE TO INCREASE PRACTICE TIME

Over the last 15 years, several retraining approaches have been proposed for promoting the recovery of locomotor skills after stroke (see Richards et al 1999 for a review; Richards and Olney 1996). Because most of the motor recovery of the lower extremity takes place within the first 6 weeks after stroke (Duncan et al 1994, Richards et al 1993), there is a general acceptance that the training of locomotor function should be initiated as early as possible (Malouin et al 1992). The intensity and the type of training are other factors to consider. In non-human primates the number of repetitions and the specificity of the activities selected for training are critical for promoting cortical reorganization associated with the recovery of movements after a cortical infarct (see Nudo et al 2001 for a review). Similar findings have been reported in human studies using transcranial magnetic stimulation (TMS), a non-invasive tool to investigate the underlying mechanisms of plasticity associated with the restitution of function (Liepert and Weiller 1999, Liepert et al 2000, Traversa et al 1997). Results from clinical studies also support the importance of repetition and training specificity in the recovery of locomotor skills (Dean et al 2000, Kwakkel et al 1999b, Richards et al 1993). For example, larger gains were obtained with more intensive practice and with training that focused on locomotor-related activities (i.e. task-specific approach) underlying the need to increase the number of repetitions (practice time) and to use a task-oriented approach for training (Dean et al 2000, Dean and Shepherd 1997, Malouin et al 1992, Richards et al 1993).

Why is it understood that Olympic athletes and virtuoso musicians must devote a large proportion of their time to practice first to acquire and then to maintain their skills, while people who must relearn a skill after stroke spend few hours practising, even when in active rehabilitation? Observational studies of rehabilitation units have found that stroke survivors in rehabilitation centres spend large proportions of the day alone and inactive (Keith 1980, Mackey et al 1996, Tinson, 1989). These findings suggest that more time could be dedicated to the practice of motor skills. Thus, because practice is critical to skill acquisition (Dean et al 2000, Nudo et al 2001, Richards et al 1993), stroke rehabilitation needs to be planned to maximize the opportunity for task-related practice, both self-monitored and under the guidance of a therapist (Carr and Shepherd 1998, Dean et al 2000). More physical practice, however, is not always possible for many patients given that the major causes of disability are weakness, fatigue, poor endurance and loss of coordination (Bohannon 1986, Burke 1988, Carr and Shepherd 1998, Tangemann et al 1990). These observations suggest that the amount of physical practice the patients can accomplish, especially in the early rehabilitation period, is limited. Further motor recovery would thus be expected if patients could practise more, both with less physical effort and on their own without endangering their safety.

Mental practice

Intrigued with the potential of mental practice as an adjunct to physical practice to enhance locomotor skill acquisition in people after stroke, in the mid-1990s the authors began to collaborate with Julien Doyon, a neuropsychologist specializing in motor learning and brain imagery techniques. This led to a series of behavioural studies using positron emission tomography (PET) and in collaboration with two doctoral students in neuropsychology (P Jackson and M Lafleur) and other researchers including a neuropsychologist specializing in working memory (S Belleville).

Mental practice as an adjunct to physical practice, used by athletes and musicians to enhance their motor skills, has been poorly exploited in rehabilitation. The results of a number of recent studies taken together have begun to reveal the potential of using mental practice techniques to promote skill acquisition by increasing the number of repetitions without the strain associated with physical repetitions.

What is mental practice? Humans have the ability to generate mental correlates of motor events without any external stimulus, a function known as motor imagery. Motor imagery corresponds to a dynamic state during which the representation of a specific action is internally reactivated within working memory without any overt motor output (Decety and Grèzes 1999). Mental practice, on the other hand, is the act of repeating the imagined movements several times with the intention of improving motor performance (Jackson et al 2001a). Several studies in sport psychology have shown that mental practice combined with physical practice can be effective in optimizing motor skills in athletes and help novice learners in the acquisition of new skilled behaviours (Driskell et al 1994, Feltz and Landers 1983, Hinshaw 1991).

A natural question is whether the neural correlates activated by mental practice compare with those activated by physical practice for the same skill. This has been answered by a series of functional brain imaging studies (for reviews see Jackson et al 2001a, Lafleur et al 2002), which have clearly demonstrated imagined and physically executed movements to share common neural networks. Because we were interested in locomotor practice, and most of the earlier studies examined hand or finger movements, we recently confirmed that similar neural networks are activated during the imagining and physical execution of sequential ankle movements (Figure 9.1, left panels) (Lafleur et al 1999, 2002). We have also shown that when healthy people imagine locomotor-related tasks (standing, walking, initiating gait and walking around obstacles) increased brain activity is found in neural networks (Figure 9.2) analogous to those activated during the execution of corresponding motor actions (Malouin et al 2003a, 2003b). A recent study by Lafleur et al (2002) has extended the anatomical association between imagined and physically executed movements to a motor learning paradigm. The pattern of dynamic changes in regional cerebral blood flow before and after practice

Figure 9.1   Brain activations during the imagining of walking. Similar brain areas activated during physical or mental rehearsal of movement sequences of the left foot. Note the similar changes at a more advanced stage of learning. Less brain areas are activated after learning and the activation is more localized. (From Lafleur et al 1999.)

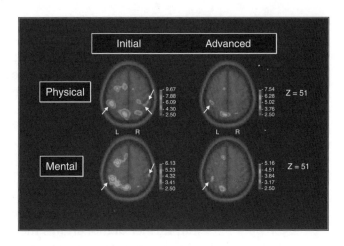

Figure 9.2   Merged positron emission tomography (PET)–magnetic resonance imaging (MRI) sections illustrating increases of regional blood flow (rCBF) associated with the imagining of walking. The images were averaged over the six subjects and presented as the imagined walking condition minus the control condition (rest). Each subtraction yielded focal changes in blood flow shown as *t*-statistic images. The range is coded by a colour scale. (From Malouin et al 2003b, with permission of EDK Publishers.)

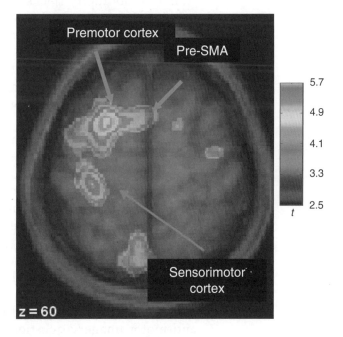

of an explicitly known sequence of foot movements was compared when executed physically and during motor imagery of the same movements. It was shown that, for both the early and late phases of learning, mental imagery and physical practice elicited a similar pattern (Figure 9.1, right panels). These data suggest that the cerebral plasticity that occurs during the acquisition of a motor skill is similar whether the skill is practised physically or mentally (Lafleur et al 2002).

Further evidence supporting the use of mental practice comes from the elegant work of Pascual-Leone et al (1995) using TMS mapping techniques to monitor brain plasticity induced by physical and mental practice of a sequence of finger movements. They not only documented that mental practice induced representational changes in the brain comparable to those yielded by physical practice, but also that subjects who had been practising mentally for five sessions could attain, with one additional physical practice session, the same level of performance as those who practised physically for five sessions. This finding suggests that part of the behavioural improvement induced by mental practice may be latent, waiting to be expressed after minimal physical practice, and further demonstrates the advantage of combining mental and physical practice. Altogether, these findings suggest that mental practice induces preparatory effects, which increase the efficiency of subsequent physical training (Pascual-Leone et al 1995). Results from our laboratory (Jackson et al 2001b, 2003) corroborate the priming effects of mental practice. Changes in brain activity, after five days of intensive mental practice, were restricted to the medial aspect of the orbito-frontal cortex, which is involved in recognition memory and reward-related learning (Rogers et al 1999). This finding supports the view that mental practice initially improves performance by acting on motor preparation and planning rather than execution.

Can all people benefit from mental practice? If so, how can we be sure that the person is engaging in the required practice? These questions are fundamental to the clinical use of mental practice. Studies show that not all people are able to engage in motor imagery, which is a prerequisite to rehearse motor actions mentally (Roure et al 1999); moreover, the location of a brain lesion may also impair imagery capacity (Sirigu et al 1996, Yaguez et al 1999). In addition, recent findings suggest the outcome of mental practice after stroke to be related to working memory performance (Malouin et al 2002, 2004a).

Motor imagery ability can be assessed with chronometric tests and motor imagery questionnaires. A number of studies have reported the temporal congruence (time taken to execute the movement) of physically and mentally simulated movements (Jackson et al 2001a). Findings from chronometric studies suggest that most patients with a cerebral lesion are able to engage in motor imagery (Decety and Boisson 1990, Malouin et al 2001a, Sirigu et al 1995). For example, people after stroke take more time when they imagine movements with their affected limb than with their unaffected limb, and the movement time for the imagined task is similar to that needed for its physical execution (Decety and Boisson 1990, Malouin et al 2001a, 2004a, 2004c, Sirigu et al 1995).

Using a motor imagery screening test, which has a construct similar to other chronometric tests involving walking (Malouin et al 2003a), and foot-tapping tasks (Lafleur et al 2002), we further investigated the motor imagery ability of a group of 29 people with chronic stroke (Malouin et al 2001a). Subjects were instructed to imagine picking up blocks from a box and to verbally signal each time they removed a block until the examiner told them to stop. Each trial terminated after varying time periods (25, 15 and 35 s) presented randomly. As expected, the number of blocks removed increased with time, and the pattern was similar in the people with stroke and in healthy control subjects, suggesting that the people with stroke were engaging in mental simulation of the task (Figure 9.3). Such chronometric tests proved useful to detect impaired motor imagery abilities as reported in some patients with lesions restricted to the basal ganglia (Yaguez et al 1999) or the parietal lobes (Sirigu et al 1996). Altogether, these findings suggest that simple chronometric measures can be used as a screening tool to assess motor imagery ability after stroke.

Questionnaires have also been used in sport psychology to assess motor imagery ability (Hall and Pongrac 1983). Their use with people with cerebral lesions, however, is relatively new. Findings from preliminary studies indicate that, contrary to healthy subjects, people after stroke find it easier to engage in visual than kinaesthetic imagery (Malouin et al 2002, 2004a). Moreover, in contrast to healthy subjects, the visual and kinaesthetic imagery scores were not correlated. Such dissociation in visual and kinaesthetic imagery is possibly related to the location of the cerebral lesion, since each type of mental representation of action depends on different brain areas (Deiber et al 1998, Naito et al 2002, Ruby and Decety 2001). Thus, further studies are needed to determine the validity of motor imagery questionnaires as a screening tool.

Figure 9.3   Motor imagery screening test. In this screening test, the subjects were instructed to imagine picking up blocks from a box and to verbally signal each time they removed a block until the examiner told them to stop. Each trial terminated after varying time periods (25, 15 and 35 s) presented randomly. As expected the number of blocks retrieved increased with time, and the increase in the number of blocks was similar in both groups, suggesting that the patients were effectively engaged in the mental simulation of the task.

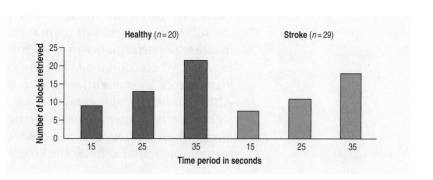

Lastly, results of our recent pilot study suggest that working memory is an important factor in the success of mental practice. Subjects with stroke were trained to increase the vertical load on their affected limb during standing-up and sitting-down tasks by combining mental and physical practice. Subjects with impaired working memory (in verbal, visuo-spatial or kinaesthetic working memory) had more difficulty in engaging in mental practice (Malouin et al 2002, 2004a). Furthermore, subjects with impaired working memory had no retention 24 hours later. The latter observation suggests that the ability to maintain and manipulate information in working memory is necessary for mental practice.

Many investigators have proposed the use of mental practice in physical rehabilitation as a cost-efficient means of promoting motor recovery after damage to the central nervous system (Decety 1993, Jackson et al 2001a, Van Leeuwen and Inglis 1998, Warner and McNeill 1988, Yue and Cole 1992). To date, however, only a few modest studies have been conducted examining the training of the upper limb after stroke using mental practice (Page 2000, Page et al 2001, Yoo et al 2001). Although findings from these studies suggest that mental practice can be beneficial, because of the global nature of the outcome measures used, it is not clear whether the effects were specific to mental practice.

The aim of our first clinical studies was thus to dissociate the effects of mental practice on the performance of a foot sequence skill in people after stroke when mental and physical practice were combined (Jackson et al 2004). An example is illustrated in Figure 9.4. The patient was a right-handed 38-year-old man who had suffered a left haemorrhagic subcortical stroke 4 months prior to the beginning of the study. He was asked to practise a serial reaction time task with the lower limb in three distinct training phases over a period of 5 weeks: 2 weeks of physical practice, 1 week of combined physical and mental practice and then 2 weeks of mental practice alone. The subject's average response time improved significantly during the first 5 days of physical practice (26%), but then fluctuated and failed to show additional improvement. The combination of mental and physical practice during the 3rd week yielded an extra 10% improvement. Finally, the following 2 weeks of mental practice resulted in a marginal increase in performance of 2%. This finding suggests that mental practice, when combined with physical practice, can improve the learning of a sequential motor skill in people after stroke. Although the use of mental practice alone might not be enough to significantly improve performance after some learning has already been achieved, it could nevertheless help in the retention of newly acquired abilities (Jackson et al 2004).

Figure 9.4   A 38-year-old man, with a left subcortical lesion, practised a serial reaction time task with the lower limb in three distinct training phases over a period of 5 weeks: 2 weeks of physical practice (PP), 1 week of combined physical and mental practice (PP and MP) and then 2 weeks of mental practice alone (MP). The motor performance reached a plateau after 10 days of physical practice (PP); it was followed by further improvement with the addition of mental practice (PP and MP) over the next week, and after 2 weeks of MP alone the motor performance was maintained. Each bar represents the mean (SD) of 30 repetitions recorded after the training sessions. Only one measure was recorded after the 10 days of MP alone (session 16; see text for further details).

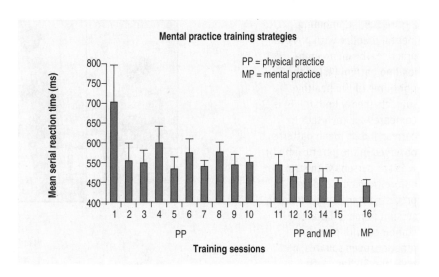

We then studied the combined effects of physical and mental practice on the retraining of limb loading during standing-up and sitting-down, a locomotor subtask that is more ecological (functional) than a foot movement sequence (Malouin et al 2002, 2004a, 2004b) in a group of 12 people with stroke. In a single session, subjects were trained with combined mental and physical practice (seven series each consisting of five mental repetitions, preceded by one physical repetition) to exert symmetrical vertical forces on the lower limbs during standing-up from a chair and sitting-down. Vertical forces were recorded using three force plates placed under each foot and the chair. The change in the per cent loading on the paretic leg was measured at baseline, after training and 24 hours later. At baseline, the patients exerted less load on the affected leg while standing-up and sitting-down and they executed both tasks 60% slower than healthy control subjects. After training, the loading on the affected leg increased for both tasks (17% and 16% respectively) and much of the improvement was retained 24 hours later, indicating a learning effect of the motor skills. In contrast, the duration of the performance did not change with training, signifying that combined mental and physical practice can lead to improved dynamic loading of the paretic leg without immediately affecting movement speed (Figure 9.5). The design of this study, however, did not permit the differentiation of the effects associated with mental practice. Thus, comparison with a group of patients trained with physical practice only would provide a measure of the additive effects of mental practice on the learning of the motor skills. Another question that needs to be addressed is whether mental practice promotes a transfer of the learned skill to

Figure 9.5 Combining mental practice with physical practice. The mean limb-loading pattern (%) of the right limb of the healthy subjects (heavy line: $n = 6$) is compared for each task to corresponding mean patterns observed in the paretic limb ($n = 12$) of persons with stroke before training (solid line: pretest), after a single training session of mental practice combined with physical practice (open squares: post test) and 24 hours after training (filled circles: follow-up). The increased loading on the paretic leg with training is maintained a day later indicating retention of the newly acquired motor skills.

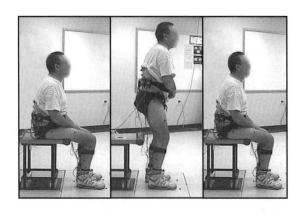

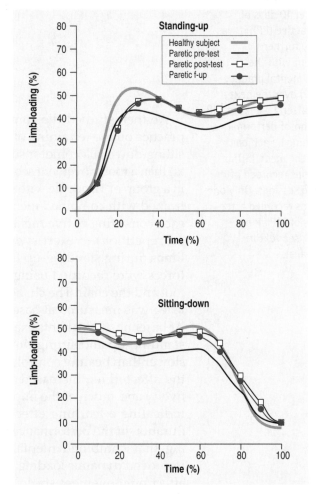

a non-practised skill, or whether it is specific to the practised task (Dean and Shepherd 1997, Winstein et al 1989). Thus, to study the specificity of mental practice, other non-practised tasks should be assessed. We are attempting to answer this question in a random-ized clinical trial.

Virtual reality (VR) training systems

Encouraged to apply technological advances to rehabilitation by the Canadian Foundation for Innovation, a multidisciplinary team has been formed to explore the potential of virtual reality (VR) systems for locomotor training. VR refers to a range of computing technologies that present artificially generated sensory information (from vision and proprioception) in a form that people perceive as similar to real-world objects and events (Rheingold 1991). The term virtual environment (VE) describes the simulation of a visual three-dimensional (3D) environment presented to the subject via a monitor, a large screen or through a helmet-mounted display (HMD). In a VE, the simulated objects and events are not only sensed, but the user can anticipate and react to them as though they were real. The user often feels, at least to some degree, 'present' in the simulated world, and this feeling of presence is arguably the defining feature of the VR experience (Steuer 1992). Walking on a treadmill in a VE allows users to walk over large virtual distances as well as practise manoeuvring (e.g. sidestep) without actually moving far in the real world (Darken et al 1997).

Specialists in stroke rehabilitation, the motor control of posture and gait and the biomechanics of gait from Quebec City (C Richards, F Malouin and B McFadyen) and Montreal (J Fung, A Lamontagne and R Forget) are collaborating with a neuropsychologist specialized in way finding (C Rainville), an electrical engineer specialized in artificial vision and the creation of VEs (D Laurendeau) and a mechanical engineer specialized in the hydraulic control of simulators (C Gosselin). This team is working with an industrial partner, the MOTEK company of Amsterdam, to develop a locomotor training system to augment the practice of locomotion. The unique advantage of training locomotion in a VE is that multiple aspects of locomotor skills can be trained safely within a confined space.

Although VR technology has long been applied to motion simulations in movies, video games, flight simulators and the training of the infantry by the US army (Darken et al 1997), its application to rehabilitation is relatively new (Deutsch et al 2001, McComas et al 1998, McComas and Sveistrup 2002, Whitney et al 2002). A basic question with regards to practice in VEs is whether the learning will be transferred to real-life situations. In rehabilitation applications, generalization from VR training to real-world environments has been reported for upper limb (Holden et al 2001) and lower limb (Deutsch et al 2001) training after stroke, and of spatial learning in children (McComas et al 1998). Of particular interest is the work of DeRugy et al (2000), demonstrating that the placement of the foot in relation to visual cues is the same in a VE as in real life. To date very little is known about the potential of VR locomotor training methods for people after stroke (Brown et al 2002).

The rationale for developing VEs for locomotor training and eventually the diagnosis of locomotor control disorders, simply put, stems from the need to increase the amount and improve the quality of locomotor practice to promote learning after stroke. Motor learning is promoted by factors (for a review see Winstein 1991) such as changing environmental contexts, alterations in the physical demands, problem solving, random presentation of practice tasks, sufficient practice and patient empowerment. It is difficult to meet these criteria for the practice of locomotor tasks in currently constrained rehabilitation settings or to practise outdoors in different weather and lighting conditions. VR technology, with the capacity for simulating environments, offers a new and safe way not only to increase practice time but also to offer the varied environments and constraints needed to maximize learning. Moreover, the 'hi-tech' nature of the practice itself can be a further motivation for the subjects. The goal is thus to design a locomotor training VR system that will be motivational, provide varied and environmentally contextual practice and allow for safe individual practice (repetitions) at ever-increasing difficulty levels while providing knowledge of results and promoting empowerment of the subject.

As shown in Figure 9.6, subjects will walk on a treadmill mounted on a six degrees of freedom movable platform and will interact with a virtual scene projected on a large screen in front of them. They will wear a safety harness and be instrumented for motion analysis using transmitters from the Polhemus electromagnetic system on the feet, trunk (estimated level of the body centre of mass), head and hands. The treadmill speed, determined by the subject, drives the movement within the virtual scene, while the programmed virtual events will dictate the platform movement. The subject will interact with the VE, controlling advancement into it and experiencing certain physical aspects (e.g. changes in surface slopes) in relation to the scene. At present, we have developed two basic VEs, one an inside corridor and the second an outdoor scene related to street crossing on the way to a shopping centre. These VEs are allowing us to test the various components of the system and will serve as the baseline for further development (Fung et al 2004, McFadyen et al 2004). Much work remains to be done on the planning and programming of the VEs, practice methods and knowledge of results before we can begin testing, first in healthy people and then in people with stroke. We then need to evaluate the potential of the developed VR-treadmill-coupled training programme to improve mobility that impacts on community ambulation by comparing it to a conventional treadmill training programme.

Figure 9.6   The top photograph illustrates the first prototype of our virtual reality system for locomotor training. A subject, wearing a safety harness, walks on a treadmill bolted to a platform capable of moving with 6 degrees of freedom while looking at a screen displaying a virtual environment (VE). A feedback system allows the subject to determine the speed of the powered treadmill. The VE is coupled to the speed of the treadmill and the movements of the platform so that the subject experiences the changes in the support surface seen in the VE. In the bottom photograph a subject is seen wearing a head-mounted display allowing him to view the VE shown on the computer screen.

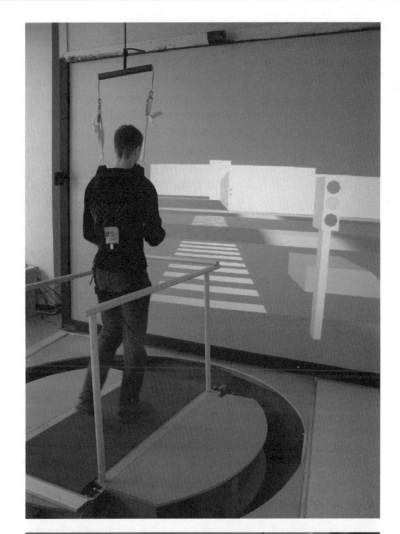

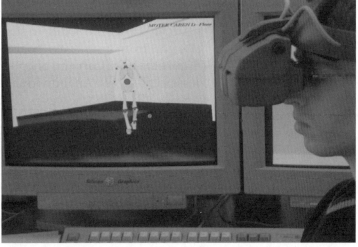

TASK-ORIENTED LOCOMOTOR-RELATED TRAINING

Rising to walk

The task-oriented concept of training of locomotor function is not exclusive to walking per se, but also requires the training of loco-motor-related activities such as standing-up from a chair and sitting-down. Following a stroke, a person's ability to stand from a seated position and to sit down from a standing position is affected to a varying degree. For example, compared with healthy subjects rising from a chair, people after stroke take 25–61% longer and put much more load on the non-paretic limb, decreasing the vertical forces on the paretic limb by 20–25% during the task (Engardt and Olsson 1992, Hesse et al 1994b, Malouin et al 2004a, 2004b). Similar disturbances in limb loading have been observed during sitting-down task (Engardt and Olsson 1992, Malouin et al 2004a, 2004b, 2004c), and these mobility tasks, which are basic parts of daily activities, are among the first to be trained in the early stage of rehabilitation (Carr and Shepherd 1998, Roorda et al 1996). Based on the task-oriented approach, the training of mobility tasks involves practice with chairs and benches having different characteristics (variable heights, shape and stability) to promote variable practice conditions (Carr and Shepherd 1998). Such practice not only improves strength and endurance, but also assists the patient in learning to adapt to environmental demands (Carr and Shepherd 1987, Dean et al 2000).

The availability of highly sophisticated equipment and specialized laboratory personnel brought together initially to study gait provided the opportunity to study other mobility tasks to gain insight into means of promoting recovery after stroke. We have thus studied different mobility tasks that we consider to be subcomponents of locomotion and essential to walking competency. Some of this work is briefly summarized below.

After a stroke, the ability to stand from a seated position or to initiate gait from a standing position is affected to varying degrees (Brunt et al 1995, Carr and Shepherd 1998, Engardt and Olsson 1992, Hesse et al 1994b). An individual assessment of the two subtasks of rise-to-walk (RTW), however, is not usually done. Instead, the task is taken as a whole and blended to other mobility tasks in the Timed Up and Go (TUG) score (Podsiadlo and Richardson 1991). While the TUG assesses the performance of an ensemble of tasks, it does not focus on the subject's performance during the rising from the chair and gait initiation, nor does it account for the motor strategies used. On the basis of in-depth biomechanical and clinical studies, we have recently proposed the use of the RTW task to assess not only mobility, or the time needed to rise from a seated position, but also locomotor coordination (Dion et al 2003, Malouin et al 2001b, 2003b). The evaluation of locomotor coordination as fluid or non-fluid is based on biomechanical measures that show that, in healthy subjects, the sit-to-stand and stand-to-walk tasks merge smoothly. Thus, RTW is characterized firstly by the initiation of stepping before reaching the full standing position, and secondly by the maintenance of the forward body momentum until the end of the task (Figure 9.7). Such a merging of the two tasks has been defined as a fluid motor strategy (Magnan et al 1996). In a recent study, we found that in contrast to healthy subjects, most subjects with stroke (16/19) were unable to merge rising-up and gait initiation in the RTW task, and had instead a non-fluid strategy as they stood-up and then initiated walking (Dion et al 1999a, 1999b, Malouin et al 2001b, 2003d). In addition, it was found that the patients took 1.6 times longer to RTW than healthy subjects (Dion et al 1999a, 1999b, 2003). Malouin et al (2001b, 2003d) further quantified the fluidity of task merging during the RTW. It was found that the maintenance of the horizontal body momentum, which characterizes the fluid motor strategy, was impaired to various degrees after stroke (Figure 9.8a). Therefore, a fluidity index (FI) was proposed to quantify the fluidity by computing the amount of change in the body forward momentum. Results indicated that only the patients with toe-off before reaching full elevation of the body had FIs that were within control values. Lastly, a four-point ordinal scale to provide a clinical measure of the fluidity of the motor strategy was developed (Malouin et al 2003d). To validate this ordinal scale (0–3: 3 = normal fluidity) FI values were compared with scores from the fluidity scale (Figure 9.8b). The FI values did not overlap across categories of the scale indicating that the descriptors of the scale provided a gradation of fluidity comparable to the gold standard measure (FI). In addition, a substantial level of agreement between raters (weighted kappa = 0.78) indicated that trained clinicians can use the fluidity scale with a substantial level of reliability. Inter-rater reliability for measurement of the RTW duration was high [intra-class correlation coefficient (ICC) = 0.95].

Altogether, the results of these studies indicate that after stroke the fluidity of body movements normally associated with the RTW task is generally lost. The drop in the centre of mass forward momentum shows that after stroke most patients separate the two tasks: they stand up and then start walking. The sequencing of tasks is consistent with the slowing of the RTW task (Dion et al 1999a, 1999b, 2003). The non-fluid strategy is also safer given the reduced capacity of the paretic limb to assist in the braking of the forward body momentum (Dion et al 1999a, Malouin et al 2001b, 2003d). In addition, the non-merging of the two tasks prevents the additional challenge of balancing on one limb while standing up and taking the first step at the same time. Clinical findings further underline that the fluidity of the body movements in the RTW task

Figure 9.7   Lack of fluidity in the rise-to-walk task after stroke. In healthy subjects (top), the heel is off (white arrow in a circle) before full body elevation (FBE) occurs, resulting in a fluid motor strategy characterized by the merging of rising-up and gait initiation. The fluid motor strategy is associated with the maintenance of the forward body momentum until the end of the task. After stroke (bottom), the FBE occurs before heel-off as the patient separates the two tasks: rising-up is followed by gait initiation.

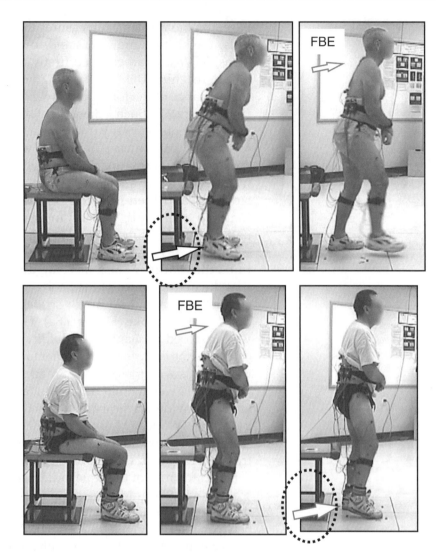

requires a higher level of motor recovery, which makes the fluidity of the motor strategy a good indicator (outcome measure) of more advanced motor control.

Initiating gait

The gait initiation process is defined as the transition from quiet stance to the cyclic movements of walking (Winter 1995). Gait initiation involves preparatory adjustments (PAs) or dynamic phenomena (Brenière et al 1987, Brenière and Do 1986) characterized by bilateral electromyographic (EMG) sequences and mechanical events that precede movements of the lower limbs (Brenière et al 1987; Crenna and Frigo 1991). These PAs are bilateral and consist of an inhibition of the soleus and an early activation burst in

Figure 9.8 (a) Patterns of forward body progression during the rise-to-walk task. The mean centre of mass (COM) horizontal momentum curve from the control group (heavy line) is compared with corresponding curves of one subject in the fluid cerebrovascular accident (CVA) subgroup (thin line) and of one subject in the non-fluid CVA subgroup (broken line). The degree of fluidity was calculated using the fluidity index (FI), which corresponds to the percentage of change in the body forward momentum. The larger FIs indicate more fluidity (merging of the tasks: initiating gait while rising-up); conversely, lower FI values indicate less fluidity (separation of the tasks: rising-up, then walking; Malouin et al 2001b). (b) Fluidity indexes (FIs) for the control (CTL) group and CVA groups. The three patients with the highest scores on the clinical fluidity scale (score 3) had the highest FI values (range: 92–72%), whereas lower FI values corresponded to lower fluidity scores. The majority (11/19) of the patients had a fluidity score of 2, with FI values ranging from 52% to 16%. The three patients with a fluidity score of 1 had near-zero FI values (8–3%), whereas in the two other patients, with a fluidity score of 0, the FI values were negative (−4% and −9%). Note that the subgroup with a fluid motor strategy (score of 3) had FI values similar to control. The FI index values for each category of the scale did not overlap indicating that the descriptors provided a gradation of the rise-to-walk (RTW) performance similar to that from the instrumented method (Malouin et al 2003d).

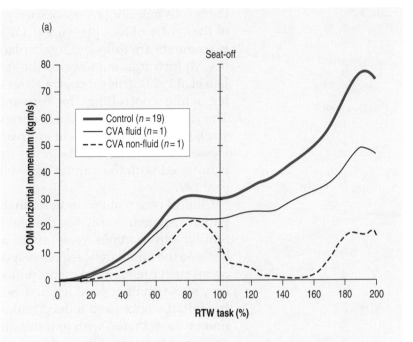

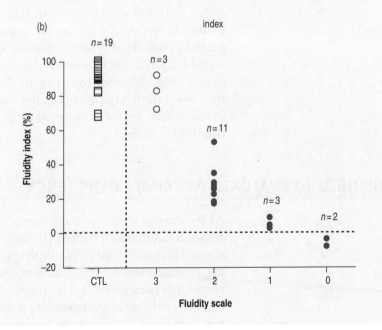

the tibialis anterior (TA) associated with a backward displacement of the centre of foot pressure (COP) (Figure 9.9a). The COP displacements are followed by displacement of the centre of mass (COM) forwards and towards the stance limb (Brenière et al 1987, Jian et al 1993). This process requires momentarily standing on one leg while controlling the forward momentum of the body. The magnitude of the PAs is correlated with gait speed. After stroke, these PAs are absent or greatly reduced (Brunt et al 1995, Hesse et al 1997) with the largest disturbances occurring when gait is initiated with the paretic leg (Malouin et al 1994, 1995, Hesse et al 1997).

Clinical observations indicate that after a stroke the majority of patients spontaneously use the paretic limb as the stepping limb. Similar observations were made for the RTW task, probably because the non-paretic leg offers more stability. When questioned about such preference patients will admit they feel more secure if they stand on their good leg first. Selecting the non-paretic leg as the initial stance limb indeed makes sense, since dynamic phenomena associated with gait initiation (Brenière et al 1987) will challenge their stability, and these phenomena are smaller when gait is initiated with the paretic leg. Thus, motivating the patients to initiate stepping with the non-paretic leg when rising-up from a seated position or when initiating gait from a standing position should contribute to improving the supporting function of the paretic leg. In addition, the finding that initiating gait with the non-paretic leg promotes the early activation of the TA burst in the paretic leg (Malouin et al 1995) further supports such a practice (Figure 9.9b).

THE NEED TO EVALUATE WALKING COMPETENCY

As discussed in the preceding sections, the concept of walking competency has not driven clinical interventions for people after stroke (Richards et al 1999). Both the quantity and quality of walking practice have been deficient, and cognitive processes have been largely neglected. The responsiveness of clinical measures used to evaluate impairments and disabilities related to locomotor function must also be questioned. For example, clinical measures such as the Balance Scale (Berg et al 1989, 1992, 1995), the Barthel Ambulation subscale (Mahoney and Barthel 1954) and the Fugl-Meyer leg subscale (Fugl-Meyer et al 1975) may be sensitive to changes in locomotor function in subjects walking very slowly but are not sensitive to changes in people walking at more than 35 cm/s (Richards et al 1995). In an in-depth study of responsiveness, Salbach et al (2001) have shown that the 5-m walk test at free

Figure 9.9   (a) A series of curves illustrating preparatory adjustments (PAs) during gait initiation. COP, displacement of the centre of foot pressure; SOL, activation of the soleus muscle; TA, activation of the tibialis anterior muscle; F_X, anteroposterior ground reaction force. Mean values in three groups of patients with stroke are compared with the 95% confidence interval around the mean from a healthy control group ($n = 11$) during gait initiation with the paretic leg. The gait initiation process (GIP) is divided into two phases and each is normalized to 100%: phase I begins with first COP backward displacement and ends with toe-off of the swing limb: (TO_1), and phase II begins with toe-off of the swing limb and ends with toe-off of the stance limb (TO_2). Heel-off (HO) is indicated by a triangle on the x-axis. The magnitude of COP_x (anteroposterior) displacement is normalized to foot length, and the F_X values are normalized in per cent of body weight. The patients in group 1 ($n = 3$) had no PAs on either side; patients in group 2 ($n = 8$) had PAs on the non-paretic leg only (not shown), and in patients of group 3 ($n = 8$) PAs were similar to that in control subjects. (b) Comparison of the TA activation when initiating gait with either the paretic (thin line: paretic swing leg, Psw) or the non-paretic leg (thick line: paretic stance leg, Pst). Note the emergence of the early TA activation burst when the paretic leg is the support limb (Pst).

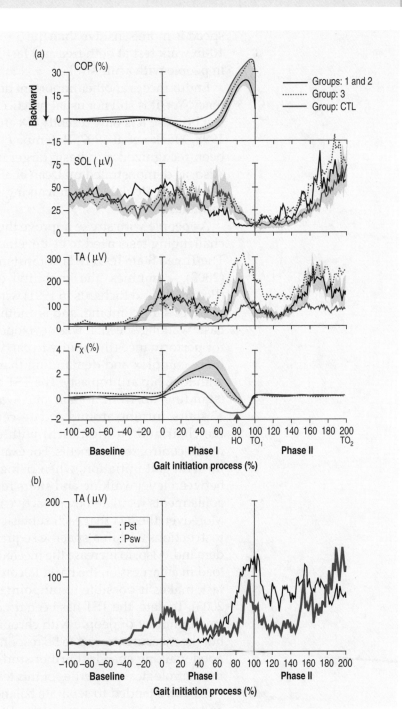

speed is more sensitive than the 5-m walk test at fast speed or the 10-m walk test at both free and fast speeds to evaluate gait speed in people with acute stroke.

Endurance is another important determinant of walking competency. Yet, it is still not usual practice to include the 6-minute walk test because it is only recently (Dean et al 2000, 2001, Duncan et al 1998, Macko et al 1997, Potempa et al 1995) that endurance has been recognized as a basic target of rehabilitation after stroke. Also, as demonstrated by Dean et al (2001), functional endurance cannot be calculated from walking speed over 10 m or reference formulas.

As people with stroke improve their walking competency, more challenging tests need to be developed to monitor improvement. The Timed Stair Test (TST), for instance, introduced by Perron et al (2003), combines the mobility characteristics of the TUG (Podsiadlo and Richardson 1991) with the added task and physical effort of stair climbing, and is another measure that goes beyond basic walking speed. It was developed to assess advanced locomotor performance (the ability to carry out locomotor-related tasks more complex and demanding than solely walking) in patients with total hip arthroplasty. The TST consists of a series of subtasks (standing up from a chair and walking, ascending a flight of 13 stairs, turning around and descending stairs, walking back to the chair and sitting down) with different biomechanical and motor control requirements. For example, the merging of standing up with gait initiation, when rising to walk, and the transitions between level walking and stairs require anticipatory locomotor adjustments regulated by proactive mechanisms of motor control. Moreover, the fact that each subtask must be completed following instructions and in a specific sequence increases the attentional demand. Also, to increase the mechanical demand, subjects carry a load in a harness on the back. Recording the duration of each subtask makes it possible to pinpoint specific deficits (Perron et al 2003). To date, the TST has been used as an outcome measure in a small number of people with chronic stroke (Richards et al 1999) but the measure proved to be responsive even in people with very good walking speeds. Further studies are required to determine the metrological properties of this test.

We have tended to separate balance from walking, and to train and evaluate them separately. The Step Test, which was developed by Hill et al (1996) and allows for the evaluation of the paretic and non-paretic legs of people with stroke when acting as the supporting or stepping leg, provides important information on dynamic balance (Dean et al 2000). We have recently examined the temporal characteristics of the Step Test, which requires stepping one foot on, then off, a 7.5-cm-high block as quickly as possible in a set time period (15 s). As with walking, the Step Test places demands on both legs. After a stroke, the stepping is slower than in normal control subjects, and the repetitions are fewer (Bernhardt et al 1998, Richards et al 1999). Neither the duration nor the number of step repetitions, however, explains whether the slowing is related to the diminished mobility of the stepping leg or to the lack of stability of the stance leg. To address this question, we recorded the time spent in bipodal and unipodal stance in two conditions: Affected Leg Stepping and Affected Leg Supporting (Malouin et al 2003c). In healthy people, the duration of the forward (576 ms ± 0.95) and backward phases (567 ms ± 103) was symmetrical when stepping with either foot, and most of the time was spent in unipodal stance (61% ± 7.7), whereas after stroke the duration was increased two- to threefold, with the largest increase in the Affected Leg Stepping condition. Moreover, the proportion of time spent in unipodal stance after stroke was smaller, with the least time spent in the Affected Leg Supporting condition (Figure 9.10). Interestingly, there was a strong correlation between time in unipodal stance and the stepping speed ($r = 0.88$). The results indicate that people with stroke spent twice as much time as healthy control subjects in bipodal stance, probably because they required more time to recover their balance. The least time spent in unilateral stance in the Affected Leg Supporting condition suggests this condition to be of greater challenge with respect to balance. Altogether these findings indicate the Affected Leg Supporting condition to be a good indicator of dynamic balance and support the construct validity of the Step Test.

The role of cognitive processes related to planning, wayfinding, obstacle avoidance and information processing are not well understood in healthy people, let alone people after stroke. Studies such as those of Gérin-Lajoie et al (2001, 2004), who examined how healthy people negotiate human-shaped obstacles, helps us better understand anticipatory locomotor adjustments and information processing, but much further work in this area remains to be done. It is anticipated that virtual reality systems will help us better approach the evaluation of these cognitive processes. Evaluation methods must keep pace with these new training methods. For example, measures such as the Dynamic Gait Index, which evaluates the ability to modify gait in response to changing task demands (Shumway-Cook et al 1997), and the Activities–Balance Completion Scale (ABC), which assesses the fear of falling or self-efficacy (Powell and Myers 1995), begin to address such factors.

If we are to measure walking competency comprehensively, the concept of handicap must be addressed. Desrosiers et al (2002, 2003) reported the recovery of locomotor skill to be, after depression,

Figure 9.10   (a) The temporal characteristic of the Step Test. Each foot and the block are placed on a force plate. The duration of the Step Test was measured in seven patients with stroke (CVA) and in 10 healthy subjects (CTL). Two conditions were studied: affected leg stepping and affected leg supporting; and for the CTL: right leg stepping and right leg supporting (middle). (b) Forward (F) and backward B) stepping duration. (c) Per cent time spent in unilateral stance in forward and backward directions for each condition. See text for further details.

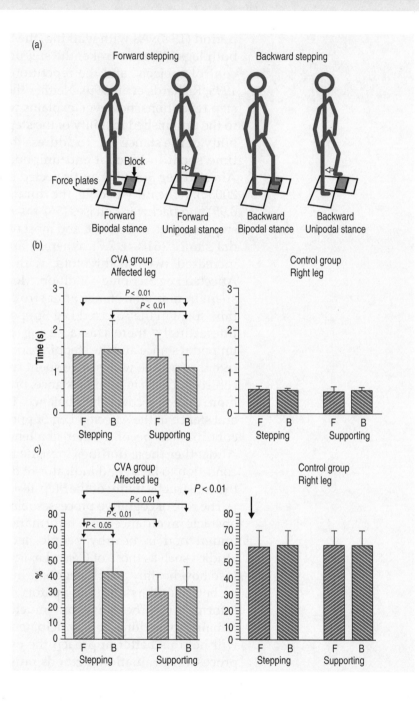

the second strongest determinant of participation in activities and social roles after a stroke. In this respect the study by Perry et al (1995) gives us reference guidelines that relate walking speed to community involvement. Another measure of interest is The Assessment of Life Habits (Life-H), a handicap measure, based on the Handicap Creation Process model (Fougeyrollas et al 1998), that evaluates many aspects of social participation of people with disabilities, regardless of the type of underlying impairment (Fougeyrollas and Noreau 2001). Such measures relating to quality of life are needed if we are to evaluate the concept of walking competency and how this impacts on quality of life – the ultimate measure of success.

SUMMARY

This chapter has reviewed a remarkable evolution in neurological rehabilitation over the last 15 years. The task-oriented approach to promote motor learning after stroke is now generally accepted, and it has been shown that this approach is not dependent on sophisticated equipment but rather on the skills of the therapist and the willingness of the patient to participate in goal-oriented and varied practice. We now accept the need to strengthen muscles, preferably during activities, and to train endurance of people after stroke and, furthermore, that we may have to modify therapy allocation to include maintenance programmes to ensure maximal recovery and maintenance of locomotor skills and endurance. The need to augment practice to promote recovery is recognized, and the potential of mental practice and virtual reality systems as adjuncts to traditional physical therapy are under study. We have greatly increased the understanding of a number of locomotor subtasks and how they are coordinated to produce smooth transitions and mobility. If we are to be able to evaluate change in these complex tasks and the concept of walking competency, assessment methods must keep pace with therapeutic developments. Finally, we must recognize the value of multidisciplinary studies and the contributions of experts from other fields, which have allowed the application of new methods and technology to the rehabilitation of people after stroke.

ACKNOWLEDGEMENTS

The authors thank colleagues and members of their research teams and graduate students who contributed to the various studies mentioned in this chapter. These studies have been supported over the years by grants from the National Health Research and Development Program, the Canadian Stroke Center for Excellence, the 'Fonds de recherche en santé du Québec' (FRSQ), the Canadian Foundation for Innovation and the 'Réseau provincial de recherché en adaptation-réadaptation' (REPAR).

References

Berg K O, Wood-Dauphinee S L, Williams J I et al 1989 Measuring balance in the elderly: preliminary development of an instrument. Physiotherapy Canada 41:304–311.

Berg K O, Wood-Dauphinee S L, Williams J I et al 1992 Measuring balance in the elderly: validation of an instrument. Canadian Journal of Public Health 83(Suppl 2):57–61.

Berg K, Wood-Dauphinee S, Williams J I 1995 The Balance Scale: reliability assessment with elderly residents and patients with acute stroke. Scandinavian Journal of Rehabilitation Medicine 27:27–36.

Bernhardt J, Ellis P, Denisenko S et al 1998 Changes in balance and locomotion measures during rehabilitation following stroke. Physiotherapy Research International 3:109–118.

Bohannon R W 1986 Strength of lower limb related to gait velocity and cadence in stroke patients. Physiotherapy Canada 38:204–210.

Brenière Y, Do M C 1986 When and how does steady state gait movement induced from upright posture begin? Journal of Biomechanics 19:1035–1040.

Brenière Y, Do M C, Bouisset S 1987 Are dynamic phenomena prior to stepping essential to walking? Journal of Motor Behavior 19:62–76.

Brown D A, Kautz S A 1998 Increased workload enhances force output during pedaling exercise in persons with poststroke hemiplegia. Stroke 29:598–606.

Brown D A, Jaffee D L, Buckley E L 2002 Use of virtual objects to improve gait velocity in individuals with post-stroke hemiplegia. Neurology Report 26:105.

Brunt D, Vander Linden D W, Berhman A L 1995 The relation between limb-loading and control parameters of gait initiation in persons with stroke. Archives of Physical Medicine and Rehabilitation 76:627–634.

Burke D 1988 Spasticity as an adaptation to pyramidal tract injury. Advances in Neurology 47:401–418.

Carr J H, Shepherd R B 1982 A motor relearning programme for stroke, 1st edn. Butterworth-Heinemann, Oxford.

Carr J H, Shepherd R B 1987 A motor learning model for rehabilitation. In: Carr J H, Shepherd R B, Gordon J et al (eds) Movement science: foundations for physical therapy in rehabilitation. Aspen, Rockville, MD, pp 31–91.

Carr J H, Shepherd R B 1998 Neurological rehabilitation: optimizing motor performance. Butterworth-Heinemann, Oxford.

Crenna P, Frigo C 1991 A motor programme for the initiation of forward-oriented movements in humans. Journal of Physiology (London) 437:635–653.

Danielsson A, Sunnerhagen K S 2000 Oxygen consumption during treadmill walking with and without body weight support in patients with hemiparesis after stroke and in healthy subjects. Archives of Physical Medicine and Rehabilitation 81:953–977.

Darken RP, Cockayne WR, Carmein D 1997 The Omni-Directional Treadmill: a locomotion device for virtual worlds. Proceedings of the 10th annual ACM symposium on User Interface Software and Technology (UIST). ACM Press, New York, pp 213–221.

Dean C M, Shepherd R B 1997 Task-related training improves the performance of seated reaching tasks after stroke. A randomized controlled trial. Stroke 28:722–728.

Dean C M, Richards C L, Malouin F 2000 Task-related circuit training improves performance of locomotor tasks in chronic stroke: a randomized, controlled pilot trial. Archives of Physical Medicine and Rehabilitation 81:409–417.

Dean C M, Richards C L, Malouin F 2001 Walking speed over 10 metres overestimates locomotor capacity after stroke. Clinical Rehabilitation 15:415–421.

Decety J 1993 Should motor imagery be used in physiotherapy? Recent advances in cognitive neurosciences. Physiotherapy Theory and Practice 9:193–203.

Decety J, Boisson D 1990 Effect of brain and spinal cord injuries on motor imagery. European Archives of Psychiatry and Clinical Neurosciences 240:39–43.

Decety J, Grèzes J 1999 Neural mechanisms subserving the perception of human actions. Trends in Cognitive Sciences 3:172–178.

Deiber M-P, Ibanez V, Honda M et al 1998 Cerebral processes related to visuomotor imagery and generation of finger movements studied with positron emission tomography. NeuroImage 7:73–85.

DeRugy A, Montagne G, Buekers M J et al 2000 The study of locomotor pointing in virtual reality: the validation of a test set-up. Behavior Research Methods, Instruments and Computers 32:515–520.

Desrosiers J, Noreau L, Rochette A et al 2002 Predictors of handicap situations following post-stroke rehabilitation. Disability and Rehabilitation 24:774–785.

Desrosiers J, Malouin F, Bourbonnais D et al 2003 Arm and leg disabilities and impairments after stroke rehabilitation: relation to handicap. Clinical Rehabilitation 17:666–673.

Deutsch J E, Latonio J, Burdca G C et al 2001 Post-stroke rehabilitation with the Rutgers ankle system A case study. Presence 10:416–430.

Dion L, Malouin F, McFadyen B J et al 1999a Modification of the sit-to-walk task after stroke. Society for Neuroscience 25:Abstr 365.2.

Dion L, Malouin F, McFadyen B J et al 1999b Assessment of the sit-to-walk capacity after stroke: a validation study. Gait and Posture Suppl 1:S24.

Dion L, Malouin F, McFadyen B J et al 2003 The Rise-to-Walk task for assessing mobility after stroke. Neurorehabilitation and Neural Repair 17:83–92.

Driskell J E, Copper C, Moran A 1994 Does mental practice enhance performance? Journal of Applied Psychology 79:481–492.

Duncan P W, Goldstein L B, Horner R D et al 1994 Similar motor recovery of upper and lower extremities after stroke. Stroke 25:1181–1188.

Duncan P, Richards L, Wallace D et al 1998 A randomized, controlled pilot study of a home-based exercise program for individuals with mild and moderate stroke. Stroke 29:2055–2060.

Eng J J, Chu K S, Dawson A S et al 2002 Functional walk tests in individuals with stroke: relation to perceived exertion and myocardial exertion. Stroke 33:756–761.

Engardt M, Olsson E 1992 Body weight-bearing while rising and sitting down in patients with stroke. Scandinavian Journal of Rehabilitation Medicine 24:67–74.

Engardt M, Knutsson E, Jonsson M et al 1995 Dynamic muscle strength training in stroke patients: effects on knee extension torque, electromyographic activity, and motor function. Archives of Physical Medicine and Rehabilitation 76:419–425.

Enright P L, Sherrill D L 1998 Reference equations for the six-minute walk in healthy adults. American Journal of Respiratory and Critical Care Medicine 158:1384–1387.

Feltz D L, Landers D M 1983 The effects of mental practice on motor skill learning and performance: a meta-analysis. Journal of Sport Psychology 5:25–57.

Finch L, Barbeau H 1985 Hemiplegic gait: new treatment strategies. Physiotherapy Canada 38:36–41.

Fougeyrollas P, Noreau L 2001 Life Habits measure–Shortened version (LIFE-H 3.0). International Network on Disability Creation Process, Lac St-Charles, (Quebec), Canada.

Fougeyrollas P, Noreau L, Bergeron H et al 1998 Social consequences of long term impairments and disabilities: conceptual approach and assessment of handicap. International Journal of Rehabilitation Research 21:127–141.

Fugl-Meyer A R, Jaaskp L, Leyman I et al 1975 The post-stroke hemiplegia patient: I a method for evaluation of physical performance. Scandinavian Journal of Rehabilitation Medicine 7:13–31.

Fung J, Barbeau H 1989 A dynamic EMG profile index to quantify muscular activation disorder in spastic paretic gait. Electroencephalography and Clinical Neurophysiology 73:233–244.

Fung J, Stewart J E, Barbeau H 1990 The combined effects of clonidine and cyproheptadine with interactive training on the modulation of locomotion in spinal cord injured subjects. Journal of Neurological Science 100:85–93.

Fung J, Malouin F, McFadyen BJ et al 2004 Locomotor rehabilitation in a complex virtual environment. Proceedings of the 26th Annual International Conference of the IEEE EMBS, pp 4859–4861.

Gentile A M 1987 Skill acquisition: action, movement, and neuromotor processes. In: Carr J H, Shepherd R B, Gordon J et al (eds) Movement science: foundations for physical therapy in rehabilitation. Aspen, Rockville, MD, pp 93–154.

Gérin-Lajoie M, Richards CL, McFadyen BJ 2001 Walking around upright obstacles: effects of obstacle mobility and division of attention on anticipatory locomotor strategies. Society for Neuroscience 27: Abstract 406.124.

Gérin-Lajoie M, McFadyen BJ, Richards CL 2004 The negotiation of stationary and moving obstruction during walking. I-Context specific anticipatory locomotor adaptations. Motor Control (submitted).

Goldie P A, Matyas T A, Evans O 1996 Deficit and change in gait velocity during rehabilitation after stroke. Archives of Physical Medicine and Rehabilitation 77:1074–1082.

Gordon J 1987 Assumptions underlying physical therapy intervention: theoretical and historical perspectives. In: Carr J H, Shepherd R B, Gordon J et al (eds) Movement science: foundations for physical therapy in rehabilitation. Aspen, Rockville, MD, pp 1–30.

Hall C R, Pongrac J 1983 Movement imagery questionnaire. Faculty of Physical Education, University of Western Ontario, London, Ontario.

Hesse S, Bertelt C, Schraffin A 1994a Restoration of gait in nonambulatory hemiparetic patients by treadmill training with partial body weight support. Archives of Physical Medicine and Rehabilitation 75:1087–1093.

Hesse S, Schauer M, Malezic M et al 1994b
Quantitative analysis of rising from a chair in
healthy and hemiparetic subjects. Scandinavian
Journal of Rehabilitation Medicine 26:161–166.

Hesse S, Bertelt C, Jahnke M T et al 1995 Treadmill
training with partial body weight support
compared with physiotherapy in nonambulatory
hemiparetic patients. Stroke 26:976–981.

Hesse S, Reiter F, Jahnke M et al 1997 Asymmetry of
gait initiation in hemiparesis stroke. Archives of
Physical Medicine and Rehabilitation 78:719–724.

Hesse S, Konrad M, Uhlenbrock D 1999 Treadmill
walking with partial body weight support versus
floor walking in hemiparetic subjects. Archives of
Physical Medicine and Rehabilitation 80:421–427.

Hesse S, Werner C, Uhlenbrock D et al 2001 An
electromechanical gait trainer for restoration of
gait in hemiparetic stroke patients: preliminary
results. Neurorehabilitation and Neural Repair
15:39–50.

Hill KD, Bernhardt J, McGann AM et al 1996 A new
test of dynamic standing balance for stroke
patients: reliability and comparison with healthy
elderly. Physiotherapy Canada 48:257–262.

Hinshaw K E 1991 The effects of mental practice on
motor skill performance: Critical evaluation and
meta-analysis. Imagin Cogn Personality
11:3–35.

Holden M, Todorov E, Callahan J et al 1999 Virtual
environment training improves motor
performance in two patients with strokes.
Neurology Report 23:57–67.

Holden M, Dyar T, Callahan J et al 2001 Quantitative
assessment of motor generalization in the real
world following training in virtual environment.
Neurology Report 25:130–131.

Horak F 1991 Assumptions underlying motor control
for neurologic rehabilitation. In: Lister M (ed)
Contemporary management of motor problems.
Proceedings of the II STEP Conference.
Foundation for Physical Therapy, Alexandria, VA,
pp 11–17.

Jackson P L, Lafleur M, Malouin F et al 1999 The effect
of mental practice in the learning of a sequence of
foot movements. Society for Neuroscience
25:Abstr 756.11.

Jackson P L, Lafleur M, Malouin F et al 2001a
Potential role of mental practice using motor
imagery in neurologic rehabilitation. Archives
of Physical Medicine and Rehabilitation
82:1133–1141.

Jackson P L, Lafleur M, Malouin F et al 2001b Mental
practice of a sequential task modulates orbitofrontal
organization. Human Brain Mapping 13:1197.

Jackson PL, Lafleurs M, Malouin F et al 2003
Functional reorganization following motor
sequence learning through mental practice with
motor imagery. Neuroimage 20:1171–1180.

Jackson PL, Richards CL, Malouin F et al 2004 The
efficacy of combined physical and mental practice
in the learning of a foot-sequence task after stroke:
a case study. Neurorehabilitation and Neural
Repair 18:106–111.

Jian Y, Winter D A, Ishac M G et al 1993 Trajectory of
the body COG and COP during initiation and
termination of gait. Gait and Posture 1:9–22.

Keith R A 1980 Activity patterns of a stroke
rehabilitation unit. Social Science and Medicine
14A:575–580.

Kim C M, Eng J J 2003 The relationship of lower
extremity muscle torque to locomotor
performance in people with stroke. Physical
Therapy 83:49–57.

Kim C M, Eng J J, MacIntyre D L et al 2001 Effects of
isokinetic strength training on walking in persons
with stroke: a double-blind controlled pilot study.
Journal of Stroke and Cerebrovascular Disease
10:265–273.

Knutsson E, Richards C L 1979 Different types of
disturbed motor control in gait of hemiparetic
patients. Brain 102:405–430.

Kwakkel G, Kollen B J, Wagenaar R C 1999a Therapy
impact on functional recovery in stroke
rehabilitation: a critical review of the literature.
Physiotherapy 85:377–391.

Kwakkel G, Wagenaar R C, Twisk JW et al 1999b
Intensity of leg and arm training after primary
middle-cerebral-artery stroke: a randomised trial.
Lancet 354:191–196.

Lafleur M, Jackson P L, Malouin F et al 1999
Functional neuroanatomy of executed and
imagined sequential movements of the foot in
humans examined with PET. Society for
Neuroscience 25:Abstr 756.12.

Lafleur M, Jackson P L, Malouin F 2002 Motor
learning produces parallel dynamic functional
changes during the execution and imagination of
sequential foot movements. NeuroImage
16:142–157.

Lamontagne A, Richards C L, Malouin F 2000a
Coactivation during gait as an adaptive behavior
after stroke. Journal of Electromyography and
Kinesiology 10:407–415.

Lamontagne A, Malouin F, Richards C L 2000b
Contribution of passive stiffness to ankle
plantarflexor moment during gait after stroke.
Archives of Physical Medicine and Rehabilitation
81:351–358.

Lamontagne A, Malouin F, Richards C L 2001 Locomotor task-specific measure of spasticity of plantarflexor muscles after stroke. Archives of Physical Medicine and Rehabilitation 82:1696–1704.

Lamontagne A, Malouin F, Richards C L et al 2002 Mechanisms of disturbed motor control in ankle weakness during gait after stroke. Gait and Posture 15:244–255.

Lerner-Frankiel M B, Vargus S, Brown M B 1986 Functional community ambulation: what are your criteria? Clinical Management of Physical Therapy 6:12–15.

Liepert J, Weiller C 1999 Mapping plastic brain changes after acute lesions. Current Opinion in Neurology 12:709–713.

Liepert J, Bauder H, Wolfgang H R 2000 Treatment-induced cortical reorganization after stroke in humans. Stroke 31:1210–1216.

McComas J, Sveistrup H 2002 Virtual reality applications for prevention, disability awareness, and physical therapy rehabilitation in neurology: our recent work. Neurology Report 26:55–61.

McComas J, Pivik J, Laflamme M 1998 Current uses of virtual reality for children with disabilities. Studies in Health Technology and Informatics 58:161–169.

McFadyen B J, Winter D A 1991 Anticipatory locomotor adjustments during obstructed walking. Neuroscience Research Communications 9:37–44.

McFadyen BJ Malouin F, Fung J et al 2004 Development of complex virtual environments for locomotor training following stroke. In: Roy SH, Bonato P, Meyer J (eds) Proceedings of 25th Congress of the International Society of Electrophysiology and Kinesiology, Boston, p 55.

MacKay-Lyons M, Makrides L 2002 Cardiovascular stress during a contemporary stroke rehabilitation program: is the intensity adequate to induce a training effect? Archives of Physical Medicine and Rehabilitation 83:1378–1383.

Mackey F, Ada L, Heard R et al 1996 Stroke rehabilitation. Are highly structured units more conducive to physical activity than less structured units? Archives of Physical Medicine and Rehabilitation 77:1066–1071.

Macko R F, DeSouza C A, Tretter L D et al 1997 Treadmill aerobic exercise training reduces the energy expenditure and cardiovascular demands of hemiparetic gait in chronic stroke patients. A preliminary report. Stroke 28: 326–330.

Macko R F, Smith G V, Dobrovolny C L et al 2001 Treadmill training improves fitness reserve in chronic stroke patients. Archives of Physical Medicine and Rehabilitation 82:879–884.

Magnan A, McFadyen B J, St-Vincent G 1996 Modification of the sit-to-stand task with the addition of gait initiation. Gait and Posture 4:232–241.

Mahoney F D, Barthel D W 1954 Rehabilitation of the hemiplegic patient: a clinical evaluation. Archives of Physical Medicine and Rehabilitation 35:359–362.

Malouin F, Potvin M, Prévost J et al 1992 Application of an intensive task-oriented gait training program: case report in a series of acute stroke patients. Physical Therapy 72:781–793.

Malouin F, Menier C, Comeau F et al 1994 Dynamic weight transfer during gait initiation in hemiparetic adults and effect of foot position. Society for Neuroscience 20: Abstr 241.3.

Malouin F, Richards C L, Dumas F et al 1995 Effect of paresis on gait initiation after stroke. Society for Neuroscience 21: Abstr 819.4.

Malouin F, Bonneau C, Pichard L et al 1997 Non-reflex changes in plantar flexors resistive torque early after stroke. Scandinavian Journal of Rehabilitation Medicine 29:147–153.

Malouin F, Desrosiers J, Doyon J et al 2001a Motor imagery ability after stroke. Society for Neuroscience 27: Abstr 950.4.

Malouin F, Dion L, McFadyen B et al 2001b Changes in the fluidity of the rise-to-walk motor strategy after stroke. In: Duysens J, Smits-Engelsman B C M, Kingma H (eds) Control of posture and gait. Symposium of the International Society for Postural and Gait Research. ISPG, Maastricht, The Netherlands, pp 671–674.

Malouin F, Belleville S, Corriveau D et al 2002 Mental practice and working memory after stroke. Society for Neuroscience 28:Abstr 169.13.

Malouin F, Richards C L, Jackson P L et al 2003a Brain activations during motor imagery of locomotor-related tasks: a PET study. Human Brain Mapping 19:47–62

Malouin F, Richards CL, McFadyen BJ et al 2003b Nouvelles perspectives en réadaptation motrice après un accident vasculaire cérébral. Médecine Science 19:994–998.

Malouin F, Corriveau D, Richards C L 2003c Temporal disorganization of the Step-test after stroke. In: Lord SR, Menz HB (eds) Proceedings of the 16th Symposium of the International Society for Postural and Gait Research, Sydney, Australia. ISPG, Abstract pp 158–159.

Malouin F, McFadyen B, Dion L et al 2003d A fluidity scale for evaluating the motor strategy of the rise-to-walk task after stroke. Clinical Rehabilitation 17:674–684.

Malouin F, Belleville F, Desrosiers J et al 2004a Working memory and mental practice after stroke. Archives of Physical Medicine and Rehabilitation 85:177–183.

Malouin F, Richards CL, Doyon J 2004b Training mobility after stroke with combined mental and physical practice: a feasibility study. Neurorehabilitation and Neural Repair 18:66–75.

Malouin F, Richards CL, Desrosiers J et al 2004c Bilateral slowing of mentally simulated actions after stroke. NeuroReport 7:1349–1353.

Naito E, Kochiyama T, Kitada R et al 2002 Internally simulated movement sensations during motor imagery activate cortical motor areas and the cerebellum. Journal of Neuroscience 22:3683–3691.

Nilsson L, Carlsson J, Danielsson A et al 2001 Walking training of patients with hemiparesis at an early stage after stroke: a comparison of walking training on a treadmill with body weight support and walking training on the ground. Clinical Rehabilitation 15:515–527.

Nudo R J, Pautz E J, Frost S B 2001 Role of adaptive plasticity in recovery of function after damage to motor cortex. Muscle and Nerve 24:1000–1019

Olney S J, Richards C L 1996 Hemiplegic gait following stroke: Part I. Characteristics. Gait and Posture 4:136–148.

Olney S J, Griffin M P, Monga T N et al 1991 Work and power in gait of stroke patients. Archives of Physical Medicine and Rehabilitation 72:309–314.

Olney S J, Nymark J, Zee B et al 1995 Effects of BioTRAC computer-assisted feedback for gait rehabilitation in subjects with stroke: interim analysis of RCT. Proceedings of the 12th International Congress of the World Confederation for Physical Therapy. American Physical Therapy Association, Alexandria, VA, p 771.

Olney S, Nymark J, Zee B et al 1997 Effects of computer-assisted gait training (BioTRAC) on early stroke – a randomised clinical trial. North American Stroke Meeting, Montreal, October 16–18. Neurology Reviews 5:38.

Page S J 2000 Imagery improves upper extremity motor function in chronic stroke: a pilot study. Occupational Therapy Journal of Research 20:200–215.

Page S J, Levine P, Sisto S A et al 2001 Mental practice combined with physical practice for upper-limb

motor deficit in sub-acute stroke. Physical Therapy 81:1455–1462.

Pascual-Leone A, Nguyet D, Cohen L G et al 1995 Modulation of muscle responses evoked by transcranial magnetic stimulation during the acquisition of new fine motor skills. Journal of Neurophysiology 74:1037–1045.

Perron M, Malouin F, Moffet H 2003 Assessing locomotor recovery after total hip arthroplasty with the Timed Stair Test. Clinical Rehabilitation 17:780–786.

Perry J, Garrett M, Gronley J K et al 1995 Classification of walking handicap in the stroke population. Stroke 26:982–989.

Podsiadlo D, Richardson S 1991 The 'timed up and go'. A test of basic functional mobility for frail elderly persons. Journal of the American Geriatric Society 39:142–149.

Potempa K, Lopez M, Braun L T et al 1995 Physiological outcomes of aerobic exercise training in hemiparetic stroke patients. Stroke 26:101–105.

Powell L E, Myers A M 1995 The Activities-specific Balance Confidence (ABC) Scale. Journals of Gerontology. Series A, Biological Sciences and Medical Sciences 50A:M28–M34.

Rheingold H 1991 Virtual reality. Secker and Warburg, London.

Richards C L, Knutsson E 1974 Evaluation of abnormal gait patterns by intermittent-light photography and electromyography. Scandinavian Journal of Rehabilitation Medicine Suppl 3:61–68.

Richards C L, Malouin F 1992 Spasticity control in the therapy of cerebral palsy. In: Forssberg H, Hirschfeld H (eds) Movement disorders in children. Med. Sports Sci. Karger, Basel, 36:217–224.

Richards C L, Malouin F 1998 Critical review of therapeutic approaches: future perspectives. Giornale di Neuropsichiatria dell'Eta Evolutiva 2(S):93–103.

Richards C L, Olney S J 1996 Hemiparetic gait following stroke. Part II: Recovery and physical therapy. Gait and Posture 4:149–162.

Richards C L, Malouin F, Wood-Dauphinee S et al 1993 Task-specific physical therapy for optimization of gait recovery in acute stroke patients. Archives of Physical Medicine and Rehabilitation 74:612–620.

Richards C L, Malouin F, Dumas F et al 1995 Gait velocity as an outcome measure of locomotor recovery after stroke. In Craik R, Oatis C (eds) Gait analysis: theory and applications. Mosby, St Louis, pp 355–364.

Richards C L, Malouin F, Dumas F et al 1998 Recovery of ankle and hip power during walking after stroke. Canadian Journal of Rehabilitation 11:271–272.

Richards C L, Malouin F, Dean C 1999 Assessment and rehabilitation. In: Duncan P (ed) Clinics in Geriatric Medicine, vol 15. WB Saunders, Philadelphia, pp 833–855.

Richards C L, Dumas F, Malouin F 2001 Hip and ankle mechanical work during walking after stroke. Society for Neuroscience 27:Abstr 831.6.

Richards CL, Malouin F, Bravo G et al 2004 The role of technology in task-oriented training in persons with sub-acute stroke: a randomized controlled trial. Neurorehabilitation and Neural Repair in press.

Robinett C S, Vondran M A 1988 Functional ambulation velocity and distance requirements in rural and urban communities. A clinical report. Physical Therapy 68:1371–1373.

Rogers R D, Owen A M, Middleton H C et al 1999 Choosing between small, likely rewards and large, unlikely rewards activates inferior and orbital prefrontal cortex. Journal of Neuroscience 20:9029–9038.

Roorda L, Roebroeck M, Lankhorst G et al 1996 Measuring functional limitations in rising and sitting down: development of a questionnaire. Archives of Physical Medicine and Rehabilitation 77:663–669.

Roure R, Collet C, Deschaumes-Molinaro C et al 1999 Imagery quality estimated by autonomic response is correlated to sporting performance enhancement. Physiology and Behavior 66:63–72.

Ruby P, Decety J 2001 Effect of subjective perspective taking during simulation of action: a PET investigation of agency. Nature Neuroscience 4:546–550.

Said C M, Goldie P A, Patla A E et al 1999 Obstacle crossing in subjects with stroke. Archives of Physical Medicine and Rehabilitation 80:1054–1059.

Said C M, Goldie P A, Patla A E et al 2001 Effect of stroke on step characteristics of obstacle crossing. Archives of Physical Medicine and Rehabilitation 82:1712–1719.

Salbach N M, Mayo N E, Higgins J et al 2001 Responsiveness and predictability of gait speed and other disability measures in acute stroke. Archives of Physical Medicine and Rehabilitation 82:1204–1212.

Salbach N M, Mayo N E, Wood-Dauphinee S et al 2004 A task-oriented intervention enhances walking distance and speed in the first year post-stroke: a randomized controlled trial. Clinical Rehabilitation 18:509–519.

Sharp S A, Brouwer B J 1997 Isokinetic strength training of the hemiparetic knee: effects on function and spasticity. Archives of Physical Medicine and Rehabilitation 78:1231–1236.

Shumway-Cook A, Baldwin M, Polissar N L 1997 Predicting the probability for falls in community-dwelling older adults. Physical Therapy 77:812–819.

Sirigu A, Cohen L, Duhamel J R et al 1995 Congruent unilateral impairments for real and imagined hand movements. NeuroReport 6:997–1001.

Sirigu A, Duhamel J R, Cohen L et al 1996 The mental representation of hand movements after parietal cortex damage. Science 273:1564–1568.

Smith G V, Silver K H, Goldberg A P et al 1999 'Task-oriented' exercise improves hamstring strength and spastic reflexes in chronic stroke patients. Stroke 30:212–219.

Steuer J 1992 Defining virtual reality: dimensions determining telepresence. Journal of Communication 42:73–93.

Tangemann P, Banaitis D, Williams A 1990 Rehabilitation for chronic stroke patients: changes in functional performance. Archives of Physical Medicine and Rehabilitation 71: 876–880.

Teixeira-Salmela L F, Olney S J, Nadeau S et al 1999 Muscle strengthening and physical conditioning to reduce impairment and disability in chronic stroke survivors. Archives of Physical Medicine and Rehabilitation 10:1211–1218.

Teixeira-Salmela L F, Nadeau S, McBride I et al 2001 Effects of muscle strengthening and physical conditioning training on temporal, kinematic and kinetic variables during gait in chronic stroke survivors. Journal of Rehabilitation Medicine 33:53–60.

Tinson D J 1989 How stroke patients spend their days: an observational study of the treatment regime offered to patients in hospital with movement disorders following stroke. International Disability Studies 11:45–51.

Traversa R, Cicinelli P, Bassi A et al 1997 Mapping of motor cortical reorganization after stroke. A brain stimulation study with focal magnetic pulses. Stroke 28:110–117.

Van Leeuwen R, Inglis J T 1998 Mental practice and imagery: a potential role in stroke rehabilitation. Physical Therapy Review 3:47–52.

Visintin M, Barbeau H, Korner-Bitensky N et al 1998 A new approach to retrain gait in stroke patients through body weight support and treadmill stimulation. Stroke 29:1122–1128.

Warner L, McNeill M E 1988 Mental imagery and its potential for physical therapy. Physical Therapy 68:516–521.

Werner C, Bardeleben A, Mauritz K H et al 2002a Treadmill training with partial body weight support and physiotherapy in stroke patients: a preliminary comparison. European Journal of Neurology 9:639–644.

Werner C, Von Frankenberg S, Treig T et al 2002b Treadmill training with partial body weight support and an electromechanical gait trainer for restoration of gait in subacute stroke patients: a randomized crossover study. Stroke 33:2895–2901.

Whitney S L, Hudak M T, Marchetti G F 2000 The dynamic gait index relates to self-reported fall history in individuals with vestibular dysfunction. Journal of Vestibular Research 10:99–105.

Whitney S L, Sparto P J, Brown K et al 2002 The potential use of virtual reality in vestibular rehabilitation: preliminary findings with the BNAVE. NeuroReport 26:72–78.

Winstein C J 1991 Knowledge of the results and motor learning: implications for physical therapy. Physical Therapy 71:140–149.

Winstein C J, Gardner E R, McNeal D 1989 Standing balance training: effects on balance and locomotion in hemiparetic adults. Archives of Physical Medicine and Rehabilitation 70:755–762.

Winter D A 1991 The biomechanics and motor control of human gait: normal, elderly and pathological, 2nd edn. University of Waterloo Press, Waterloo, ON

Winter D A 1995 ABC of balance during standing and walking. Waterloo Biomechanics, Waterloo, ON.

Wood-Dauphinee S, Kwakkel G 2004 The impact of rehabilitation on stroke outcomes: a review of the evidence. In: Bogousslavsky J, Barnes M P, Dobkin B (eds) Recovery after stroke. Cambridge University Press (in press).

Yaguez L, Canavan A G, Lange H W et al 1999 Motor learning by imagery is differentially affected in Parkinson's and Huntington's diseases. Behavioral Brain Research 102:115–127.

Yoo E, Park E, Chung B 2001 Mental practice effect on line-tracing accuracy in persons with hemiparesis stroke: a preliminary study. Archives of Physical Medicine and Rehabilitation 82:1213–1218.

Yue G, Cole K J 1992 Strength increases from the motor program: comparison of training with maximal voluntary and imagined muscle contractions. Journal of Neurophysiology 67:1114–1123.

Chapter **10**

Strategies to minimize impairments, activity limitations and participation restrictions in parkinson's disease

Meg Morris, Victoria Jayalath, Frances Huxham, Karen Dodd and Jennifer Oates

Parkinson's disease (PD) is common in older people, affecting around 200 per 100 000 people over the age of 65 years. With the growing proportion of older people in national populations worldwide, the need for expert clinicians with specialist skills in the treatment of impairments, activity limitations and participation restrictions arising from PD will rapidly increase. Disorders in movement performance are a key feature of PD, and much of the emphasis of treatment is directed towards minimizing their disabling effects so that individuals can participate more fully in activities of daily life. Although medical management using pharmacological therapy is usually the initial form of treatment, most individuals are referred to physiotherapists, speech pathologists and occupational therapists soon after diagnosis, so that movement strategies can be learned before severe disabilities and cognitive impairment occur.

The early signs of PD can include a general slowing in movement, micrographic handwriting, a forward stooped posture, small footsteps and reduced speech volume (Morris 2000). These changes can occur very gradually, and sometimes it is a family member, friend or therapist who first notices that something is abnormal, rather than the person themselves. The disease then typically progresses slowly over periods of 15–25 years, with typical occurrence of resting tremor, postural instability, gait disturbance and speech disturbance. In the latter stages, and after many years of pharmacological therapy, dyskinesias, dystonia, thoracic kyphosis, severe hypokinesia and swallowing difficulties often arise. Multitasking becomes extremely challenging, and the person can also experience difficulty in performing long movement sequences. It is at this stage that slips, trips and falls frequently occur.

In this chapter we use the international classification of health and functioning (ICF) framework (WHO 2001) to explore the ways in which the pathology associated with PD leads to impairments of body structure and body function, limitations in the ability to perform activities of daily living and restrictions in participation in societal roles. The impact of PD on quality of life for the person and their 'significant others', such as family members and friends, is also discussed. Treatment options are then reviewed. A brief overview of medical and surgical management is followed by a critical evaluation of the evidence for physiotherapy, speech pathology and occupational therapy. Although it is acknowledged that the cognitive and psychosocial sequelae of PD are associated with marked disability in some individuals, this chapter focuses on motor control.

IMPAIRMENTS OF BODY STRUCTURE AND FUNCTION

In PD, impairments of body structure and function can be considered in relation to the primary neurological features of the disease as well as secondary adaptations that occur as the disease progresses. The key pathological feature of idiopathic PD is necrosis of dopamine-producing cells in the substantia nigra pars compacta, which occurs for reasons that are not known and steadily progresses over time (Alexander and Crutcher 1990). This region of the brainstem has output projections to the caudate nucleus, globus pallidus and subthalamic nucleus. As well as a diminution of dopamine in the nigrostriatal pathways, receptor sites for the uptake of dopamine in the caudate nucleus can be affected, compounding the neurotransmitter imbalance in the basal ganglia (Alexander and Crutcher 1990). In addition to dopamine insufficiency, abnormalities occur in the levels of gamma-aminobutyric acid (GABA), acetylcholine, substance P and glutamate (Alexander and Crutcher 1990). As a result, the 'classical' impairments of movement arise, namely hypokinesia, akinesia, rigidity, resting tremor, dyskinesia, dystonia and postural instability. Hypokinesia refers to reduced movement size and speed (Morris et al 1994a, 1994b). Akinesia refers to an 'absence' of movement, which can present as difficulty in initiating movement or motor blocks during the performance of long or complex movement sequences (Giladi et al 1992, 1997). Rigidity presents as increased stiffness in muscles because of overactivity of agonist and antagonist muscles. Dyskinesias are 'extra movements' that are writhing in nature and occur in the latter stages of the disease, as with abnormal dystonic postures. Postural instability eventually occurs in the majority of people with PD and contributes in a major way to morbidity and mortality, particularly via fall-related incidents (Bloem et al 2001a, 2001c, Hely et al 1999).

In addition to the primary neurotransmitter impairment, people with PD can experience impairments of musculoskeletal and cardiopulmonary structures secondary to disuse. Thoracic kyphosis is frequently seen after many years of PD and may be a primary deficit associated with dystonia or shortening of the forward trunk flexors. Alternatively, it could be argued that the forward stooped posture in people with PD is a compensation, to reverse their natural tendency to fall backwards. Decreased muscle length and contractures, particularly of the triceps surae and hip flexors, are common in those with reduced activity levels. Although muscle weakness is not a feature of the primary pathology, impaired trunk muscle performance is present even in early disease (Bridgewater and Sharpe 1998), perhaps resulting from habitual low levels of activity. Cardiopulmonary deterioration may result from a combination of reduced activity and disease-related changes. Both sympathetic and parasympathetic autonomic function may be impaired as a result of the condition, causing changes in cardiovascular regulation (Haapaniemi et al 2001) and decreased baroreceptor sensitivity (Szili-Torok et al 2001). Pneumonia remains the most common ultimate cause of death in advanced PD (Hely et al 1999) but there is also an increased incidence of concurrent cerebrovascular and cardiovascular disease secondary to an inactive lifestyle (Hely et al 1999). Other secondary impairments include weight loss and anxiety.

Because most people with idiopathic PD are older than 65 years, normal age-related impairments of body structure and function can add to disability. For example, skeletal muscle weakness can be a major health problem for older people. With age, the number of muscle fibres and the size of each individual fibre reduces, particularly type II 'fast twitch' fibres (see review by Dodd et al 2004). As a result, after the age of 50 years muscle mass decreases by more than 6% each decade, while strength decreases by more than 10% each decade (Lynch et al 1999). Other age-related changes include loss of bone mass and changes in fibrous cartilage and ligaments, which are associated with decreased joint range of movement throughout the body (Nigg et al 1992). The sensory systems responsible for posture and balance also undergo age-related changes. The visual system is less adept at picking up contours and depth cues due to a decline in contrast sensitivity. The vestibular system loses hair cells, which are important for detecting changes in direction of endolymph flow within the semicircular canals, saccule and utricle. Vibratory sense in the lower limbs diminishes, which contributes to a reduction in somatosensory feedback from the support surface and from the joints of the lower limbs. The cardiovascular and pulmonary systems also undergo age-related changes. Changes include structural alterations in the heart and cardiac cells and increasing amounts of elastic tissue, fat and collagen in the myocardium, which contribute to increased stiffness and decreased compliance of the ventricles. With age there is also loss of elastic recoil and chest wall compliance, and a reduction in lung alveolar surface area. These cardiovascular and pulmonary system changes are important factors in reducing an older individual's aerobic capacity, particularly for those with PD (Canning et al 1997).

Impairments of movement always occur in people with PD. According to Iansek et al (1995), a key role of the basal ganglia is to enable the smooth and efficient execution of well-learned movement sequences, removing the need for conscious control or constant visual guidance of movement trajectories. More specifically, the basal ganglia enable the size and speed of movements to be matched to the context in which movement occurs (Houk et al 1995). Repetitive or complex movements in people with PD are frequently under-scaled in size and speed, and there can be progressive diminution of movement size and speed as a sequential action proceeds. The basal ganglia also appear to play a role in enabling people to shift motor set from one mode to another, such as changing from fast walking to slow walking or changing from straight-line walking to walking and turning. Therefore, when basal ganglia function is compromised, movements are often performed in a fixed way, even if this is not energy efficient or well suited to the task demands. For example, footsteps can remain small despite the need to walk quickly (Bagley et al 1991, Morris et al 1999), and voice volume can be severely reduced even though the person needs to talk loudly for effective conversation in a noisy social environment. Similarly, people with advanced PD typically use a stereotyped pattern of movement 'en bloc' when turning during gait (Yekutiel et al 1991), whereas able-bodied people adjust intersegmental coordination according to the magnitude of the turning angle (Huxham et al 2003). Thus, characteristic features of motor disturbance in people with PD are inflexibility of motor responses, poor matching to context and a lack of variability in performance. The limited repertoire of motor responses is argued to increase the risk of falls as well as slow performance to inefficient levels.

One of the issues of contention in research circles is whether movement disturbance in people with PD is due to disordered proprioceptive mechanisms. For static clinical tests of limb proprioception such as matching the angle of a joint to a criterion, or dynamic tests such as matching the movement pattern of one limb to the other, people with PD do not show abnormalities. Nevertheless, they do have decreased limb-load sensitivity affecting extensor activity in the lower limbs (Dietz and Colombo 1998). Moreover, when they are required to integrate proprioceptive and visual information in order to match different environmental contexts during actions such as walking, they can experience difficulty (Almeida et al 2003). One suggestion is that the basal ganglia might play a role in integrating proprioceptive and visual input to control movement towards a target. Partial support for this hypothesis was found in a study by Almeida et al (2003), who showed that when people with PD had to locate themselves to a target in the dark using a wheelchair (which thus removed proprioceptive input from the legs) or by walking (where proprioception could be used) they were less accurate than control subjects. Thus, at this stage the idea that people with PD have a disorder in the central integration of proprioceptive information cannot be discounted.

Impairments of balance and postural control are usually seen in the latter stages of disease progression and permeate every layer of postural responses. Anticipatory postural adjustments tend to be inadequate and their effectiveness reduced by increased levels of stiffness (Bloem 1994). This is particularly so when faster focal movements are required. Postural adjustments are often inflexible, failing to respond appropriately when a movement or perturbation changes because of problems changing motor set (Chong et al 2000). When required to respond to perturbations of a moving platform in standing, people with PD demonstrate both increased destabilizing and reduced stabilizing responses (Bloem et al 1996). Further, the latencies and amplitudes of voluntary postural responses may also be impaired (Bloem 1994). Finally, when unexpectedly perturbed, they have difficulty executing corrective stepping responses. This may result from a combination of under-scaled amplitude together with slowed response times. People with PD are more likely to fall when walking in unfamiliar environments where unpredictable or multiple threats to balance challenge the postural control system. When pushed off balance during standing or walking, people with advanced PD do not always generate precautionary stepping responses, further increasing their risk of falls.

LIMITATIONS IN ACTIVITIES OF DAILY LIVING

In the early stages of disease progression, many of the symptoms of PD can be controlled by medication, thereby enabling the individual to continue with their usual daily self-care, work, family and leisure activities. In the later stages, motor, cognitive and communication impairments can severely impact upon the performance of daily activities. Dressing, grooming, household duties such as cleaning and meal preparation, as well as gardening tasks are performed much more slowly and with greater effort than usual. Impairments of speech, voice, swallowing and facial expression can affect functional activities, such as talking, eating and drinking, and impinge on community activities such as shopping, banking and public speaking.

Handwriting is one of the few functional activities studied extensively in people with PD. Approximately 20% of people exhibit micrographia, a phenomenon whereby the writing becomes slower and size of letters become progressively smaller with the length of text. When people with PD write in cursive script, the size of sequential strokes progressively diminishes, eventually resulting in perfectly formed yet very small handwriting (Oliveira et al 1997). The provision of lined paper or instructions to think about writing with large strokes can temporarily increase stroke size (Morris 2000). Nevertheless, when attention is diverted to a secondary task, such as taking a telephone message or speaking, micrographia re-emerges (Morris 2000).

Another theme to emerge recently from the disability literature is that people with PD have particular difficulty in the performance of activities that require multitasking. Multitasking requires a person to focus his or her attention on performing more than one motor or cognitive task at a time or in series. Our research group has conducted a line of experiments showing that when people with PD do more than one thing at a time, performance deteriorates in either the primary task, the secondary task or both (e.g. Bond and Morris 2000, Morris et al 1996b, O'Shea et al 2002). The extent to which the primary or secondary task becomes slower and smaller than usual or is performed with more errors is a product of attentional demands, the instructions given and the motivation of the person to perform in a given way. Attention can involve the selection and filtering of information, focusing of thought and shifting, dividing or sustaining thought (Brauer and Morris 2004). Brauer and Morris (2004) have shown that people with PD have particular difficulty in the selection, dividing and shifting of attention, whereas they can sustain attention on simple thoughts for prolonged periods. In agreement with this finding, O'Shea et al (2002) showed that stride length and walking speed in people with PD were severely compromised when they were required to perform either a secondary motor task (transferring coins from one pocket to another) or a secondary cognitive task (subtracting digits from a number sequence). As shown by Figures 10.1–10.3, secondary task performance per se was a greater determinant of gait deterioration than whether the task was motor or cognitive in type. Bloem et al (2001a, 2001b) demonstrated that multitasking deficits in people with PD were a product of the number of tasks or subtasks performed and the level of difficulty of each task.

Figure 10.1   Mean (SE) stride length for preferred walking (free) and walking with dual motor task (coin) and dual cognitive task (digit). (After O'Shea et al 2002, with permission of the American Physical Therapy Association.)

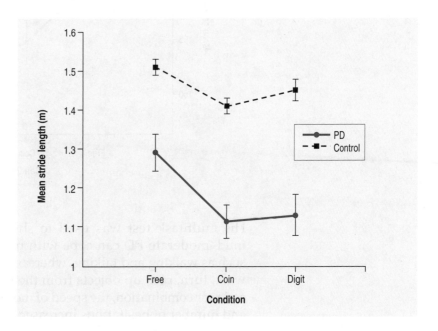

Figure 10.2 Mean (SE) walking speed for preferred walking (free) and walking with dual motor task (coin) and dual cognitive task (digit). (After O'Shea et al 2002, with permission of The American Physical Therapy Association.)

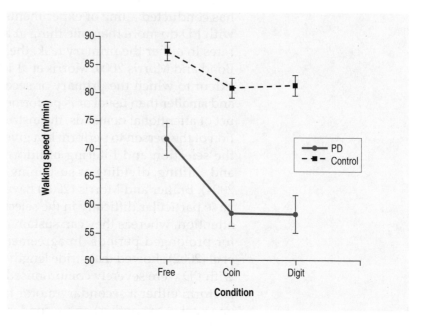

Figure 10.3 Mean (SE) cadence for preferred walking (free) and walking with dual motor task (coin) and dual cognitive task (digit). (After O'Shea et al 2002, with permission of The American Physical Therapy Association.)

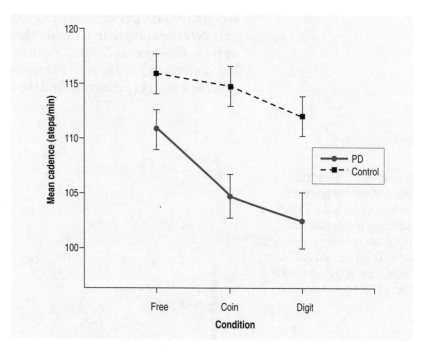

His multitask test was used to show that some people with mild–moderate PD can cope with relatively simple dual tasks, such as walking and talking, whereas when they were required to walk, turn, pick up objects from the floor and cross obstacles in series or combination, the speed of movement reduced much more and number of hesitations increased further than in control subjects. Again, these difficulties with performance were more marked as the complexity of the secondary task increased.

Locomotor dysfunction is one of the hallmark features of PD. The experimental literature has mainly reported locomotor control disorders for straight-line walking in laboratory settings, even though community ambulation, stair climbing, obstacle negotiation and turning are affected. The studies of straight-line walking show the majority of people with PD to have gait hypokinesia, with short strides, asymmetrical arm swing and little variability in the pattern of locomotor movements (Morris et al 1994b, 1996a, 1998). Kinematic analyses from three-dimensional motion studies indicate that lower limb, trunk and arm movements are scaled down in size across all joints, with asymmetry in the amplitude of movements (Morris et al 1999, Munneke et al 2003). Kinetic analyses have subsequently shown that power generation is abnormally low at the hip and ankle, with particular difficulty in generating a sufficiently large moment of force at push-off (Morris et al 1999). This is one reason why stride length is reduced in people with PD, because reduced push-off power reduces the momentum of the swinging leg. Around one-fifth of people with PD have akinesia and experience difficulty initiating locomotor sequences. In particular they have difficulty in weight-shifting to unload the stance leg in order to take the first step forwards. Once the walking sequence is initiated, they can then experience difficulty in terminating locomotion, due to their difficulty in shifting motor set. People with akinesia or who experience freezing episodes frequently have a footstep timing disorder in addition to the stride length regulation problem. Locomotor timing disorders are also evident in people with dyskinesia, which produces an erratic footstep pattern with variability in timing, amplitude and force control.

The ability to turn while walking is nearly always compromised in people with PD. Difficulties reported range from a lack of fluency through to motor blocking (Bloem et al 2001c, Giladi et al 1992) and frequent falls. Turning is the activity most commonly associated with PD falls (Bloem et al 2001c, Stack and Ashburn 1999). As noted previously, movement is slow and turning is often executed en bloc (Bloem et al 2001a, Stack and Ashburn 1999, Yekutiel et al 1991). A recent study noted that loss of arm swing during walking, which is generally related to reduced trunk rotation, was an independent predictor of falling (Wood et al 2002). Normal turning is accomplished by a complex combination of head and trunk rotation and lateral translation of the body onto the new path (Patla et al 1999). The pathognomonic under-scaling of movement sequences in PD may underlie the rigid appearance of the trunk when turning. People with mild-to-moderate PD [Hoehn and Yahr (1967) status II–III] have much lower peak velocities for both trunk rotation (yaw) and trunk lateral translation (roll) than age-matched control subjects (Munneke 2003). Underlying the joint and segmental angular changes that characterize turning are the kinetics, or moments and powers, that drive those angular alterations. In straight walking, people with PD appear to generate lower ankle power during push-off in the sagittal plane. Normal turning requires an accelerated braking component followed by a reduction in push-off power in that plane, together with marked changes in mediolateral forces to drive the centre of mass around the corner and onto the new path (Patla et al 1991). Although the kinetics of turning have not been reported for PD, the alterations reported in straight-line walking (Koozekani et al 1987, Morris et al 1999a, 2001) could be expected to impact on turning ability as well. A further factor contributing to turning difficulties is difficulty in changing motor set (Chong et al 2000). This would particularly apply when turns must be executed quickly. The movement difficulties of people with PD are further aggravated by dual or multiple task performance, in particular because they appear to have difficulty prioritizing the most important components, such as maintaining balance (Bloem et al 2001a, 2001b).

Speech and voice disorders in people with PD are classified as dysarthric impairments. The dysarthria associated with PD is hypokinetic in type and is generally attributed to hypokinesia and rigidity of the speech, voice and respiratory musculature (Darley et al 1969). Vocal impairments in PD have been attributed to incomplete closure of the vocal folds and rigidity of the laryngeal and respiratory muscles. More recently, speech and voice impairments in people with PD have been associated with disorders of central planning and control of learned motor sequences (Sapir et al 2001). In addition, the depression and neurocognitive dysfunction seen in subsets of people with PD is hypothesized to contribute to their speech and voice disorders (Rao et al 1992, Sapir et al 2001). Dysarthria increases in frequency and intensity with the severity of PD (Holmes et al 2000) and prevalence rates for dysarthric speech and voice impairments range from 70% to 89% (Logemann et al 1978). The primary speech manifestations are imprecise articulation of speech sounds, inappropriate silences, slow or fast rate and festinated speech (short rushes of speech) (Hartelius et al 1993, Logemann et al 1978). The common vocal impairments include reduced loudness, mono-loudness (reduced stress) and mono-pitch (reduced intonation), breathiness, roughness and strained voice quality (i.e. hoarseness) (Darley et al 1969, Holmes et al 2000, Johnson and Pring 1990).

Hypomimia (also termed 'Parkinsonian facies') is also common and is associated with poverty of movement in the muscles of the face for both volitional and emotional expression. Although individuals with PD may be impaired in expressing emotions using the muscles of the face, their perception of facially expressed emotions is not affected (Borod et al 1990). The prevalence of hypomimic symptoms in people with PD is not well established, although it appears to be proportional to the severity of the disease. Hypokinesia and rigidity of facial musculature may be contributing factors.

Dysphagia, or swallowing impairment, also increases in severity with the progress of PD. The prevalence of dysphagic symptoms in people with PD is thought to be approximately 46% (Bushmann et al 1989). Abnormal bolus formation, disturbed motility in the oral phase of swallowing, aspiration and oesophageal dysmotility are common findings in people with this condition (Bushmann et al 1989, Nagaya et al 1998). Parkinsonian dysphagia is generally attributed to rigidity and hypokinesia of swallowing musculature, as well as to the influence of the basal ganglia on the sensory components of the swallowing mechanism (Robbins et al 1986).

RESTRICTIONS TO PARTICIPATION IN SOCIETAL ROLES

As PD progresses, activity limitations arising from impairments of movement may restrict participation in societal roles such as work, family life, community life, education and leisure. Participation in various life situations may be particularly restricted by hypokinesia, akinesia, dyskinesia, dysarthria, dysphagia and hypomimia. Such impairments potentially result in reduced social contact, reduced employment opportunities and reduced ability to participate in leisure activities (Baatile et al 2000, Damiano et al 1999, GPDS 2002, Trend et al 2002). In addition, swallowing limitations are often associated with weight loss, high levels of anxiety with each meal, disturbed medication intake and self-consciousness. Participation restrictions such as this can impact on health-related quality of life and incur significant costs to the individual and society (Rubenstein et al 2001).

TREATMENT OF IMPAIRMENTS

Because the cause of PD remains unknown, current forms of treatment can only address the symptoms of the disease. In the early stages, levodopa and other forms of anti-PD medication can be very effective for treating hypokinesia, tremor and rigidity. When coupled with allied health interventions promoting physical activity and continued participation in societal roles, the person with newly diagnosed PD can experience very little disturbance to movement and function (Morris 2000). As the disease progresses, the efficacy of medication reduces and the person finds that at times when they are 'on' movement disorders are minimal, yet at the end or beginning of dose slowness, tremor and rigidity can be a problem. In the advanced stages of disease progression, postural instability compounds the stiffness and slowness, and falls are common. Parkinsonian medications typically have little impact on postural instability, and physiotherapists play a major role in teaching the person how to prevent loss of balance and falls at this stage. After many years of PD, dyskinesia can arise despite all attempts to refine the medication schedule. Pharmacotherapy and physiotherapy have not been shown to have long-lasting effects on dyskinesia, and surgery is one of the few options that remains. Systematic reviews of the literature (e.g. Morris et al 2001, Polgar et al 2003) have shown that pallidotomies, deep brain stimulation or reconstructive neurosurgery can sometimes reduce dyskinesia although they have little effect on postural instability.

The Cochrane collaboration has recently published several systematic reviews of randomized controlled clinical trials of therapy outcomes for people with PD (Deane et al 2001a–d). A synthesis of this material by Deane et al (2002) critically evaluated the results of 23 randomized trials of physiotherapy, occupational therapy and speech pathology in 637 people with PD. Although insufficient evidence was available to recommend definitively any particular type of allied health intervention, this was not interpreted as a lack of benefit. Instead, the methodological flaws inherent in previous studies may have masked underlying effects of therapy. Rather than considering only randomized controlled trials, in the remainder of this chapter we evaluate allied health studies that have used a range of designs and allied health interventions to quantify therapy outcomes. Most of the literature centres around the effects of traditional exercise therapy or movement strategy training on mobility. A small number of articles have explored the effects of speech and language therapy and several have reported the outcomes of a multidisciplinary approach for minimizing impairments, activity limitations and participation restrictions.

Exercise therapy

Many studies have investigated the effects of exercise therapy on impairments in people with PD (Banks and Caird 1989, Doshay 1964, Dunne et al 1987, Formisano et al 1992, Hurwitz 1989, Kamsma et al 1995, Levine 2000, Scandalis et al 2001, Szekely et al

1982, Toole et al 2000, Viliani et al 1999). The results have, however, been somewhat equivocal, and there are only a few randomized controlled clinical trials. Palmer et al (1986) compared the effectiveness of karate training and stretching exercises in PD using a parallel group design. As discussed by Deane et al (2002), participants were assigned into either group by an unstated method of randomization and treated as out-patients for 36 hours over 12 weeks. In addition to the PD motor battery (which measured gait, arm tremor, rigidity, pursuit performance and pronation–supination rates), grip strength, motor coordination and speed were assessed at baseline and immediately after treatment by assessors blinded to the patient's treatment. Data were analysed on an intention-to-treat basis. Since the two interventions produced very similar results despite using conceptually different approaches, it can be suggested that placebo, medication or other non-specific treatment effects were responsible for the results, rather than the specific elements of the novel and standard approaches. Nevertheless, it is difficult to conclude which intervention was superior.

Hurwitz (1989), also using a parallel group design, evaluated the outcomes of head-to-toe range of movement exercises for ambulatory people with PD. People were randomly assigned into either a home-supervised exercise regimen for 16 hours over 8 months or a home visit without an exercise regimen. At baseline and immediately after intervention they were assessed for memory, nausea, incontinence and rigidity. Because the assessors were not blinded to the aims of the study, there was the potential to unknowingly under-report or discount symptoms if they believed that a particular intervention was more effective than another (Deane et al 2002). Nevertheless, the author reported significant changes in 5 of the 53 items after the 8-month course of therapy.

More recently, Bridgewater and Sharpe (1997) investigated the effects of trunk muscle training in the early stages of PD using a parallel group design. Subjects were allocated alternately to a group that received 12 weeks of half-weekly exercise classes or a group that participated in an 'interest talk' every 3 weeks. Range of motion, torque and velocity of trunk flexors, extensors and rotators were examined by blinded assessors using a dynamometer 1 week before the intervention, following completion of the programme and 4 weeks later. Isometric torque production and velocity against resistance improved in both groups to a similar extent and no between-group differences were found for range of motion. The possibility that the Hawthorne effect contributed to the results cannot be discounted. In addition, trunk strength training did not incorporate a progressive increase in the amount of resistance used, hence not optimizing the potential for strengthening to occur.

Schenkman et al (1998) studied the use of spinal flexibility exercises using a parallel group design. Participants were stratified according to gender and then randomized to either the experimental group, who were treated as out-patients for 30 hours over 10–13 weeks, or to a control group, who received no treatment but were put on a waiting list for a future exercise programme. Assessors blinded to the treatment allocation of subjects tested performance on the functional reach test and for functional axial rotation at baseline and immediately after treatment. Functional reach was the only outcome measure to have statistical significance and the amount of change was small (1.85 cm), drawing into question the clinical significance of the results.

Although not strictly defined as exercise therapy, the effects of neuromuscular facilitation and Bobath training on motor performance in people with PD were evaluated by Cerri et al (1994) and Homann et al (1998). Whereas Cerri et al (1994) investigated the effectiveness of neuromuscular facilitation on posture, rigidity and conscious movement control, Homann et al (1998) measured the effects of Bobath training on posture and gait. Both methods use handling techniques to inhibit abnormal muscle tone and facilitate more normal patterns of movement. Cerri (1994) reported that, as a result of therapy, participants were able to reduce their levodopa to levels previously insufficient to control symptoms. Homann found that axial symptoms improved in people who received neuromuscular training yet deteriorated in comparison subjects. Despite widespread use, 'traditional therapies' such as stretching, strengthening and range of motion exercises as well as karate, Bobath and neuromuscular facilitation do not have strong scientific evidence for their efficacy in treating impairments in people with PD. This is possibly because exercise and alternative therapies are not always directed towards the underlying central deficit in PD, which is a disorder of motor planning and execution that results from basal ganglia dysfunction (Marsden 1994).

Movement strategies

In clinical circles many allied health professionals now use movement rehabilitation strategies to teach people with PD how to move more quickly and easily (Schenkman et al 1989, 1998). A 'strategy' in this context is a method used to bypass defective neural networks in order to move in a desired way. In PD this can, for example, involve using conscious attention to control movements that are normally performed with little thought, or using visual, auditory or proprioceptive stimuli ('cues') to guide performance. Other movement strategies aim to enhance motor set, avoid simultaneous task performance and break movement down into short 'chunks' (Morris 2000). Abbruzzese and Berardelli (2003) recently evaluated the literature on the effects of external cues on motor performance in PD. Although there are small studies (e.g. Lewis et al 2000, McIntosh et al 1997, Scandalis et al 2001, Stefaniwsky and Bilowit 1973, Waterston et al 1993), few randomized controlled trials have evaluated the effects of movement strategy training on impairments.

The use of visual cues for overcoming gait hypokinesia and akinesia in people with PD was investigated by Kompoliti et al (2000). Participants attempted to walk on a 60-ft (18.2 m) track under three conditions in a randomized order: unassisted walking, walking with a modified inverted stick and walking with a visual laser beam stick. Instructions were provided on how to hold the modified inverted stick and laser beam stick so that the slat or beam projected in front of their feet, so as to visually cue longer steps. The results failed to show any differences between conditions for walking time or number of freezing episodes, although the low power of this study makes it difficult to draw firm conclusions.

The effectiveness of auditory cues for improving gait hypokinesia and akinesia in people with PD was evaluated by Thaut et al (1996). Participants were randomly assigned to a group that received rhythmic auditory stimulation, standard self-paced walking or no training. As pointed out by Deane et al (2002), they all received 10.5 hours of out-patient treatment over 3 weeks. People who received rhythmic auditory stimulation spent 30 minutes per day walking to music with a tempo that progressively increased in rate. The self-paced group spent 30 minutes each week walking at normal, quick and fast speeds. Gait speed, cadence, stride length and EMG analysis of leg muscles were made at baseline and immediately after treatment. Those who trained with rhythmic auditory stimulation improved their gait speed, stride length, step cadence and EMG patterns in the anterior tibialis and vastus lateralis muscles to a greater extent than people who did not. Those who did not receive training showed reduced gait speed over the course of the study.

Mohr et al (1996) found that visual cue training was superior to standard therapy for people with PD. The standard treatment consisted of breathing and physical exercises without cues, relaxation, and discussion of disease-related problems. The experimental treatment ('behavioural therapy') involved progressive muscle relaxation aimed at reducing tremor, motor training with the use of external cues and internal commands, and social interactions training using role playing and aiming at reducing stress. Although clinical psychologists conducted the therapy, these types of interventions are also used by occupational therapists and physiotherapists. The study found statistically significant differences in favour of the cued group on all outcome measures.

More recently, Miyai et al (2000) used a crossover design to compare the effectiveness of body weight-supported treadmill training and conventional physical therapy. Using an unstated method of randomization, people with PD received either a 4-week conventional therapy programme or a programme of treadmill training with up to 20% of their body weight supported during locomotion followed by 4 weeks of conventional physical therapy that included general conditioning, range of motion exercises, ADL training and gait training. Ambulation endurance and walking speed were measured before and immediately after treatment, as well as the number of steps taken to complete a 10-m walk. The authors reported a significant improvement in gait speed and stride length difference in favour of treadmill training, although a Rosenthal effect was again present.

Treatment of speech and swallowing

Treatment approaches for speech disturbance include behavioural techniques, instrumental aids, medication and surgery. Medical and surgical management of Parkinsonian dysarthria has a limited role, especially in later stages of the disease. Non-medical approaches to dysarthria in PD found in the literature include prosodic exercise with and without visual feedback (Johnson and Pring 1990, Scott and Caird 1983), respiration therapy (Ramig et al 1995), Lee Silverman Voice Therapy (LSVT) (Ramig et al 2001) and voice production and intelligibility exercises (Robertson et al 1984). All trials found speech therapy to have a positive effect on dysarthria in PD. However, there were limitations in these studies, including the use of very small sample sizes, lack of random allocation to treatment groups and lack of no-treatment control groups. There is therefore no consensus in the literature as to 'best practice' for treating dysarthria in this population, although the Cochrane collaboration review group have recently synthesized much of the evidence (see Deane et al 2002 for a summary).

Levodopa has been found to improve the speed of swallowing in people with PD with less severe impairments. Although non-pharmacological approaches may affect dysphagia in later stages of the disease, only two studies were found that investigated its effectiveness. El-Sharkawi et al (1998) found LSVT had a positive effect on the swallowing disorders of eight patients with PD. However, because of the uncontrolled and non-randomized research design, the efficacy of this approach to treating dysphagia in PD is questionable. In a randomized controlled trial (RCT), Marks et al (2000) assessed the efficacy of specific speech and language therapy (including a portable metronome brooch to cue swallowing) to reduce the amount of saliva produced. Participants showed reduction in drooling severity using the drooling rating scale, as compared with the baseline scores and the age-matched control subjects.

Pharmacological treatment of Parkinsonian hypomimia has a limited role, particularly in patients with more severe deficits. Although non-medical approaches have the potential to facilitate the display of facial expression, only one study was found. In an RCT, Katisikitis and Polowsky (1996) investigated the effects of techniques such as brushing muscles, applying ice to muscles and blowing through a straw to stimulate facial muscles. Although there was a significant improvement on one measure (mouth-opening) in the intervention group, the Webster scores for items describing facial expression did not change after therapy.

Despite the sound theoretical basis for using movement strategies in treating Parkinsonian dysarthria, dysphagia and hypomimia, no studies investigating their effectiveness were found. Some aspects of LSVT may be described as movement strategies. LSVT is a high-effort intensive treatment (four times a week for 16 individual sessions in 1 month) designed to improve speech and swallowing by increasing vocal loudness, vocal tract coordination and sensory perception of effort. Increasing vocal loudness is attempted through increasing vocal adduction, 'thinking loud' and increasing respiratory effort (Ramig et al 1995, 2001). One study investigating LSVT for swallowing was found, but this was presented only as an abstract, and the mechanism for improving swallowing was not described (El-Sharkawi et al 1998).

TREATMENT OF ACTIVITY LIMITATIONS

Several studies have investigated the effects of allied health interventions on activity limitations using outcome measures such as the United Parkinson's Disease Rating Scale, Webster Scale, the Hoehn and Yahr Scale, the Northwestern University Disability Scale and the Columbia University Disability Scale.

Exercise therapy

Although the studies by Hurwitz (1989) and Miyai et al (2000) discussed earlier found that exercise therapy had a positive effect on some functional activities, the external validity of both experiments was questionable. For example, in the study by Hurwitz, subjects in the experimental group who underwent exercises to improve range of movement improved with respect to sucking and eating, but not the other items of the Parkinson's Home Visiting Assessment tool. Palmer et al (1986), Bridgewater and

Sharpe (1997) and Schenkman et al (1998) found that exercise therapy interventions had no effect on physical activity. Likewise Schenkman et al (1998) did not find any changes in activity on the supine-to-sit time following a programme of spinal flexibility exercises. In the study by Bridgewater and Sharpe (1997), no change in activity was found on the Webster Disability Rating Scale, NUDS or Human Activity Profile following a trunk muscle strength regime.

Cerri et al (1994) and Homann et al (1998) used the Webster Scale and Unified Parkinson's Disease Rating Scale (UPDRS) to assess the effects of physiotherapy on functional activity. Fundamental to the approach used in both studies was the assumption of carryover from passive non-functional treatment sessions into activities of daily living. Currently, there is no scientific evidence for using neurofacilitation for the treatment of movement disorders in people with PD. Furthermore, there is no evidence to support the use of traditional exercise therapy for long-term activity limitations in people with PD. The short-term improvements observed with exercise therapy were arguably due to changes in the musculoskeletal and cardiopulmonary systems, because these effects were not sustained once normal activity was resumed (Bridgewater and Sharpe 1996).

Movement strategies

There has been little attempt to use RCT experimental designs to quantify the effects of movement strategies on activity limitations despite many small non-randomized experiments (e.g. Bagley et al 1991, Ball 1967, Behrman et al 1998, Crossley 1986, Dam et al 1996, Doshay 1964, Dunne et al 1987, Eni 1988, Koseoglu et al 1997, Krasilovsky and Gianutsos 1991, McIntosh et al 1997, Pedersen et al 1990, Stefaniwsky and Bilowit 1973, Sunvisson et al 1997, Weissenborn 1993). The effectiveness of visual and auditory cues for improving functional activity was investigated by Marchese et al (2000) using a parallel group design. Participants were randomly assigned into either a 'cued' training group or a 'non-cued' treatment group, according to a pseudo-random number list. All subjects received training as out-patients over 6 weeks. The 'cued' group underwent a strategy training programme including visual and auditory cues. The 'non-cued' group underwent a similar programme but without the cues. The ADL and motor subsections of the UPDRS were administered at baseline, immediately after treatment and also 6 weeks after treatment. The study found a statistically significant improvement following both interventions although changes were only significant at follow-up in the 'cued' group. The difference was in favour of the cued therapy group and appeared to be of sufficient magnitude to be clinically significant.

Thus, as pointed out by Deane et al (2002), there is limited evidence to suggest that augmenting therapy with cues improves therapy efficacy.

Several small RCTs have evaluated the effectiveness of occupational therapy on activity limitations. For example, Homann et al (1998) compared PNF with Bobath therapy to improve locomotion and postural stability, although no data were available in this abstract. Using a parallel group design with 20 out-patients with PD, Fiorani et al measured the effects of occupational therapy sessions provided 12 hours per week for 1 month. Therapy incorporated handicrafts, picture drawing, basketry, folk singing, dancing and ball games. Although the outcome was positive, mean change over the course of therapy was small and lacked clinical significance. In contrast, a larger study of 64 out-patients by Gauthier et al (1987) found that occupational therapy sessions provided for 20 hours per week for five weeks enabled people to improve their movement initiation and speed. Therapy included the use of visual stimuli from mirrors, imitation of target movement patterns and auditory cues (moving to a rhythmical beat). Participants continued to receive physiotherapy treatment throughout the trial. Neither of these studies documented blinding procedures, handling of missing data or intention-to-treat analyses. Thus, currently there is scant scientific evidence demonstrating the positive effects of occupational therapy for people with PD, although it may be very beneficial.

TREATMENT OF PARTICIPATION RESTRICTIONS

Although literature comparing the effectiveness of physical therapies for impairments and activity limitations is growing, few studies have explored the effects of allied health interventions on participation in societal roles (Baatile et al 2000, Chandler and Plant 1999). These showed that people with advanced PD can have major restrictions to their family life, work roles, education, leisure and participation in community life. In some cases, participation restrictions can be alleviated with timely service provision from speech pathologists, occupational therapists and physiotherapists, although the long-term effects of therapy on this domain of health and disability remain open to question (Baatile et al 2000, Chandler and Plant 1999, Damiano et al 1999). Therapy also has the potential to enhance societal participation, quality of life and well-being for care-givers, such as husbands, wives, children and close friends, although the extent to which major benefits can be achieved and maintained needs to be determined with controlled research (GPDS 2002, Montgomery et al 1994).

MULTIDISCIPLINARY REHABILITATION

Few RCTs have investigated the effectiveness of multidisciplinary approaches to the treatment of movement disorders in PD. In an early investigation, Gibberd et al (1981) compared the effectiveness of out-patient multidisciplinary rehabilitation – based on neurofacilitatory therapies such as proprioceptive neuromuscular facilitation (PNF), Bobath and Peto interventions – with placebo therapy (infrared radiation, table games and crafts) for people with PD. Physiotherapy aimed to improve rotation, balance, walking, range of movement, festination and rigidity. The goal of occupational therapy was to improve the ability to perform activities of daily living such as feeding, dressing and cooking. Whilst speech therapy was available, the aims were not described. No significant change in any of the variables was found. In addition the study did not provide direct evidence that a multidisciplinary approach was more successful than therapies provided in isolation.

Comella et al (1994) investigated the effectiveness of an intensive traditional exercise programme for PD administered by both physiotherapists and occupational therapists compared with a comparison group that was not treated. The programme included repetitive exercises to improve range of motion, endurance, balance, gait and fine motor dexterity. Although the study found improvement in the motor subsection of the UPDRS following intensive exercise, the performance of timed motor tasks did not improve. Further, the UPDRS scores returned to baseline when patients resumed their normal activities. Again, no evidence was provided that a multidisciplinary approach was more successful than therapies provided in isolation.

Patti et al (1996) examined the effectiveness of in-patient multidisciplinary rehabilitation that emphasized strategy training compared with no intervention. Physiotherapy intervention included the use of auditory cues, rhythmic repetitive movements and exercises to improve gait and balance. Occupational therapy consisted of teaching compensatory strategies, providing assistive devices and discharge home visits. In speech therapy, patients were advised about strategies to improve speech and swallowing. An intensive, multidisciplinary, personalized in-patient rehabilitation programme delivered twice per year was associated with improvements in many people with PD. Moreover, many of the gains achieved immediately after therapy were stable over the 5-month span examined.

More recently, Trend et al (2002) evaluated the short-term effectiveness of multidisciplinary rehabilitation for people with PD and their care-givers using a pre–post design. Over 100 people with PD who did not have cognitive impairment attended day-hospital therapy with their care-givers, once per week for 6 weeks. After therapy, improvements were noted for gait, mobility, speech, depression and health-related quality of life. Those with more advanced disease made the greatest gains. Subsequent replication using a randomized controlled trial design in 144 subjects demonstrated a steady decline in quality of life, disability and care-giver strain over a 6-month period of treatment, although an intensive burst of multidisciplinary therapy improved mobility in some individuals (Wade et al 2003). Further studies with different contents and dosages of therapy are now needed to determine which elements of treatment have the greatest impact on outcome.

CONCLUSION

Acquired progressive neurological conditions such as PD can have a major effect on the quality of life of individuals, their families and society. The progressive impairments of movement, cognition and autonomic function pathognomonic to PD can limit the ability of individuals in functional activities of daily living and restrict their capacity to participate in a range of societal roles. As a result, well-being can be affected in both people with PD and the other significant people in their lives. The burden of care for families can be substantial, particularly in the latter stages of the disease, when immobility, falls, locomotor freezing, micrographia and swallowing disturbance are common. In addition, the economic effects of PD are profound (Rubenstein et al 2001). Although physiotherapy, speech pathology and occupational therapy cannot cure PD, there is preliminary evidence that some allied health interventions can enable people to maintain physical activity, movement and function for longer and at a higher level than is usually the case. The extent to which a multidisciplinary team environment optimizes recovery awaits confirmation with controlled clinical trials.

ACKNOWLEDGEMENTS

Parts of the sections of this chapter on treatment of impairments and activity limitations are adapted from the Parkinson's disease section of the following report: *Therapy Outcomes for Adults with Acquired, Progressive, Neurological Conditions and Lifelong Developmental Disabilities*, by M Morris, A Perry and S Duckett (2003), Faculty of Health Sciences, La Trobe University, published by the Victorian Government Department of Human Services, Melbourne, Victoria. A small portion is adapted from an honours thesis by V Jayalath (2002), School of Physiotherapy, La Trobe University, Australia, with permission from the author.

References

Abbruzzese G, Berardelli A 2003 Sensorimotor integration in movement disorders. Movement Disorders 18(3):231–240.

Alexander G E, Crutcher M D 1990 Functional architecture of basal ganglia circuits: neural substrates of parallel processing. Trends in Neuroscience 13:266–271.

Almeida QJ, Frank JS, Jenkins M et al 2003 Relative contributions of visual and proprioceptive inputs during locomotion towards a target in Parkinson's disease. In: Proceedings International Society for Postural and Gait Research XVI th conference, Sydney, Australia.

Baatile J, Langbein W E, Weaver F et al 2000 Effect of exercise on perceived quality of life of individuals with Parkinson's disease. Journal of Rehabilitation Research and Development 37(5):529–534.

Bagley S, Kelly B, Tunnicliffe N et al 1991 The effect of visual cues on the gait of independently mobile Parkinson's disease patients. Physiotherapy 77(6):415–420.

Ball J M 1967 Demonstration of the traditional approach in the treatment of a patient with parkinsonism. American Journal of Physical Medicine 46:1034–1036.

Banks M A, Caird F I 1989 Physiotherapy benefits patients with Parkinson's disease. Clinical Rehabilitation 3(1):11–16.

Behrman A L, Teitelbaum P, Cauraugh J H 1998 Verbal instructional sets to normalise the temporal and spatial gait variables in Parkinson's disease. Journal of Neurology, Neurosurgery and Psychiatry 65:580–582.

Behrman A L, Cauraugh J H, Light K E 2000 Practice as an intervention to improve speeded motor performance and motor learning in Parkinson's disease. Journal of Neurological Science 174(2):127–136.

Bloem B R 1994 Postural reflexes in Parkinson's disease. PhD dissertation. Cip-Gegevens Koninklijke, The Hague.

Bloem B R, Beckley D J, van Dijk J G 1993 Pathophysiology of balance impairment in Parkinson's disease. Focus on Parkinson's Disease.

Bloem BR, Beckley DJ, van Dijk JG et al 1996 Influence of dopaminergic medication on automatic postural responses and balance impairments in Parkinson's disease. Movement Disorders 11(50):509–521.

Bloem B R, van Vugt J P, Beckley D J 2001a Postural instability and falls in Parkinson's disease. In: Ruzicka E, Hallet M, Jankovic J (eds) Gait disorders. Lippincott, Williams and Wilkins, Philadelphia, pp 209–223.

Bloem B R et al 2001b The multiple tasks test. Strategies in Parkinson's disease. Experimental Brain Research 137(3–4):478–486.

Bloem B R et al 2001c Prospective assessment of falls in Parkinson's disease. Journal of Neurology 248(11):950–958.

Bond J M, Morris M 2000 Goal-directed secondary motor tasks: their effects on gait in subjects with Parkinson disease. Archives of Physical Medicine and Rehabilitation 81(1):110–116.

Borod J C, Welkowitz J, Alpert M et al 1990 Parameters of emotional processing in neuropsychiatric disorders: conceptual issues and a battery of tests. Journal of Communication Disorders 23:247–271.

Brauer S, Morris M E 2004 Dual task interference in older people. In: Morris M E, Schoo A (eds) Optimizing physical activity and exercise in older people. Elsevier, London, pp 267–287.

Bridgewater K J, Sharpe M H 1996 Aerobic exercise and early Parkinson's disease. Journal of Neurologic Rehabilitation 10(4):233–241.

Bridgewater K J, Sharpe M H 1997 Trunk muscle training and early Parkinson's disease. Physiotherapy Theory and Practice 13(2):139–153.

Bridgewater K J, Sharpe M H 1998 Trunk muscle performance in early Parkinson's disease. Physical Therapy 78(6):566–576.

Burleigh-Jacobs A, Horak F B, Nutt J G et al (1997) Step initiation in Parkinson's disease: influence of levodopa and external sensory triggers. Movement Disorders 2:206–215.

Bushmann M, Dobmyer S, Leeker L et al 1989 Swallowing abnormalities and their response to treatment in Parkinson's disease. Neurology 39: 1309–1314.

Canning C G, Alison J A, Allen N E et al 1997 Parkinson's disease: an investigation of exercise capacity, respiratory function, and gait. Archives of Physical Medicine and Rehabilitation 78(2):199–207.

Cerri C, Arosio A, Biella AM et al 1994 Physical exercise therapy of Parkinson's. Movement Disorders 9 (Suppl 1):68

Chandler C, Plant R 1999 A targeted physiotherapy service for people with Parkinson's disease from diagnosis to end stage: a pilot study. In: Percival R, Hobson P (eds) Parkinson's disease: Studies in psychological and social care. BPS Books, Leicester, pp 256–269.

Chong R K, Horak F, Woollacott M 2000 Parkinson's disease impairs the ability to change set quickly. Journal of the Neurological Sciences 175:57–70.

Comella C L, Stebbins G T, Brown-Toms N et al 1994 Physical therapy and Parkinson's disease: a controlled clinical trial. Neurology 44(3 I): 376–378.

Crossley S M 1986 Intensive physiotherapy for Parkinson's disease in a holiday environment. Physiotherapy 72(8):383–384.

Dam M, Tonin P, Casson S et al 1996 Effects of conventional and sensory-enhanced physiotherapy on disability of Parkinson's disease patients. Advanced Neurology 69:551–555.

Damiano A M, Snyder C, Strausser B et al 1999 A review of health-related quality-of-life concepts and measures for Parkinson's disease. Quality of Life Research 8:235–243.

Darley FL, Aronson AE, Brown JR 1969 Differential diagnostic patterns of dysarthria. Journal of Speech and Hearing Research 12:246–269.

Deane KH, Jones D, Ellis-Hill C et al 2001a A comparison of physiotherapy techniques for patients with Parkinson's disease. Cochrane Database Syst Rev 1CD002815.

Deane KH, Ellis-Hill C, Clarke CE et al 2001b Occupational therapy for Parkinson's disease. Cochrane Database Syst Rev 1CD002813.

Deane KH, Whurr R, Clarke CE et al 2001c Speech and language therapy techniques for dysarthria in Parkinson's disease. Cochrane Database Syst Rev 2CD002812.

Deane KH, Whurr R, Clarke CE et al 2001d A comparison of speech and language therapy techniques for patients with Parkinson's disease. Cochrane Database Syst Rev 2CD002814.

Deane KHO, Ellis-Hill C, Jones D et al 2002 Systematic review of paramedical therapies for Parkinson's disease. Movement Disorders 17:984–991.

Dietz V, Colombo G 1998 Influence of body load on the gait pattern in Parkinson's disease. Movement Disorders 13(2):255–261.

Dodd K, Taylor N, Bradley S 2004 Strength training for older people. In: Morris M E, Schoo A (eds) Optimising physical activity and exercise in older people. Elsevier, London, pp 125–157.

Doshay L J 1964 Method and value of physiotherapy in Parkinson's disease. New England Journal of Medicine 266:465–480.

Dunne J W, Hankey G J, Edis R H 1987 Parkinsonism: upturned walking stick as an aid to locomotion. Archives of Physical Medicine and Rehabilitation 68(6):380–381.

El-Sharkawi A, Ramig L, Logeman J et al 1998 Voice treatment (LSVT) and swallowing in Parkinson's disease. Movement Disorders 13 (Suppl. 2):121.

Eni G O 1988 Gait improvement in Parkinsonism: the use of rhythmic music. International Journal of Rehabilitation Research 11(3):272–274.

Fiorani C, Mari F, Bartolini M et al 1997 Occupational therapy increases ADL score and quality of life in Parkinson's disease. Movement Disorders 12 (Suppl. 1):135.

Formisano R, Pratesi L, Modarelli F T et al 1992 Rehabilitation and Parkinson's disease. Scandinavian Journal of Rehabilitation Medicine 24(3):157–160.

Gauthier L, Dalziel S, Gauthier S 1987 The benefits of group occupational therapy for patients with Parkinson's disease. The American Journal of Occupational Therapy 41(6):360–365.

Gibberd F B, Page N G, Spencer K M et al 1981 Controlled trial of physiotherapy and occupational therapy for Parkinson's disease. British Medical Journal Clinical Research Edition 282(6271):1196.

Giladi N et al 1992 Motor blocks in Parkinson's disease. Neurology 42(2):333–339.

Giladi N, Kao R, Fahn, S 1997 Freezing phenomenon in patients with parkinsonian syndromes. Movement Disorders 12:302–305.

GPDS (The global Parkinson's disease survey steering committee) 2001 Factors impacting on quality of life in Parkinson's disease: results from an international survey. Movement Disorders 17(1):60–67.

Haapaniemi T H, Pursiainen V, Korpelainen JJ et al 2001 Ambulatory ECG and analysis of heart rate variability in Parkinson's disease. Journal of Neurology, Neurosurgery and Psychiatry 70(3):305–310.

Hartelius L, Svensson P, Bubach A 1993 Clinical assessment of dysarthria: performance on dysarthria test by normal adult subjects and by individuals with Parkinson's disease or with multiple sclerosis. Scandinavian Journal of Logopedics and Phoniatrics 18:131–141.

Hely M A et al 1999 The Sydney multicentre study of Parkinson's disease: progression and mortality at 10 years. Journal of Neurology, Neurosurgery and Psychiatry 67(3):300–307.

Hoehn M M, Yahr M 1967 Parkinsonism: onset, progression, and mortality. Neurology 17: 427–442.

Holmes RJ, Oates JM, Phyland DJ et al 2000 Voice characteristics in the progression of Parkinson's disease. International Journal of Language and Communication Disorders 35:407–418.

Homann CN, Crevenna H, Kojnig B et al 1998 Can physiotherapy improve axial symptoms in parkinsonian patients? Movement Disorders 13 (Suppl 2):234.

Houk J C, Davis J L, Beiser DG 1995 Models of information processing in the basal ganglia. The MIT Press, London.

Hurwitz A 1989 The benefit of a home exercise regimen for ambulatory Parkinson's disease patients. Journal of Neuroscience Nursing 21(3):180–184.

Huxham F et al 2003 Trunk position relative to the inside foot during online turns: the effect of turn magnitude. In: Proceedings ISPGR, 2003, Sydney, Australia.

Iansek R et al 1995 Interaction of the basal ganglia and supplementary motor area in the elaboration of movement. In: Glencross B, Piek J (eds) Motor control and sensorimotor integration. Elsevier Science, Amsterdam, pp 49–60.

Iansek R, Bradshaw J, Phillips J et al 1997 Review article: the functions of the basal ganglia and the paradox of stereotaxic surgery in Parkinson's disease. Brain 117:1613–1615.

Johnson J A, Pring T R 1990 Speech therapy in Parkinson disease: a review and further data. British Journal of Disorders of Communication 25:183–194.

Kamsma Y P T, Brouwer W H, Lakke J 1995 Training of compensational strategies for impaired gross motor skills in Parkinson's disease. Physiotherapy Theory and Practice 11(4):209–229.

Katsikitis M, Pilowsky I 1997 A controlled study of facial mobility treatment in Parkinson's disease. Journal of Psychosomatic Research 40:4387–4396.

Kinsman R 1986 Conductive education for the patient with Parkinson's disease. Physiotherapy 72(8).

Kompoliti K, Goetz C G, Leurgans S et al 2000 On freezing in Parkinson's disease: resistance to visual cue walking devices. Movement Disorders 15(2):309–312.

Koozekanani S 1987 Ground reaction forces during ambulation in parkinsonism: pilot study. Archives of Physical Medicine and Rehabilitation 68(1): 28–30.

Koseoglu F, Inan L, Ozel S et al 1997 The effects of a pulmonary rehabilitation program on pulmonary function tests and exercise tolerance in patients with Parkinson's disease. Functional Neurology 12(6):319–325.

Krasilovsky G, Gianutsos J 1991 Effect of video feedback on the performance of a weight shifting controlled tracking task in subjects with parkinsonism and neurologically intact individuals. Experimental Neurology 113(2):192–201.

Levine S 2000 A strenuous exercise program benefits patients with mild to moderate Parkinson's disease. Clinical Exercise Physiology 2(1):43–48.

Lewis G N, Byblow W D, Walt S E 2000 Stride length regulation in Parkinson's disease: the use of extrinsic, visual cues. Brain 123(10):2077–2090.

Logemann JA, Fisher HB, Boshes B et al 1978 Frequency and concurrence of vocal tract dysfunctions in the speech of a large sample of Parkinson patients. Journal of Speech and Hearing Disorders 43:47–57.

Lynch N A, Metter E J 1999 Muscle quality: age-associated differences between arm and leg muscle groups. Journal of Applied Physiology 86(1):188–194.

McIntosh G C, Brown S H, Rice R R et al 1997 Rhythmic auditory-motor facilitation of gait patterns in patients with Parkinson's disease. Journal of Neurology, Neurosurgery and Psychiatry 62(1):22–26.

Marchese R, Diverio M, Zucchi F et al 2000 The role of sensory cues in the rehabilitation of parkinsonian patients: a comparison of two physical therapy protocols. Movement Disorders 15(5):879–883.

Marks L, Turner K, O'Sullivan J et al 2001 Drooling in Parkinson's disease: a novel speech and language therapy intervention. International Journal of Language & Communication Disorders 36 (Suppl. 2001):282–287.

Marsden C D 1994 Parkinson's disease. Journal of Neurology, Neurosurgery and Psychiatry 57:672–681.

Miyai I, Fujimoto Y, Ueda Y et al 2000 Treadmill training with body weight support: its effect on Parkinson's disease. Archives of Physical Medicine and Rehabilitation 81(7):849–852.

Mohr B, Muller V, Mattes R et al 1996 Behavioural treatment of Parkinson's disease leads to improvement of motor skills and to tremor reduction. Behaviour Therapy 27:235–255.

Montgomery EB Jr, Lieberman A, Singh G, Fries JF 1994 Patient education and health promotion can be effective in Parkinson's disease: a randomized controlled trial. PROPATH Advisory Board. American Journal of Medicine 97(5):429–435.

Morris M E 2000 Movement disorders in people with Parkinson's disease: a model for physical therapy. Physical Therapy 80(6):578–597.

Morris M E, Iansek R, Matyas T A et al 1994a Ability to modulate walking cadence remains intact in Parkinson's disease. Journal of Neurology, Neurosurgery and Psychiatry 57(12):1532–1534.

Morris M E, Iansek R, Matyas T A et al 1994b The pathogenesis of gait hypokinesia in Parkinson's disease. Brain 117(5):1169–1181.

Morris M E, Iansek R, Matyas T A et al 1996a Stride length regulation in Parkinson's disease:

normalization strategies and underlying mechanisms. Brain 119(2):551–568.

Morris M E, Iansek R, Matyas T A 1997 Gait disorders in Parkinson's disease: a framework for physical therapy practice. Neurology Report 21(4):125–131.

Morris M E, McGinely J, Huxham F 1999 Kinetic, kinematic and spatiotemporal constraints of gait in Parkinson disease. Human Movement Science 18:461–483.

Morris M E et al 2001 The biomechanics and motor control of gait in Parkinson disease. Clinical Biomechanics 16(6):459–470.

Munneke M 2003 Quantification of trunk movements during turning in Parkinson's disease. In: International Society for Postural and Gait Research XVIth Conference, 2003, Sydney.

Nagaya M, Kachi T, Yamada T et al 1998 Videofluorographic study of swallowing in Parkinson's disease. Dysphagia 13:95–100.

Nieuwboer A, Feys P, De Weerdt W et al 1997 Clinical problem solving. Is using a cue the clue to the treatment of freezing in Parkinson's disease? Physiotherapy Research International 2(3):125–134.

Nigg B, Fisher V, Allinger T et al 1992 Range of motion of the foot as a function of age. Foot and Ankle 13: 336–343.

Oliveira R M, Gurd J M, Nixon P 1997 Micrographia in Parkinson's disease: the effect of providing external cues. Journal of Neurology, Neurosurgery and Psychiatry 63:429–433.

O'Shea S, Morris M E, Iansek R 2002 Dual task interference during gait in people with Parkinson disease: effects of motor versus cognitive secondary tasks. Physical Therapy 82:888–897.

Palmer S S, Mortimer J A, Webster D D et al 1986 Exercise therapy for Parkinson's disease. Archives of Physical Medicine and Rehabilitation 67(10):741–745.

Patla A E, Prentice SD, Robinson C et al 1991 Visual control of locomotion: strategies for changing direction and for going over obstacles. Journal of Experimental Psychology, Human Perception and Performance 17(3):603–634.

Patla A E, Adkin A, Ballard T 1999 Online steering: coordination and control of body center of mass, head and body reorientation. Experimental Brain Research 129(4):629–634.

Patti F, Reggio A, Nicoletti F et al 1996 Effects of rehabilitation therapy on Parkinson's disability and functional independence. Journal of Neurologic Rehabilitation 10(4):223–231.

Pedersen S W, Oberg B, Insulander A et al 1990 Group training in parkinsonism: quantitative

measurements of treatment. Scandinavian Journal of Rehabilitation Medicine 22(4):207–211.

Polgar S, Morris M E, Reilly S et al 2003 Reconstructive surgery for Parkinson's disease: a systematic review and preliminary meta-analysis. Brain Research Bulletin 60:1–24

Ramig L, Countryman S, Thompson IL et al 1995 A comparison of two forms of intensive speech treatment for Parkinson disease. Journal of Speech and Hearing Research 38:1232–1251.

Ramig L, Sapir S, Fox C et al 2001 Changes in vocal loudness following intensive voice treatment (LSVT) in individuals with Parkinson's disease: a comparison with untreated patients and normal age-matched controls. Movement Disorders 16: 79–83.

Rao SM, Huber SJ, Bornstein RA 1992 Emotional changes with multiple sclerosis and Parkinson's disease. Journal of Consulting and Clinical Psychology 60:369–378.

Robbins JA, Logemann JA, Kirshner HS 1986 Swallowing and speech production in Parkinson's disease. Annals of Neurology 19:283–287.

Robertson SJ, Thompson F 1984 Speech therapy in Parkinson's disease; a study of the long-term effects of intensive treatment. British Journal of Disorders of Communication 23:213–224.

Rubenstein L M, DeLeo A, Chrischilles E A 2001 Economic and health-related quality of life considerations of new therapies in Parkinson's disease. Pharmacoeconomics 19(7):729–752.

Sapir S, Pawlas AA, Ramig LO et al 2001 Voice and speech abnormalities in Parkinsonian disease: relation to severity of motor impairment, duration of disease, medication, depression, gender and age. Journal of Medical Speech Language Pathology 9:213–226.

Scandalis T A, Bosak A, Berliner J C et al 2001 Resistance training and gait function in patients with Parkinson's disease. American Journal of Physical Medicine and Rehabilitation 80(1):38–43.

Schenkman M, Donovan J, Tsubota J et al 1989 Management of individuals with Parkinson's disease: rationale and case studies. Physical Therapy 69(11):944–955.

Schenkman M, Cutson T M, Kuchibhatla M et al 1998 Exercise to improve spinal flexibility and function for people with Parkinson's disease: a randomized, controlled trial. Journal of the American Geriatrics Society 46(10):1207–1216.

Scott S, Caird FI 1983 Speech therapy for Parkinson's disease. Journal of Neurology, Neurosurgery and Psychiatry 46:140–144.

Stack E, Ashburn A 1999 Fall events described by people with Parkinson's disease: implications for clinical interviewing and the research agenda. Physiotherapy Research International 4(3):190–200.

Stallibrass C 1997 An evaluation of the Alexander Technique for the management of disability in Parkinson's disease – a preliminary study. Clinical Rehabilitation 11(1):8–12.

Stefaniwsky L, Bilowit D S 1973 Parkinsonism: facilitation of motion by sensory stimulation. Archives of Physical Medicine and Rehabilitation 266:75–90

Sunvisson H, Lokk J, Ericson K et al 1997 Changes in motor performance in persons with Parkinson's disease after exercise in a mountain area. Journal of Neuroscience Nursing 29(4):255–260.

Szekely B C, Kosanovich N N, Sheppard W 1982 Adjunctive treatment in Parkinson's disease: physical therapy and comprehensive group therapy. Rehabilitation Literature 43:72–76.

Szili-Torok T et al 2001 Depressed baroreflex sensitivity in patients with Alzheimer's and Parkinson's disease. Neurobiology of Aging 22(3):435–438.

Thaut M H, McIntosh G C, Rice R R et al 1996 Rhythmic auditory stimulation in gait training for Parkinson's disease patients. Movement Disorders 11(2):193–200.

Toole T, Hirsch M A, Forkink A et al 2000 The effects of a balance and strength training program on equilibrium in Parkinsonism: a preliminary study. Neurorehabilitation 14(3):165–174.

Trend P, Kaye J, Gage H et al 2002 Short-term effectiveness of intensive multi-disciplinary rehabilitation for people with Parkinson's disease and their carers. Clinical Rehabilitation 16:717–725.

Viliani T, Pasquetti P, Magnolfi S et al 1999 Effects of physical training on straightening-up processes in patients with Parkinson's disease. Disability and Rehabilitation 21(2):68–73.

Wade D T, Gage H, Owen C et al 2003 Multidisciplinary rehabilitation for people with Parkinson's disease: a randomised controlled study. Journal of Neurology, Neurosurgery and Psychiatry 74:18–162.

Waterston J A, Hawken M B, Tanyeri S 1993 Influence of sensory manipulation on postural control in Parkinson's disease. Journal of Neurology, Neurosurgery and Psychiatry 56:1276–1281.

Weissenborn S 1993 The effect of using a two-step verbal cue to a visual target above eye level on the Parkinsonian gait: a case study. Physiotherapy 79(1):26–31.

Wood B H 2002 Incidence and prediction of falls in Parkinson's disease: a prospective multidisciplinary study. Journal of Neurology, Neurosurgery and Psychiatry 72(6):721–725.

World Health Organization 2001 International classification of functioning disability and health. WHO, Geneva.

Worringham C J, Stelmach G E 1990 Practice effects on the pre-programming of discrete movements in Parkinson's disease. Journal of Neurology, Neurosurgery and Psychiatry 53(8):702–704.

Yekutiel M, Pinhasov A, Shahar G et al 1991 A clinical trial of the re-education of movement in patients with Parkinson's disease. Clinical Rehabilitation 5(3):207–214.

Index